The Intersection of Dermatology and Oncology

Editor

LINDSAY C. STROWD

DERMATOLOGIC CLINICS

www.derm.theclinics.com

Consulting Editor

BRUCE H. THIERS

October 2019 • Volume 37 • Number 4

ELSEVIER

1600 John F. Kennedy Boulevard • Suite 1800 • Philadelphia, Pennsylvania, 19103-2899

http://www.theclinics.com

DERMATOLOGIC CLINICS Volume 37, Number 4
October 2019 ISSN 0733-8635, ISBN-13: 978-0-323-70894-4

Editor: Jessica McCool
Developmental Editor: Laura Kavanaugh

Dermatologic Clinics (ISSN 0733-8635) is published quarterly by Elsevier Inc., 360 Park Avenue South, New York, NY 10010-1710. Months of publication are January, April, July, and October. Business and editorial offices: 1600 John F. Kennedy Blvd., Suite 1800, Philadelphia, PA 19103-2899. Customer service office: 11830 Westline Drive, St. Louis, MO 63146. Periodicals postage paid at New York, NY, and additional mailing offices. Subscription prices are USD 404.00 per year for US individuals, USD 736.00 per year for US institutions, USD 456.00 per year for Canadian individuals, USD 898.00 per year for Canadian institutions, USD 510.00 per year for international individuals, USD 898.00 per year for international institutions, USD 100.00 per year for US students/residents, and USD 240.00 per year for Canadian and international students/residents. International air speed delivery is included in all *Clinics* subscription prices. All prices are subject to change without notice. **POSTMASTER:** Send address changes to *Dermatologic Clinics*, Elsevier Health Sciences Division, Subscription Customer Service, 3251 Riverport Lane, Maryland Heights, MO 63043. **Customer Service: 1-800-654-2452 (U.S. and Canada); 314-447-8871 (outside U.S. and Canada). Fax: 314-447-8029. E-mail: journalscustomerservice-usa@elsevier.com (for print support); journalsonlinesupport-usa@elsevier.com (for online support).**

Reprints. For copies of 100 or more, of articles in this publication, please contact the Commercial Reprints Department, Elsevier Inc., 360 Park Avenue South, New York, New York 10010-1710. Tel.: 212-633-3874; Fax: 212-633-3820; Email: reprints@elsevier.com.

The *Dermatologic Clinics* is covered in *MEDLINE/PubMed (Index Medicus), Current Contents/Clinical Medicine, Excerpta Medica, Chemical Abstracts,* and *ISI/BIOMED.*

Contributors

CONSULTING EDITOR

BRUCE H. THIERS, MD
Professor and Chairman Emeritus, Department of Dermatology and Dermatologic Surgery, Medical University of South Carolina, Charleston, South Carolina, USA

EDITOR

LINDSAY C. STROWD, MD, FAAD
Assistant Professor, Department of Dermatology, Wake Forest School of Medicine, Winston-Salem, North Carolina, USA

AUTHORS

ADEWOLE S. ADAMSON, MD, MPP
Division of Dermatology, Department of Internal Medicine, The University of Texas at Austin, Dell Medical School, Austin, Texas, USA

CHRISTINE AHN, MD
Assistant Professor Departments of Dermatology and Pathology, Wake Forest School of Medicine, Winston-Salem, North Carolina, USA

ZEYNEP M. AKKURT, MD
Department of Dermatology, Wake Forest School of Medicine, Winston-Salem, North Carolina, USA

AUBREY ALLEN, BA
Brody School of Medicine, East Carolina University, Greenville, North Carolina, USA

BENJAMIN BECKER, MD
Department of Neurology, Wake Forest Baptist Health, Winston-Salem, North Carolina, USA

LEONORA BOMAR, MD
Department of Dermatology, Wake Forest School of Medicine, Winston-Salem, North Carolina, USA

ADELA R. CARDONES, MD, MHSc
Department of Dermatology, Duke University, Duke Cancer Institute, Durham VA Medical Center, Durham, North Carolina, USA

PEI-LING CHEN, MD, PhD
Department of Cutaneous Oncology, Moffitt Cancer Center, Tampa, Florida, USA

EVAN ALEXANDER CHOATE, BA
Medical Student, David Geffen School of Medicine, University of California, Los Angeles, Los Angeles, California, USA

JENNIFER N. CHOI, MD
Associate Professor, Department of Dermatology, Chief, Division of Oncodermatology, Robert H. Lurie Comprehensive Cancer Center, Northwestern University Feinberg School of Medicine, Chicago, Illinois, USA

ALEXANDRA COLLINS, BS
Wake Forest School of Medicine, Winston-Salem, North Carolina, USA

ANNA K. DEWAN, MD, MHS
Department of Dermatology, Vanderbilt University Medical Center, Nashville, Tennessee, USA

LAURA DOERFLER, MD
Assistant Professor, Department of Dermatology, Wake Forest Baptist Hospital, Wake Forest School of Medicine, Winston-Salem, North Carolina, USA

DEBORAH N. DORRELL, MD
Medical Student, Wake Forest School of Medicine, Winston-Salem, North Carolina, USA

JESSICA DOWLING, BS
Center for Dermatology Research, Department of Dermatology, Wake Forest School of Medicine, Winston-Salem, North Carolina, USA

DREW A. EMGE, MD, MSc
Department of Dermatology, Duke University, Durham, North Carolina, USA

SHERVIN A. ETEMAD, BS
Department of Dermatology, Vanderbilt University Medical Centre, Nashville, Tennessee, USA

NICOLE M. FETT, MD
Oregon Health & Science University, Portland, Oregon, USA

RAMIZ N. HAMID, MD, MPH
Department of Dermatology, Wake Forest School of Medicine, Winston-Salem, North Carolina, USA

VALERIE M. HARVEY, MD, MPH
Hampton University Skin of Color Research Institute, Hampton, Virginia, USA; TPMG Hampton Roads Center for Dermatology, Newport News, Virginia, USA

LATRICE HOGUE, BA
Department of Dermatology, Wake Forest School of Medicine, Winston Salem, North Carolina, USA

BENJAMIN H. KAFFENBERGER, MD
Ohio State Dermatology, Columbus, Ohio, USA

SUBUHI KAUL, MBBS, MD
Senior Resident, Department of Dermatology, All India Institute of Medical Sciences, New Delhi, India

JESSE J. KELLER, MD
Oregon Health & Science University, Portland, Oregon, USA

SREE S. KOLLI, BA
Center for Dermatology Research, Department of Dermatology, Wake Forest School of Medicine, Winston-Salem, North Carolina, USA

SHAWN G. KWATRA, MD
Assistant Professor, Johns Hopkins School of Medicine, Baltimore, Maryland, USA

JO-ANN LATKOWSKI, MD
The Ronald O. Perelman Department of Dermatology, Associate Professor of Dermatology, Chief of Dermatology, New York Harbor VA Healthcare System, Director, Dermatology Residency Training Program, New York, New York, USA

KRISTEN LO SICCO, MD
Assistant Professor of Dermatology, Associate Director of NYU Skin and Cancer Unit, The Ronald O. Perelman Department of Dermatology, New York, New York, USA

SOPHIA MA, MD
Department of Dermatology and Cutaneous Surgery, University of South Florida Morsani College of Medicine, Tampa, Florida, USA

STEPHEN J. MALACHOWSKI, MD, MS
Department of Dermatology and Cutaneous Surgery, University of South Florida Morsani College of Medicine, Tampa, Florida, USA

SEAN P. McGREGOR, DO, PharmD
Center for Dermatology Research, Department of Dermatology, Wake Forest School of Medicine, Winston-Salem, North Carolina, USA

LYNNE H. MORRISON, MD
Oregon Health & Science University, Portland, Oregon, USA

ADRIAN MOY, MS
Department of Dermatology and Cutaneous Surgery, University of South Florida Morsani College of Medicine, Tampa, Florida, USA

ALEXANDER NOBORI, MD
Department of Pathology and Laboratory Medicine, David Geffen School of Medicine, University of California, Los Angeles, Los Angeles, California, USA

ERIK PETERSON, BA, BS
Research Fellow, The Ronald O. Perelman Department of Dermatology, New York, New York, USA

VIGNESH RAMACHANDRAN, BS
Baylor College of Medicine, Houston, Texas, USA

OMAR P. SANGÜEZA, MD
Professor, Departments of Dermatology and Pathology, Wake Forest School of Medicine, Winston-Salem, North Carolina, USA

JESSICA SAVAS, MD
Assistant Professor, Department of Dermatology, Wake Forest Baptist Hospital, Wake Forest School of Medicine, Winston-Salem, North Carolina, USA

LUCIA SEMINARIO-VIDAL, MD, PhD
Department of Dermatology and Cutaneous Surgery, University of South Florida Morsani College of Medicine, Department of Cutaneous Oncology, Moffitt Cancer Center, Tampa, Florida, USA

ADITI SENITHILNATHAN, BA
Department of Dermatology, Wake Forest School of Medicine, Winston-Salem, North Carolina, USA

MEGAN E. SHELTON, MD
Division of Dermatology, Department of Internal Medicine, The University of Texas at Austin, Dell Medical School, Austin, Texas, USA

LINDSAY C. STROWD, MD, FAAD
Assistant Professor, Department of Dermatology, Wake Forest School of Medicine, Winston-Salem, North Carolina, USA

ROY E. STROWD III, MD, MEd
Departments of Neurology and Internal Medicine, Section on Hematology and Oncology, Translational Science Institute, Wake Forest Baptist Health, Winston Salem, North Carolina, USA

JAMES SUN, MD
Department of Cutaneous Oncology, Moffitt Cancer Center, Tampa, Florida, USA

JASON WEED, MD
The Ronald O. Perelman Department of Dermatology, New York, New York, USA

PHILIP WILLIFORD, MD
Department of Dermatology, Wake Forest School of Medicine, Winston-Salem, North Carolina, USA

SCOTT WORSWICK, MD
Associate Professor, Department of Dermatology, Keck School of Medicine of USC, University of Southern California, Los Angeles, California, USA

Contents

Primary cutaneous melanoma describes any primary melanoma lesion of the skin that does not have evidence of metastatic disease. This article reviews the current workup, treatment, and follow-up recommendations for primary cutaneous melanoma (stages 0, I, and II). Specific attention is focused on recent updates with regard to staging, sentinel lymph node biopsy, and surgical modalities.

The incidence of metastatic melanoma continues to increase each decade. Although surgical treatment is often curative for localized stage I and stage II disease, the median survival for patients with distant metastases is less than 1 year. The last 2 decades have witnessed a breakthrough in therapeutic options with the development of immune checkpoint inhibitors, small molecule targeted therapy, and oncolytic viral therapy. This article provides an overview of the treatment options available for advanced melanoma, including chemotherapy, targeted therapy, immunotherapy, interleukin-2, and oncolytic viral agents.

Nonmelanoma skin cancer (NMSC) is the most commonly diagnosed malignancy in the United States. Surgery is considered the gold standard treatment. Techniques include curettage and electrodesiccation, surgical excision, and Mohs micrographic surgery. While each is effective, there are relative advantages and disadvantages with respect to cost, time, quality of life, and role in patients with limited life expectancy. Preventing local tumor recurrence is the primary objective; however, recurrence rates are based on retrospective data, and high-quality comparator studies assessing effectiveness are scarce. Prospective and randomized controlled trials are imperative to create comprehensive, evidence-based recommendations for the surgical management of NMSC.

Although surgical intervention remains the standard of care for nonmelanoma skin cancer, other treatment modalities have been studied and used. Nonsurgical treatment methods include cryotherapy, topical medications, photodynamic therapy, radiation therapy, Hedgehog pathway inhibitors, programmed cell death protein 1 inhibitors, and active nonintervention. Despite the favorable efficacy of surgical treatment methods, many factors, including but not limited to patient age, preference, and severity of disease, must be taken into consideration when choosing the most appropriate, patient-centered treatment approach.

Primary cutaneous B-cell lymphomas are a group of diseases with indolent and aggressive behavior. The goal of the initial workup is to evaluate for systemic involvement, provide adequate staging, and guide therapy. Histopathological studies are a critical part of the workup for classification of these lymphomas because they are similar to their nodal counterparts. There are limited data for treatment guidelines, and thus, therapy differs among institutions. Overall, localized therapies are preferred for indolent types and chemotherapy or immunotherapy for the aggressive forms.

Cutaneous T cell lymphoma (CTCL) represents a heterogeneous group of extranodal non-Hodgkin lymphomas in which monoclonal T lymphocytes infiltrate the skin. The mechanism of CTCL development is not fully understood, but likely involves dysregulation of various genes and signaling pathways. A variety of treatment modalities are available, and although they can induce remission in most patients, the disease may recur after treatment cessation. Owing to relatively low incidence and significant chronicity of disease, and the high morbidity of some therapeutic regimens, further clinical trials are warranted to better define the ideal treatment option for each subtype of CTCL.

Pityriasis lichenoides et varioliformis acuta and pityriasis lichenoides chronica are the 2 main subtypes of pityriasis lichenoides. They represent the acute and chronic forms of the disease; both may have clonal T cells. Several treatment modalities are used, but it has been difficult to determine efficacy because of the possibility of spontaneous remission. Cutaneous CD30+ lymphoproliferative disorders constitute many cutaneous T-cell lymphomas and comprise lymphomatoid papulosis and primary cutaneous anaplastic large cell lymphoma (ALCL). Both have an excellent prognosis. Lymphomatoid papulosis often only requires observation or treatment of symptoms. First-line therapies for primary cutaneous ALCL are surgical excision or radiotherapy.

Dermatofibrosarcoma protuberans (DFSP) is an uncommon dermal neoplasm that exhibits a high rate of local recurrence and infiltrative behavior, but has a low risk of metastasis. It arises as a slowly progressive, painless pink or violet plaque. Histologically, DFSP is characterized by a monomorphous spindle cell proliferation in a storiform pattern. The gold standard of treatment is surgical resection with negative margins. In cases where obtaining clear margins is not possible, radiation and systemic therapy with tyrosine kinase inhibitors, such as imatinib mesylate, has been shown to be effective.

Drew A. Emge and Adela R. Cardones

Merkel cell carcinoma (MCC) is a rare but aggressive skin cancer associated with the Merkel cell polyoma virus. Its incidence and mortality are increasing. There have been many advances in the last several decades in the etiology, detection, and management of MCC, but much about its natural history and most effective treatment remains unknown. Surgical excision with margins of 1 to 2 cm remains first-line therapy for early-stage MCC, but robust evidence supporting immunotherapy for patients with advanced disease has led to recent approval of immune checkpoint inhibitors in the treatment of advanced MCC.

Shervin A. Etemad and Anna K. Dewan

Kaposi sarcoma (KS) is an angioproliferative mesenchymal neoplasm caused by Kaposi sarcoma-related herpesvirus. This review outlines our current understanding of the epidemiology, pathogenesis, clinical presentation, and staging for this disease. Recent research has informed a more comprehensive understanding of the epidemiology of KS in the post-antiretroviral therapy era, and highlights the continued need to better characterize the African endemic subtype. Advances in clinical oncology, including checkpoint inhibitors and new skin-directed therapies, have translated into exciting new developments for the future of KS treatment options.

Latrice Hogue and Valerie M. Harvey

Skin cancers are relatively rare in patients with skin of color; however, they are an important public health concern because of disparities in patient outcomes. Gaps in skin cancer knowledge exist because of lack of large-scale studies involving people of color, and limitations in data collection methods and skin classification paradigms. Additional research is needed to address questions regarding risk and reasons for disparate skin cancer outcomes in these patients. We summarize the clinical and epidemiologic features for basal cell carcinoma, squamous cell carcinoma, and melanoma and touch on some of their unique features in patients with skin of color.

Deborah N. Dorrell and Lindsay C. Strowd

Skin cancer is the most common malignancy in the United States. Health care providers and patients alike are tasked with identifying suspicious skin lesions in order to diagnose skin cancers early and treat them quickly. The normal pathway to skin cancer diagnosis is visual, with dermoscopic assessment of the lesion followed by biopsy and histopathologic evaluation. Recently, many innovative skin cancer detection technologies have been developed to increase diagnostic accuracy for skin cancers. These noninvasive technologies offer benefits over biopsy but are limited by expense, training, and poor specificity. The skin cancer detection techniques are reviewed in this article.

nodules, and tumors including neurofibromas, malignant peripheral nerve sheath tumors, and gliomas. Tuberous Sclerosis Complex is characterized by benign hamartomas presenting with hypomelanotic macules, shagreen patches, angiofibromas, confetti lesions and tumors including cortical tubers, subependymal nodules, subependymal giant cell astrocytomas and tumors of the kidney, lung, and heart. Managing these disorders requires disease specific supportive care, tumor monitoring, surveillance for selected cancers, and treatment of comorbid conditions.

Cutaneous findings that appear in childhood may be the first sign of a hereditary tumor syndrome. Early detection of genodermatoses allows the patient and at-risk family members to be screened for associated malignancies. This article provides a brief description of the pathogenesis and clinical manifestations of various inherited disorders with skin involvement, along with treatment updates. Advances in molecular-based therapy have spurred development of novel treatment methods for various genodermatoses such as xeroderma pigmentosum (XP) and Gorlin-Goltz syndrome. Further studies are needed to better assess the efficacy of many of these new treatment options.

DERMATOLOGIC CLINICS

SERIES OF RELATED INTEREST

Facial Plastic Surgery Clinics
Available at: http://www.facialplastic.theclinics.com/
Surgical Oncology Clinics
Available at: https://www.surgonc.theclinics.com/

THE CLINICS ARE AVAILABLE ONLINE!
Access your subscription at:
www.theclinics.com

Erratum

An error was made in the July 2019 issue of *Dermatologic Clinics* (Volume 37, Issue 3) in article titled *Extramammary Paget Disease,* by Drs. Bradley Merritt, Catherine Degesys, and David Brodland regarding Figures 1 and 2.

Figures 1 and 2 should be swapped. Figure 1 is the clinical image and Figure 2 should be the H&E stain. Figure 3 is correct.

The print and online versions of the Figures have now been corrected to reflect the correct Figure legends.

Dermatol Clin 37 (2019) xiii
https://doi.org/10.1016/j.det.2019.07.001
0733-8635/19/© 2019 Published by Elsevier Inc.

Preface
Standing at a Crossroads: Dermatology and Oncology

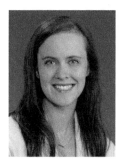

Lindsay C. Strowd, MD, FAAD
Editor

Dermatology as a specialty is uniquely positioned to interface with multiple other areas of medicine; there is significant overlap in the disease states dermatologists manage and those of our physician colleagues. Dermatologists often find themselves collaborating with infectious disease experts or comanaging connective tissue disease patients with rheumatology. Dermatology plays a critical role in diagnosing and managing facets of oncologic disease. While most physicians consider dermatologists to be experts in managing skin cancer, our role as a specialty extends far beyond to include diagnosing paraneoplastic disease, managing cutaneous side effects of cancer and its treatment, and leading research efforts to develop innovative diagnostic methods and trial novel oncologic therapeutics. This issue attempts to cover the breadth of diseases relevant to oncology and dermatology while updating readers on the newest topical literature. The issue begins with updating readers on the latest guidelines for surgical and nonsurgical management of melanoma and nonmelanoma skin cancers. This is followed by a review of less common cutaneous malignancies, including Kaposi sarcoma and cutaneous lymphomas. A section on special topics in skin cancer covers diagnosis and management of skin cancer in patients with skin of color as well as emerging cancer detection technology. The issue transitions to discuss dermatology's role in both diagnosis and management of cutaneous complications of internal malignancy and finishes with a review of genetic diseases associated with neoplasms and skin findings.

Lindsay C. Strowd, MD, FAAD
Department of Dermatology
Wake Forest University School of Medicine
Medical Center Boulevard
Winston-Salem, NC 27157, USA

E-mail address:
lchaney@wakehealth.edu

Dermatol Clin 37 (2019) xv
https://doi.org/10.1016/j.det.2019.06.003
0733-8635/19/

Update on Current Treatment Recommendations for Primary Cutaneous Melanoma

Jessica Dowling, BS[a], Sean P. McGregor, DO, PharmD[a,b,*], Philip Williford, MD[b]

KEYWORDS

• Melanoma • Primary • Staging • Sentinel • Mohs • Excision

KEY POINTS

• The American Joint Committee on Cancer has updated the tumor (T)-category staging criteria.
• There are new indications for the management of melanoma and sentinel lymph node biopsy.
• The surgical treatment of primary cutaneous melanoma is updated.

INTRODUCTION

Definition and Epidemiology

Primary cutaneous melanoma describes any primary melanoma lesion of the skin that does not have evidence of metastatic disease (**Figs. 1–3**).[1] Melanoma is a malignancy arising from melanocytes that most commonly occurs in the skin.[2] There are 4 major subtypes of malignant melanoma based on growth patterns, including superficial spreading, nodular, lentigo maligna, and acral lentiginous melanoma. Most melanomas are diagnosed while still confined to the primary cutaneous location.[3] With the highest mortality rate among all skin cancers and a rising incidence, malignant melanoma is a significant public health problem, although it accounts for less than 5% of skin cancer diagnoses overall.[3,4] There are expected to be about 91,270 cases of cutaneous melanoma diagnosed in 2018 alone, leading to an estimated 9320 deaths.[5] The probability of developing melanoma in one's lifetime is 1 in 27 in male individuals and 1 in 42 in female individuals.[5]

Risk factors for the development of primary cutaneous melanoma include tanning bed use, sun exposure, residence nearer to the equator, male sex, immunosuppression, increasing age, family history of cutaneous melanoma, germline genetic mutations and polymorphisms predisposing to melanoma (ie, CDKN2A, CDK4, Mc1r), personal history of dysplastic nevi, fairer colored hair and eyes, increased common nevi count, and increased tendency to sunburn.[4,6]

Cutaneous melanoma is classified as localized disease (stage I–II), regional disease (stage III), and distant metastatic disease (stage IV).[6] The initial management of cutaneous melanoma is often surgical excision with recommended margins based on tumor thickness; additional modalities can be used based on staging. Patients with regional or metastatic melanoma, whether nonnodal locoregional, nodal, or distant metastases, can be treated with a variety of local, regional, and systemic options. Recently, immunotherapy and targeted therapy has changed the landscape of treatment decisions in stage III and stage IV

Disclosure: The authors have nothing to disclose.
[a] Center for Dermatology Research, Department of Dermatology, Wake Forest School of Medicine, Winston-Salem, NC, USA; [b] Department of Dermatology, Wake Forest School of Medicine, Winston-Salem, NC, USA
* Corresponding author. Department of Dermatology, Wake Forest School of Medicine, Medical Center Boulevard, Winston-Salem, NC 27157-1071.
E-mail address: smcgrego@wakehealth.edu

Dermatol Clin 37 (2019) 397–407
https://doi.org/10.1016/j.det.2019.06.001

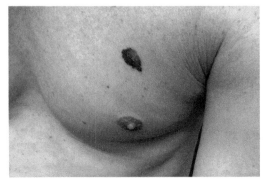

Fig. 1. Primary melanoma located on the chest. (*Courtesy of* P. Kosari, MD, Charlotte, NC.)

melanoma. Although these advances are exciting, a detailed analysis of these treatments is beyond the scope of this article. The primary objective of this article is to review the current workup, treatment, and follow-up recommendations for primary cutaneous melanoma (stages 0, I, and II).

METHODS

The authors searched PubMed, Embase, and Google Scholar databases for literature published in English pertaining to primary cutaneous melanoma. Keywords included: primary cutaneous melanoma, malignant melanoma, treatment, adjuvant

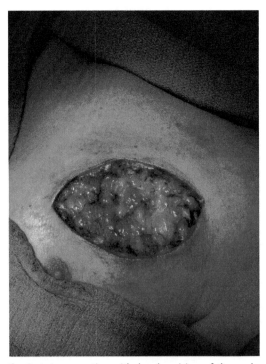

Fig. 2. Intraoperative wide local excision of the melanoma. (*Courtesy of* P. Kosari, MD, Charlotte, NC.)

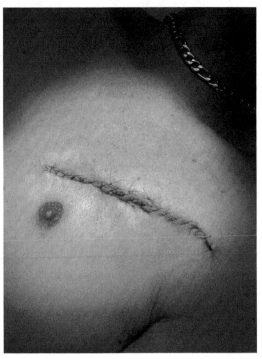

Fig. 3. Postoperative primary closure of the excision site. (*Courtesy of* P. Kosari, MD, Charlotte, NC.)

treatment, biopsy, workup, follow-up, sentinel lymph node biopsy (SLNB), and Mohs micrographic surgery (MMS). Keywords were searched both individually and combined. Articles identified were then narrowed down by abstract, with an emphasis on papers that focused on treatment options, both medical and surgical, for cutaneous melanoma. Studies that reviewed recommendations for staging, workup, and follow-up were also included.

BIOPSY

Lesions suspicious for cutaneous melanoma must always be biopsied for an accurate diagnosis. Full-thickness biopsy via excision, punch, or saucerization with clinically negative 1-mm to 3-mm margins is preferred.[6,7] Superficial biopsies are not recommended because they may lead to difficulty assessing Breslow thickness and microsatellitosis.[6–9] In anatomic locations where excisional biopsy is difficult, a full-thickness biopsy of the thickest or most atypical portion of the lesion may be performed.[7] The pathology report for all malignant melanoma should include Breslow thickness, ulceration status, microsatellitosis, mitotic rate, and margin for accurate microstaging.[6] Additionally, vertical growth phase, presence of tumor-infiltrating lymphocytes, and regression may be included in the pathology report.[1]

STAGING

Staging of cutaneous melanoma is important with regard to treatment and patient outcomes. Staging is based on the American Joint Committee on Cancer (AJCC) eighth edition manual and there have been some changes since the seventh edition (2010).[10] Stages 0, I, and II melanoma are defined by tumor (T-)category thickness in the absence of regional lymph node and distant metastases. Changes in T-category are important to recognize because dermatologists are often involved in the initial diagnosis and there are implications regarding treatment decisions and prognosis. T-categories are still based on tumor thickness ranging from less than 1 mm to greater than 4 mm but should now be reported to the nearest 0.1 mm.[10] Additionally, the T1-category is further subdivided based on tumor thickness greater than or less than 0.8 mm and the presence or absence of ulceration.[10] This is based on a multivariate analysis in which tumors less than 0.8 mm with ulceration and tumors 0.8 mm to 1.0 mm with or without ulceration were predictive of melanoma-specific survival (MSS).[10] Ulceration is still designated with the letter b and represents loss of the epidermis above the tumor with an associated inflammatory response.[10] The mitotic rate was previously included in the T-category in the seventh edition of the AJCC manual but has been removed from the staging criteria in the eighth edition of the AJCC manual. Although the mitotic rate is no longer included in staging criteria, it should be reported because an increasing mitotic rate is associated with poorer prognosis.[10]

PROGNOSIS

Generally, the earlier primary cutaneous melanoma is detected, the better the prognosis. Later detection increases the risk of metastatic disease, which occurs in up to 20% of melanoma cases.[7] The histologic features of Breslow thickness, ulceration, and mitotic rate also have all been shown to be predictive of prognosis.[10–13] The 5-year survival rate for localized melanoma less than 4.0 mm in thickness is typically greater than 90%.[5] For tumors greater than 4.0 mm in thickness, the 5-year and 10-year survival rates range from 82% to 90%, depending on ulceration status (**Table 1**).[10] However, the presence of regional and distant metastases results in 5-year survival rates of 63% and 20%, respectively.[5] It is estimated that 2% to 10% of patients with primary cutaneous melanoma will develop a recurrence at the primary site and are also at increased risk of developing a second primary malignancy.[14]

WORKUP

Patient workup should include a complete history and physical examination. History should include both personal and family history of skin cancer and melanoma, as well as any personal history of dysplastic nevi.[6] The physical examination should include a full-body skin examination, as well as palpation of lymph nodes, with special care taken to examine regional lymph nodes near the site of the primary cutaneous tumor.[6]

Patients are staged clinically after microstaging of the primary tumor is done from the initial biopsy specimen. Stage 0 primary cutaneous melanoma is synonymous with melanoma in situ (MIS). It encompasses cutaneous melanoma lesions that are confined to the epidermis without evidence of regional or distant metastases. SLNB, routine imaging, and laboratory evaluations are not recommended based on the low rates of metastasis seen in this population of patients.[6,13,15,16]

Table 1
Primary tumor classification and melanoma-specific survival in patients with stage I and II disease

T-Category	Tumor Thickness	Ulceration Status	T-Subcategory	MSS (10-y)
T1	<0.8 mm	No	T1a	98%
	<0.8 mm	Yes	T1b	96%
	0.8–1.0 mm	Yes or no	T1b	
T2	>1.0–2.0 mm	No	T2a	92%
		Yes	T2b	88%
T3	>2.0–4.0 mm	No	T3a	88%
		Yes	T3b	81%
T4	>4.0 mm	No	T4a	83%
		Yes	T4b	75%

Adapted from Gershenwald JE, Scolyer, RA, Hess KR, et al. Melanoma staging: Evidence-based changes in the American Joint Committee on Cancer eighth edition cancer staging manual. CA Cancer J Clin. 2017 Nov;67(6):472–492; with permission.

Stages I and II cutaneous melanoma include patients with T-category tumor thickness (T1–T4) without evidence of regional or distant metastases. As in stage 0 disease, routine imaging (computed tomography [CT], PET-CT, or MRI) and laboratory evaluation are not recommended in asymptomatic patients and should only be considered when there are concerning signs or symptoms on history and physical examination.[6,17–19] Ultrasonography of the nodal basin can be considered if there are equivocal findings on the physical examination. Certain patients may benefit from or require SLNB, and ultrasonography of regional lymph nodes may be used before SLNB to further evaluate lymph nodes for areas concerning for metastatic disease.[6,19] Screening regional lymph nodes with ultrasonography before SLNB has been shown to have a high sensitivity and specificity, 60% and 97%, respectively.[19] Patients with tumors of greater thickness and with features of ulceration and high mitotic rate are more likely to have a positive sentinel lymph node (SLN), with increasing tumor thickness being the strongest predictor.[6,20]

SENTINEL LYMPH NODE BIOPSY

SLNB is a procedure used to establish the presence or absence of nodal metastases. It is important for dermatologists to understand the indications for SLNB in patients with cutaneous melanoma. The SLN is the first draining lymph node from the site of the primary tumor and is identified via lymphatic mapping with lymphoscintigraphy following injection of radioisotope and/or blue dye.[1,3,21] The procedure is useful for determining prognosis and helps to guide future treatment, whether regional disease control or adjuvant therapy.[21] Guidelines on the indications for SLNB have been established by the American Society of Clinical Oncology and the Society of Surgical Oncology.[21] Indications for SLNB are based on Breslow tumor thickness and T-category.

Thin Melanoma

For patients with T1a melanomas (<0.8 mm without ulceration), SLNB is not recommended. However, it may be considered in patients with T1b melanomas (0.8–1.0 mm or <0.8 mm with ulceration). Approximately 5% of patients with thin melanomas have SLN metastases.[21–23] Patients with melanomas greater than 0.75 mm in Breslow thickness have been found to have an SLN positivity rate between 6.3% and 8.8%.[22,23] Additionally, similar SLN positivity rates have been seen in patients with melanomas greater than Clark level IV, those with greater than 1 mitoses/mm^2, and those

with ulceration.[22,23] The eighth edition of the AJCC staging manual incorporates these changes in the classification of T1b melanomas, and there is an improved prognosis in patients with a negative SLNB.[21] In comparison, patients with a positive SLNB have significantly worse MSS.[23] Ultimately, an individualized approach with attention to the aforementioned clinicopathologic risk factors is recommended when considering SLNB in patients with T1b disease.[21]

Intermediate-Thickness Melanoma

For patients with intermediate-thickness melanomas, defined as T2 to T3 (Breslow thickness >1.0–4.0 mm), SLNB is recommended. This recommendation helps improve regional disease control and decisions regarding adjuvant therapy.[21] Overall, the rate of nodal metastases in this patient population ranges from 16% to 20%, and the rate of complications from SLNB is approximately 5%.[21,24,25] With regard to intermediate-thickness melanoma, the Multicenter Selective Lymphadenectomy Trial I (MSLT-I) data deserve specific attention.

According to MSLT-I data, there was no significant difference in MSS after 10 years in subjects with intermediate-thickness melanomas, with or without nodal metastases, who underwent SLNB as opposed to nodal observation (hazard ratio [HR] for death from melanoma 0.84%; 95% CI 0.64–1.09; $P = .18$).[24] However, there was significantly higher 10-year disease-free survival (DFS) in subjects who underwent SLNB as opposed to nodal observation (HR for recurrence or metastasis 0.76%; 95% CI 0.62–0.94; $P = .01$).[24] Among subjects who underwent SLNB, those with metastases had poorer outcomes. The MSS rate at 10 years was 62% in those with a positive SLNB as opposed to 85% in those with a negative SLNB (HR for death from melanoma 3.09%; 95% CI 2.12–4.49; $P<.001$).[24] The estimated cumulative incidence of nodal metastasis at 10 years was 19.5% and 21.9% for subjects in the observation group and SLNB group, respectively. A total of 31 subjects (4.8%) who were found to have a negative SLNB ultimately developed metastases in the subsequent observation period.[24] In subjects with intermediate-thickness melanomas and nodal metastases, the MSS rate at 10 years was approximately 62% in those who underwent SLNB in comparison with 42% in those randomized to observation (HR for death from melanoma 0.56%; 95% CI 0.37–0.84; $P = .006$).[24] Despite this, the cumulative data failed to demonstrate a survival advantage for SLNB.

Surveillance Epidemiology and End Result (SEER) tumor registry data were used in another study in an attempt to clarify the results seen in MSLT-I.[26] The 5-year survival rate in the unmatched cohort of subjects who underwent SLNB was 87.9% in comparison with 83.9% in subjects who underwent nodal observation ($P<.0001$).[26] In the matched cohort, there was a small but significant difference in 5-year MSS in subjects who underwent SLNB in comparison with those who underwent nodal observation (85.7 vs 84%; $P = .02$).[26] Given the 1.7% improvement in MSS in subjects who underwent SLNB in this study, it could be inferred that MSLT-1 was underpowered to detect this small survival advantage.[26] Conversely, a Cochrane review of SLNB versus observation for localized primary cutaneous melanoma found no significant difference in overall survival (OS) between the groups.[3]

Certain features may be associated with higher rates of SLN positivity. Thickness seems to be the largest predictor of SLN positivity, and a positive SLNB can be seen in 21.2% of patients with tumors greater than 1.5 mm in thickness.[25] Additionally, the presence of lymphovascular invasion (LVI) is associated with higher rates of SLNB positivity in patients with tumors greater than 1.5 mm in thickness (40.8%).[25] In contrast, tumor thickness greater than 1.5 mm, absence of LVI, and absence of satellitosis are factors associated with decreased rates of SLN positivity.[25] The rate of SLNB positivity in patients with tumors greater than 1.5 mm in thickness is 6.6% (95% CI 3.8%–9.4%) and is similar to patients with thin melanomas.[25]

Thick Melanoma

For patients with thick melanomas, defined as T4 (Breslow thickness >4.0 mm), SLNB may be recommended. MSLT-I data revealed no significant difference in 10-year MSS between subjects who underwent SLNB in comparison with those who underwent nodal observation (48% vs 45.8%; HR 0.92%; 95% CI 0.53–1.6; $P = .78$).[24] However, 10-year DFS rates were significantly higher in the SLNB cohort (50.7% vs 40.5%; HR 0.7%; 95% CI 0.5–0.96; $P = .03$).[24] In subjects with thick melanomas and a positive SLNB, the 10-year MSS was 48% in comparison with 65% in those with a negative SLNB (HR 1.75%; 95% CI 1.07–2.87; $P = .03$).[24] A total of 57 subjects (32.9%) who underwent SLNB had nodal metastases and the cumulative incidence of nodal metastases in this subject population was 42% at 10 years.[24] Based on SEER data in subjects with thick melanomas, approximately 32% of subjects who underwent SLNB had nodal metastases.[26] Similar to the MSLT-I data, subjects with a positive SLNB had

a disease-specific survival (DSS) of 44.1% at 5 years in comparison with 75% in subjects with a negative SLNB.[26] As a result, SLNB does offer prognostic value and may be recommended for staging purposes and regional disease control.[21,26]

TREATMENT
Wide Excision

The recommended treatment modality for primary cutaneous melanoma is wide excision (WE). The recommended surgical margins are predicated on tumor thickness (T1–T4) and derived from randomized controlled trials in conjunction with expert consensus opinion (**Table 2**). It is well known that melanoma can spread subclinically and the goal of excision is to obtain negative margins to prevent recurrence.[1,27]

The recommended surgical margin for MIS is 0.5 cm to 1.0 cm around the visible lesion (see **Table 2**).[6] In clinical trials, there has not been an improvement in survival or a reduction in local recurrence with surgical margins exceeding 1 cm in subjects with MIS.[28–30] However, the lentigo maligna subtype of MIS has a greater risk of superficial spreading and thus may require greater than 0.5-cm margins to adequately clear.[31,32]

The recommended treatment of melanoma less than 1.0 mm in thickness is WE of the lesion with 1.0-cm margins (see **Table 1**).[1,6] When 1.0-cm margins have been compared with wider surgical margins, DFS and OS rates, as well as the development of metastatic disease, were similar.[32–35] However, margins less than 1.0 cm are associated with increased rates of local recurrence. For tumors that are 1.0 mm to 2.0 mm in thickness, surgical margins should be 1.0 cm to 2.0 cm

Table 2
Recommended surgical excision margins for primary cutaneous melanoma based on tumor thickness

Tumor Thickness	Recommended Surgical Excision Margins
In situ	0.5–1.0 cm
≤1.0 mm	1.0 cm
1.0–2.0 mm	1.0–2.0 cm
>2.0 mm	2.0 cm

Data from Bichakjian CK, Halpern AC, Johnson TM, et al. Guidelines of care for the management of primary cutaneous melanoma. American Academy of Dermatology. J Am Acad Dermatol 2011;65:1032–1047 and Coit DG, Thompson JA, Albertini MR. Melanoma. National Comprehensive Cancer Network Clinical Guidelines. 3.2018. Available at: www.NCCN.org. Accessed: October 9th 2018.

(see **Table 1**). This recommendation is derived from multiple prospective, randomized trials in which no significant differences with regard to local recurrence or OS were observed between 1.0-cm to 2.0-cm margins and margins greater than 3 cm for tumors less than 2.0 mm in thickness.[36–40] For tumors that are greater than 2.0 mm in thickness, surgical margins should be 2.0 cm (see **Table 1**).[6] This recommendation is based on prior studies that found no significant survival advantage when wider margins are used for melanomas less than 2 mm in thickness.[40–42] Specifically, a randomized controlled trial of 936 subjects with cutaneous melanoma greater than 2 mm in thickness showed no difference in OS at 5 years between 2-cm and 4-cm margins (65% vs 65%; $P = .69$).[43]

Exact margins within these parameters should be based on provider judgment, taking into account the location of the lesion, as well as cosmetic and functional issues.[1,6] The surgical excision depth for the removal of cutaneous melanoma of any stage should reach the deep subcutaneous tissue. The American Academy of Dermatology (AAD) recommends an excisional depth to at least the level of the muscular fascia, when feasible.[1] However, this recommendation is based on limited evidence.[1] Surgical sections are routinely processed in paraffin rather than as frozen sections if there is suspected subclinical extension of the tumor because permanent paraffin sections typically allow for better evaluation of surgical margins.[44] However, the use of frozen sections with MMS is increasingly being used for the treatment of MIS and invasive melanoma.

Mohs Micrographic Surgery

The recommendations for surgical margins based on Breslow thickness (see previous discussion) include several methods to achieve this goal, including WE, staged excision, and MMS. The advantage of MMS for melanoma is tissue conservation with more effective margin control and complete margin assessment histologically.[45] The rationale for more effective margin control is based on differences in histologic processing techniques. Traditional vertical sectioning examines less than 1% of the margin and MMS examines 100% of the surgical margin.[45] There is a 19% chance of detecting a positive margin if vertical sections are performed at 4-mm intervals.[46] However, vertical sections need to be performed at 0.1-mm intervals to detect 100% of positive margins, and this is clinically impractical.[45,46] As a result, MMS is an effective and practical modality

for complete margin assessment. However, the use of MMS in the treatment of melanoma is somewhat controversial.

In comparison with historical controls, MMS offers similar rates of survival to traditional WE, with similar or lower rates of metastases, and smaller surgical margins for thicker melanomas.[45,47,48] However, larger margins are often required for MIS and thinner melanomas when evaluated with the Mohs technique.[47,48] In a trial of 1246 subjects with MIS, 9-mm margins were required for 98.9% tumor clearance and the 10-year cancer-specific survival was 99.2%.[49] These results have been reproduced in other studies on MMS for MIS, with 6-mm margins required for 83% tumor clearance and 9-mm margins for 97% tumor clearance.[50]

Despite the advantages of margin control with MMS in the treatment of melanoma, difficulty in interpreting melanocytic proliferations on frozen sections has led some to question its utility, especially if not routinely performed.[45,47] As a result, immunostaining with melanocytic markers has been incorporated to aid in interpretation.[45]

Immunostaining has been used successfully with MMS for the treatment of MIS and invasive melanoma. There have been multiple studies establishing the efficacy of melanoma-associated antigen recognized by T cells (MART-1) immunostaining during MMS, resulting in similar rates of MSS, recurrence, and metastases. Local recurrence following MMS with MART-1 immunostaining ranges from less than 1% to 2%.[45,51,52] Approximately 5% of cases are upstaged at the time of extirpation and this is consistent with upstaging observed following WE.[51,53]

When used on frozen sections, MART-1 immunostaining allows for identification and evaluation of melanocytes and is equivalent to traditional permanent sections, whether stained with hematoxylin-eosin (H&E) stain or MART-1.[54] However, it is still difficult to differentiate from chronic sun damage and specific criteria for positive margins have been described. Indicators of tumor presence include: greater than 3 nests of atypical melanocytes, presence of melanocytes above the dermal-epidermal junction, confluence of melanocytes with greater than 9 adjacent melanocytes, vertical melanocytic stacking, nonuniform melanocytic hyperplasia, and the presence of atypical nests in the dermis.[45]

A study that used MART-1 staining in the treatment of 1982 subjects with melanoma revealed DSS rates of 100% for primary MIS and 96.42% for primary invasive melanoma.[45] When adjusted for thickness, MSS at 5 years was 98.7% for tumors less than 1 mm, 93.5% for tumors between

1.0 mm and 2.0 mm, and 85.4% for tumors between 2.0 mm and 4.0 mm, and 67.5% for tumors greater than 4 mm.[45] In a retrospective study of invasive melanomas, predominantly less than 1 mm in thickness and treated with MMS, local recurrence was 1.67% and MSS was 100% at 3.5 years.[52] Approximately 60% of these cases were on the head and neck, which are locations with historically higher rates of local recurrence. In comparison, a retrospective study of 151 subjects with invasive melanoma located on the face found no significant difference between MMS and WE with regard to local recurrence, MSS, and OS.[55] Additionally, another retrospective review of 662 subjects with MIS found no significant difference in recurrence rates at 5, 10, and 15 years between MMS and WE.[56] These studies did not use immunostaining with MMS and it could be argued that a difference may have been seen if this modality was used. Additionally, staged excision with en face margin assessment of permanent sections may allow for better histologic assessment of melanocytic lesions with similar surgical defects in comparison with MMS.[44,57] Similar findings were also seen in an analysis of SEER data from 2003 to 2012, which did not reveal a difference in MSS between MMS, narrow margin excision, and WE.[58] However, most melanomas treated with MMS throughout this time period were MIS. Overall, the treatment of MIS and invasive melanoma with MMS is evolving, with reduced to similar rates of local recurrence and survival in comparison with traditional modalities. The AAD recently updated their guidelines of care and it was published online on November 1, 2018. They affirm, "The general 1 cm minimum surgical margin for invasive cutaneous melanoma as espoused in all international guidelines and cautions strongly against the routine use of narrower surgical margins."[59]

ADJUVANT TREATMENT

Although surgical excision is the gold standard for treatment of all primary cutaneous melanomas, adjuvant treatments can be considered in specific situations. There is evidence for the use of imiquimod 5% cream as the primary treatment of the lentigo maligna subtype of MIS. However, there is an increased risk of recurrence with imiquimod treatment compared with surgical excision.[60–63] Specifically, a retrospective review of 12 subjects with MIS treated with imiquimod found a 17% recurrence rate at 5 years.[64] Imiquimod may also be used as an adjuvant treatment following surgical excision and may help to decrease the risk of subclinical extension and treat residual disease.[65]

A retrospective review of 22 subjects treated with imiquimod 5% cream following excision with residual MIS showed 95% clearance after posttreatment biopsy.[66] As stated, lentigo maligna often requires larger margins for clearance and is more common in the elderly. Imiquimod may be a reasonable option for such patients, or those with significant comorbidities, who are unwilling or unable to undergo surgical excision.

Radiation therapy and cryosurgery may also be used for treatment of the lentigo maligna subtype when complete surgical excision is not feasible. Similar to imiquimod, radiotherapy and cryotherapy may be used to treat lentigo maligna but with an increased risk of recurrence when compared with surgical excision.[67–71]

Patients should be educated that, if adjuvant therapy is used alone as the primary treatment, there is an increased risk of local recurrence due to potential undertreatment of the tumor because subclinical margins cannot be accurately assessed. There is up to a 25% risk of persistent tumor following treatment with imiquimod alone and up to a 14% risk following radiation therapy alone.[1,72] Additionally, there are no current treatment guidelines available for the use of these adjuvant therapies in the treatment of primary cutaneous melanoma.

FOLLOW-UP

The primary goal of follow-up and surveillance is to detect cutaneous melanoma, recurrent disease, and additional melanomas at an early phase of development, which is associated with improved survival.[73–75] Physical examination can detect up to 50% of recurrences and more frequent examinations may lead to earlier detection.[76] Following excision, 80% of recurrences occur within the first 3 years following diagnosis, with less than 8% of recurrences occurring after 5 years from diagnosis.[73] Therefore, the most critical follow-up period for these patients is within the first few years following treatment. Recurrent disease is most likely to occur in distant skin sites or nodes, followed by distant metastases.[77] If lymph node disease is suspected, lymph nodes should first be evaluated with ultrasonography.[19]

The AAD and the National Comprehensive Cancer Network guidelines recommend that patients with stage Ia to IIa disease be followed every 6 to 12 months for the first 5 years following diagnosis, then annually.[6,59] Patients with stage IIb to IV disease should be followed every 3 to 6 months for the first 2 years following diagnosis, then every 3 to 12 months for an additional 3 to 5 years, and then annually.[6,59] All patients should at least have a yearly dermatologic examination for life because recurrent disease discovered more than 10 years after initial diagnosis is documented.[6,78] In particular, a study of 1372 subjects with stage I to II melanoma found that 5.6% of subjects relapsed after more than 10 years following their primary diagnosis.[78]

Routine surveillance with imaging or laboratory studies in asymptomatic patients with stage Ia to IIa disease is not recommended.[1,79–81] For patients with stage IIb to IIc disease, there are no recommendations for imaging or laboratory studies if asymptomatic. Chest radiograph, CT, and/or brain MRI may be used at physicians' discretion within the first 3 to 5 years after diagnosis to screen for asymptomatic recurrent disease, although there are no specific guidelines for the use of these tests owing to conflicting evidence in the literature.[6,82,83] When routine imaging is used, ultrasonography has the highest sensitivity and specificity when used for surveillance of lymph node metastases, whereas PET-CT had the highest sensitivity and specificity when used for surveillance of distant metastases.[19] However, routine imaging in asymptomatic patients is not recommended beyond 3 to 5 years following initial diagnosis.[6]

At each follow-up visit, patients should receive a full-body skin examination, as well as a thorough history and review of systems to assess for signs of disease recurrence. Providers should take into account patient anxiety, personal and family history of skin cancer, history of dysplastic nevi, number of nevi overall, and ability to self-detect suspicious lesions to devise individualized follow-up schedules.[8] Patients should be educated on how to self-identify suspicious lesions and palpate regional lymph nodes to help detect recurrences and potential metastases. Almost half of melanoma recurrences are detected by the patient themselves, followed by physical examination, and then constitutional symptoms.[73,74,79–82] As a result, all patients should also be encouraged to come in earlier than scheduled if a suspicious lesion is discovered.[84]

SUMMARY

Overall, the management of primary cutaneous melanoma is evolving. Earlier detection and better characterization of management strategies have led to improvements in prognosis and survival. Collaboration among specialties is essential to delivery of high-quality cancer care and dermatologists play an important role in the detection and management of melanoma.

REFERENCES

1. Bichakjian CK, Halpern AC, Johnson TM, et al. Guidelines of care for the management of primary cutaneous melanoma. American Academy of Dermatology. J Am Acad Dermatol 2011;65:1032–47.
2. Kibbi N, Kluger H, Choi JN. Melanoma: clinical presentations. Cancer Treat Res 2016;167:107–29.
3. Kyrgidis A, Tzellos T, Mocellin S, et al. Sentinel lymph node biopsy followed by lymph node dissection for localised primary cutaneous melanoma. Cochrane Database Syst Rev 2015;(5):CD010307.
4. Chen ST, Geller AC, Tsao H. Update on the epidemiology of melanoma. Curr Dermatol Rep 2013;2:24–34.
5. Siegel RL. Cancer statistics, 2018. CA Cancer J Clin 2018;68(1):7–30.
6. Coit DG, Thompson JA, Albertini MR. Melanoma. National Comprehensive Cancer Network clinical guidelines. 3 2018. Available at: www.NCCN.org. Accessed October 9, 2018.
7. Stell VH, Norton HJ, Smith KS, et al. Method of biopsy and incidence of positive margins in primary melanoma. Ann Surg Oncol 2007;14:893–8.
8. Ng JC, Swain S, Dowling JP, et al. The impact of partial biopsy on histopathologic diagnosis of cutaneous melanoma: experience of an Australian tertiary referral service. Arch Dermatol 2010;146:234–9.
9. Armour K, Mann S, Lee S. Dysplastic nevi: to shave, or not to shave? A retrospective study of the use of the shave biopsy technique in the initial management of dysplastic nevi. Australas J Dermatol 2005;46:70–5.
10. Gershenwald JE, Scolyer RA, Hess KR, et al. Melanoma staging: evidence-based changes in the American Joint Committee on Cancer eighth edition cancer staging manual. CA Cancer J Clin 2017;67(6):472–92.
11. Oliveira Filho RS, Ferreira LM, Biasi LJ, et al. Vertical growth phase and positive sentinel node in thin melanoma. Braz J Med Biol Res 2003;36:347–50.
12. Xu X, Chen L, Guerry D, et al. Lymphatic invasion is independently prognostic of metastasis in primary cutaneous melanoma. Clin Cancer Res 2012;18:229–37.
13. Balch CM, Soong SJ, Gershenwald JE, et al. Prognostic factors analysis of 17,600 melanoma patients: validation of the American Joint Committee on Cancer melanoma staging system. J Clin Oncol 2001;19:3622–34.
14. Caini S, Boniol M, Botteri E, et al. The risk of developing a second primary cancer in melanoma patients: a comprehensive review of the literature and meta-analysis. J Dermatol Sci 2014;75:3–9.
15. Ho Shon IA, Chung DK, Saw RP, et al. Imaging in cutaneous melanoma. Nucl Med Commun 2008;29:847–76.

16. Andtbacka RH, Gershenwald JE. Role of sentinel lymph node biopsy in patients with thin melanoma. J Natl Compr Canc Netw 2009;7:308–17.

17. Wang TS, Johnson TM, Cascade PN, et al. Evaluation of staging chest radiographs and serum lactate dehydrogenase for localized melanoma. J Am Acad Dermatol 2004;51:399–405.

18. Yancovitz M, Finelt N, Warycha MA, et al. Role of radiologic imaging at the time of initial diagnosis of stage T1b-T3b melanoma. Cancer 2007;110: 1107–14.

19. Xing Y, Bronstein Y, Ross MI, et al. Contemporary diagnostic imaging modalities for the staging and surveillance of melanoma patients: a meta-analysis. J Natl Cancer Inst 2011;103:129–42.

20. Statius Muller MG, van Leeuwen PA, de Lange-De Klerk ES, et al. The sentinel lymph node status is an important factor for predicting clinical outcome in patients with Stage I or II cutaneous melanoma. Cancer 2001;91:2401–8.

21. Wong SL, Kennedy EB, Lyman GH. Sentinel lymph node biopsy and management of regional lymph nodes in melanoma: American Society of Clinical Oncology and Society of Surgical Oncology clinical practice guideline update summary. J Oncol Pract 2018;14(4):242–5.

22. Cordeiro E, Gervais MK, Shah PS, et al. Sentinel lymph node biopsy in thin cutaneous melanoma: a systematic review and meta-analysis. Ann Surg Oncol 2016;23(13):4178–88.

23. Han D, Zager JS, Shyr Y, et al. Clinicopathologic predictors of sentinel lymph node metastasis in thin melanoma. J Clin Oncol 2013;31(35): 4387–93.

24. Morton DL, Thompson JF, Cochran AJ, et al, MSLT Group. Final trial report of sentinel-node biopsy versus nodal observation in melanoma. N Engl J Med 2014;370(7):599–609.

25. Bartlett EK, Peters MG, Blair A, et al. Identification of patients with intermediate thickness melanoma at low risk for sentinel lymph node positivity. Ann Surg Oncol 2016;23(1):250–6.

26. Kachare SD, Brinkley J, Wong JH, et al. The influence of sentinel lymph node biopsy on survival for intermediate-thickness melanoma. Ann Surg Oncol 2014;21(11):3377–85.

27. McKenna DB, Lee RJ, Prescott RJ, et al. A retrospective observational study of primary cutaneous malignant melanoma patients treated with excision only compared with excision biopsy followed by wider local excision. Br J Dermatol 2004; 150:523–30.

28. Akhtar S, Bhat W, Magdum A, et al. Surgical excision margins for melanoma in situ. J Plast Reconstr Aesthet Surg 2014;67:320–3.

29. Welch T, Reid J, Knox ML, et al. Excision of melanoma in situ on nonchronically sun-exposed skin using 5-mm surgical margins. J Am Acad Dermatol 2014;71:834–6.

30. Duffy KL, Truong A, Bowen GM, et al. Adequacy of 5-mm surgical excision margins for non-lentiginous melanoma in situ. J Am Acad Dermatol 2014;71(4): 835–8.

31. Felton S, Taylor RS, Srivastava D. Excision margins for melanoma in situ on the head and neck. Dermatol Surg 2016;42:327–34.

32. Anderson KW, Baker SR, Lowe L, et al. Treatment of head and neck melanoma, lentigo maligna subtype: a practical surgical technique. Arch Facial Plast Surg 2001;3:202–6.

33. Veronesi U, Cascinelli N. Narrow excision (1-cm margin). A safe procedure for thin cutaneous melanoma. Arch Surg 1991;126:438–41.

34. Veronesi U, Cascinelli N, Adamus J, et al. Thin stage I primary cutaneous malignant melanoma. Comparison of excision with margins of 1 or 3 cm. N Engl J Med 1988;318(18):1159–62.

35. Lens MB, Nathan P, Bataille V. Excision margins for primary cutaneous melanoma: updated pooled analysis of randomized controlled trials. Arch Surg 2007;142:885–93.

36. Ringborg U, Andersson R, Eldh J, et al. Resection margins of 2 versus 5 cm for cutaneous malignant melanoma with a tumor thickness of 0.8 to 2.0 mm: randomized study by the Swedish melanoma study group. Cancer 1996;77:1809–14.

37. Cohn-Cedermark G, Rutqvist LE, Andersson R, et al. Long term results of a randomized study by the Swedish Melanoma Study Group on 2-cm versus 5-cm resection margins for patients with cutaneous melanoma with a tumor thickness of 0.8-2.0 mm. Cancer 2000;89:1495–501.

38. Khayat D, Rixe O, Martin G, et al. Surgical margins in cutaneous melanoma (2 cm versus 5 cm for lesions measuring less than 2.1-mm thick). Cancer 2003;97:1941–6.

39. Haigh PI, DiFronzo LA, McCready DR. Optimal excision margins for primary cutaneous melanoma: a systematic review and meta-analysis. Can J Surg 2003;46:419–26.

40. Hayes AJ, Maynard L, Coombes G, et al, UK Melanoma Study Group; British Association of Plastic; Reconstructive and Aesthetic Surgeons, and the Scottish Cancer Therapy Network. Wide versus narrow excision margins for high-risk, primary cutaneous melanomas: long-term follow-up of survival in a randomised trial. Lancet Oncol 2016;17(2): 184–92.

41. Balch CM, Soong SJ, Smith T, et al, Investigators from the Intergroup Melanoma Surgical Trial. Long-term results of a prospective surgical trial comparing 2 cm vs. 4 cm excision margins for 740 patients with 1-4 mm melanomas. Ann Surg Oncol 2001;8(2):101–8.

42. Balch CM, Urist MM, Karakousis CP, et al. Efficacy of 2-cm surgical margins for intermediate-thickness melanomas (1 to 4 mm). Results of a multi-institutional randomized surgical trial. Ann Surg 1993;218(3):262–7.

43. Gillgren P, Drzewiecki KT, Niin M, et al. 2-cm versus 4-cm surgical excision margins for primary cutaneous melanoma thicker than 2 mm: a randomised, multicentre trial. Lancet 2011;378(9803):1635–42.

44. Prieto VG, Argenyi ZB, Barnhill RL, et al. Are en face frozen sections accurate for diagnosing margin status in melanocytic lesions? Am J Clin Pathol 2003; 120:203–8.

45. Valentín-Nogueras SM, Brodland DG, Zitelli JA, et al. Mohs micrographic surgery using MART-1 immunostain in the treatment of invasive melanoma and melanoma in situ. Dermatol Surg 2016;42(6): 733–44.

46. Kimyai-Asadi A, Katz T, Goldberg LH, et al. Margin involvement after the excision of melanoma in situ: the need for complete en face examination of the surgical margins. Dermatol Surg 2007;33(12): 1434–9 [discussion: 1439–41].

47. Zitelli JA, Brown C, Hanusa BH. Mohs micrographic surgery for the treatment of primary cutaneous melanoma. J Am Acad Dermatol 1997;37(2 Pt 1): 236–45.

48. Bricca GM, Brodland DG, Ren D, et al. Cutaneous head and neck melanoma treated with Mohs micrographic surgery. J Am Acad Dermatol 2005;52(1): 92–100.

49. Kunishige JH, Brodland DG, Zitelli JA. Surgical margins for melanoma in situ. J Am Acad Dermatol 2012;66(3):438–44.

50. Stigall LE, Brodland DG, Zitelli JA. The use of Mohs micrographic surgery (MMS) for melanoma in situ (MIS) of the trunk and proximal extremities. J Am Acad Dermatol 2016;75(5):1015–21.

51. Etzkorn JR, Sobanko JF, Elenitsas R, et al. Low recurrence rates for in situ and invasive melanomas using Mohs micrographic surgery with melanoma antigen recognized by T cells 1 (MART-1) immunostaining: tissue processing methodology to optimize pathologic staging and margin assessment. J Am Acad Dermatol 2015;72(5):840–50.

52. Degesys CA, Powell HB, Hsia LB, et al. Outcomes for invasive melanomas treated with mohs micrographic surgery: a retrospective cohort study. Dermatol Surg 2019;45(2):223–8.

53. Etzkorn JR, Sharkey JM, Grunyk JW, et al. Frequency of and risk factors for tumor upstaging after wide local excision of primary cutaneous melanoma. J Am Acad Dermatol 2017;77(2):341–8.

54. Cherpelis BS, Moore R, Ladd S, et al. Comparison of MART-1 frozen sections to permanent sections using a rapid 19-minute protocol. Dermatol Surg 2009; 35(2):207–13.

55. Chin-Lenn L, Murynka T, McKinnon JG, et al. Comparison of outcomes for malignant melanoma of the face treated using Mohs micrographic surgery and wide local excision. Dermatol Surg 2013; 39(11):1637–45.

56. Nosrati A, Berliner JG, Goel S, et al. Outcomes of melanoma in situ treated with Mohs micrographic surgery compared with wide local excision. JAMA Dermatol 2017;153(5):436–41.

57. Walling HW, Scupham RK, Bean AK, et al. Staged excision versus Mohs micrographic surgery for lentigo maligna and lentigo maligna melanoma. J Am Acad Dermatol 2007;57(4):659–64.

58. Trofymenko O, Bordeaux JS, Zeitouni NC. Melanoma of the face and Mohs micrographic surgery: nationwide mortality data analysis. Dermatol Surg 2018;44(4):481–92.

59. Swetter SM, Tsao H, Bichakjian CK, et al. Guidelines of care for the management of primary cutaneous melanoma. J Am Acad Dermatol 2018. https://doi.org/10.1016/j.jaad.2018.08.055.

60. Buettiker UV, Yawalkar NY, Braathen LR, et al. Imiquimod treatment of lentigo maligna: an open-label study of 34 primary lesions in 32 patients. Arch Dermatol 2008;144:943–5.

61. Spenny ML, Walford J, Werchniak AE, et al. Lentigo maligna (melanoma in situ) treated with imiquimod cream 5%: 12 case reports. Cutis 2007;79:149–52.

62. Cotter MA, McKenna JK, Bowen GM. Treatment of lentigo maligna with imiquimod before staged excision. Dermatol Surg 2008;34:147–51.

63. Gautschi M, Oberholzer PA, Baumgartner M, et al. Prognostic markers in lentigo maligna patients treated with imiquimod cream: a long-term follow-up study. J Am Acad Dermatol 2016;74(1):81–7.e1.

64. Park AJ, Paul J, Chapman MS, et al. Long-term outcomes of melanoma in situ treated with topical 5% imiquimod cream: a retrospective review. Dermatol Surg 2017;43(8):1017–22.

65. Swetter SM, Chen FW, Kim DD, et al. Imiquimod 5% cream as primary or adjuvant therapy for melanoma in situ, lentigo maligna type. J Am Acad Dermatol 2015;72:1047–53.

66. Pandit AS, Geiger EJ, Ariyan S, et al. Using topical imiquimod for the management of positive in situ margins after melanoma resection. Cancer Med 2015;4(4):507–12.

67. Fogarty GB, Hong A, Scolyer RA, et al. Radiotherapy for lentigo maligna: a literature review and recommendations for treatment. Br J Dermatol 2014;170:52–8.

68. Schmid-Wendtner MH, Brunner B, Konz B, et al. Fractionated radiotherapy of lentigo maligna and lentigo maligna melanoma in 64 patients. J Am Acad Dermatol 2000;43:477–82.

69. Farshad A, Burg G, Panizzon R, et al. A retrospective study of 150 patients with lentigo

maligna and lentigo maligna melanoma and the efficacy of radiotherapy using Grenz or soft X-rays. Br J Dermatol 2002;146:1042–6.

70. Kuflik EG, Gage AA. Cryosurgery for lentigo maligna. J Am Acad Dermatol 1994;31:75–8.

71. Collins P, Rogers S, Goggin M, et al. Cryotherapy for lentigo maligna. Clin Exp Dermatol 1991;16:433–5.

72. Kai AC, Richards T, Coleman A, et al. Five-year recurrence rate of lentigo maligna after treatment with imiquimod. Br J Dermatol 2016;174(1):165–8.

73. Dicker TJ, Kavanagh GM, Herd RM, et al. A rational approach to melanoma follow-up in patients with primary cutaneous melanoma. Scottish Melanoma Group. Br J Dermatol 1999;140:249–54.

74. Hofmann U, Szedlak M, Rittgen W, et al. Primary staging and follow-up in melanoma patients-monocenter evaluation of methods, costs and patient survival. Br J Cancer 2002;87:151–7.

75. Leiter U, Buettner PG, Eigentler TK, et al. Is detection of melanoma metastasis during surveillance in an early phase of development associated with a survival benefit? Melanoma Res 2010;20:240–6.

76. Garbe C, Paul A, Kohler-Spath H, et al. Prospective evaluation of a follow-up schedule in cutaneous melanoma patients: recommendations for an effective follow-up strategy. J Clin Oncol 2003;21:520–9.

77. Salama AK, de Rosa N, Scheri RP, et al. Hazard-rate analysis and patterns of recurrence in early stage melanoma: moving towards a rationally designed surveillance strategy. PLoS One 2013;8: e57665.

78. Osella-Abate S, Ribero S, Sanlorenzo M, et al. Risk factors related to late metastases in 1,372 melanoma patients disease free more than 10 years. Int J Cancer 2015;136:2453–7.

79. Basseres N, Grob JJ, Richard MA, et al. Cost-effectiveness of surveillance of stage I melanoma. A retrospective appraisal based on a 10-year experience in a dermatology department in France. Dermatology 1995;191:199–203.

80. Mooney MM, Kulas M, McKinley B, et al. Impact on survival by method of recurrence detection in stage I and II cutaneous melanoma. Ann Surg Oncol 1998; 5(1):54–63.

81. Moore Dalal K, Zhou Q, Panageas KS, et al. Methods of detection of first recurrence in patients with stage I/II primary cutaneous melanoma after sentinel lymph node biopsy. Ann Surg Oncol 2008; 15:2206–14.

82. Meyers MO, Yeh JJ, Frank J, et al. Method of detection of initial recurrence of stage II/III cutaneous melanoma: analysis of the utility of follow-up staging. Ann Surg Oncol 2009;16:941–7.

83. Podlipnik S, Carrera C, Sanchez M, et al. Performance of diagnostic tests in an intensive follow-up protocol for patients with American Joint Committee on Cancer (AJCC) stage IIB, IIC, and III localized primary melanoma: a prospective cohort study. J Am Acad Dermatol 2016;75: 516–24.

84. Pollitt RA, Geller AC, Brooks DR, et al. Efficacy of skin self-examination practices for early melanoma detection. Cancer Epidemiol Biomarkers Prev 2009;18:3018–23.

Systemic Therapies for Advanced Melanoma

Leonora Bomar, MD*, Aditi Senithilnathan, BA, Christine Ahn, MD

KEYWORDS

- Melanoma • Metastatic • Advanced • BRAF inhibitors • MEK inhibitors • Anti-PD1 agents
- Ipilimumab • Chemotherapy

KEY POINTS

- Although systemic therapy is the treatment of choice for metastatic melanoma, there is no standard regimen at this time.
- Current systemic therapies include chemotherapy, interleukin-2, small molecule targeted therapy (BRAF and MEK inhibitors, immune checkpoint inhibitors (cytotoxic T lymphocyte–associated antigen-4 and programmed cell death-1 inhibitors), interferon alfa, and viral oncolytic therapy.
- Each therapy comes with unique cutaneous and extracutaneous side effects and requires management strategies to deal with these effects.

INTRODUCTION

Metastatic melanoma is the sixth most prevalent cancer in the United States and accounts for more than 80% of skin cancer mortalities.[1] Surgical resection is the standard of care for localized disease, with 5-year survival rates of 98% and 90% for American Joint Commission on Cancer (AJCC) stages I and II, respectively.[2] Stage III melanoma, defined by regional metastases at the time of diagnosis, is managed by surgical resection and adjuvant chemotherapy. Although stage III has a higher risk of recurrence compared with stage I and II melanoma, stage IV melanoma, defined by distant metastases at diagnosis, has a median survival of less than 1 year. Advanced (stage IV) melanoma is treated with systemic therapy, and traditional cytotoxic chemotherapy was the standard until the early 2000s. Five-year survival rates with chemotherapy are around 16%.[3,4] In the last decade several new therapeutic options, including immune checkpoint inhibitors, small molecule targeted therapy, and oncolytic viral agents, have been approved by the US Food and Drug Administration (FDA) for advanced melanoma and have significantly altered the treatment landscape.

CHEMOTHERAPY

Before the development of targeted and immunotherapy, chemotherapy was the mainstay of treatment of widespread melanoma. Chemotherapeutic agents used to treat advanced-stage melanoma include dacarbazine (DTIC), temozolamide, carboplatin, cisplatin, vincristine, vinblastine, carmustine, fotemustine, paclitaxel, and docetaxel. DTIC was approved by the FDA in 1975 for the treatment of melanoma and remains the only FDA-approved cytotoxic chemotherapy agent for melanoma to date (**Table 1**).[5,6] DTIC is given intravenously at a dosage of 850 mg/m^2/d for 1 day or 150 to 250 mg/m^2/d for 5 days repeated every 3 weeks.[5] In a large meta-analysis of patients with metastatic melanoma, only 15% of patients responded to DTIC, and the progression-free survival (PFS) was 5 to 6 months.[7] Studies have failed to show any survival benefit with DTIC.[6,7] The main adverse effects (AEs) include nausea,

Disclosures: Dr L. Bomar, A. Senithilnathan, and Dr C. Ahn have no conflicts to disclose.
Department of Dermatology, Wake Forest School of Medicine, Winston-Salem, NC, USA
* Corresponding author. 4618 Country Club Road, Winston-Salem, NC 27104.
E-mail address: lculp@wakehealth.edu

Dermatol Clin 37 (2019) 409–423
https://doi.org/10.1016/j.det.2019.05.001
0733-8635/19/© 2019 Elsevier Inc. All rights reserved.

Table 1
Systemic therapies for advanced melanoma

Cytotoxic Chemotherapy	DTIC
	Temozolamide
	Carboplatin/cisplatin
	Vincristine/vinblastine
	Carmustine/fotemustine
	Paclitaxel
	Docetaxel
Small Molecule Targeted Therapy	
BRAF Inhibitors	Vemurafenib
	Dabrafenib
	Encorafenib
MEK Inhibitors	Trametinib
	Cobimetinib
	Binimetinib
BRAF + MEK Inhibitors	Dabrafenib + trametinib
	Vemurafenib + cobimetinib
	Encorafenib + binimetinib
Immunotherapy	
CTLA-4 Inhibitors	Ipilimumab
PD-1 Inhibitors	Nivolumab
	Pembrolizumab
Combination Immunotherapy	Nivolumab + ipilimumab
Other Therapies	Interleukin-2
	Oncolytic viral therapy
	Interferon alfa

Abbreviations: CTLA-4, cytotoxic T lymphocyte–associated antigen-4.

vomiting, fatigue, flulike symptoms, and myelosuppression.[5,7] Severe complications include liver failure from hepatic necrosis and venoocclusive disease (Budd-Chiari syndrome).

Temozolomide, an oral analogue of DTIC, failed to show improved response rates (RRs) or overall survival (OS) compared with DTIC in 2 phase III trials.[5,6] Despite good central nervous system penetrance, temozolomide in combination with cisplatin and interleukin-2 (IL-2) showed no benefit in preventing recurrence of melanoma brain metastases compared with DTIC with cisplatin and IL-2.[5] Vinca alkaloids (vincristine and vinblastine), taxanes (paclitaxel and docetaxel), nitrosoureas (carmustine, lomustine, and fotemustine), and platinum analogues (cisplatin and carboplatin) have failed to show improved RR or OS for stage IV melanoma compared with DTIC monotherapy.[5]

Combination chemotherapy initially showed promise for stage IV melanoma with RR of 50% to 55% in one single institution study with the Dartmouth regimen (cisplatin, DTIC, carmustine, and tamoxifen).[8] A large, phase III, multicenter trial failed to replicate these robust responses, finding no significant difference in RR compared with DTIC monotherapy.[9] Although various other combination chemotherapy regimens have shown slightly higher RR compared with DTIC, they are not routinely used because of lack of survival advantage and a more severe side effect profile compared with DTIC.[5–7,10] Common AEs of these combination regimens include nausea, vomiting, fatigue, and myelosuppression.[6,7]

INTERLEUKIN-2

IL-2, or aldesleukin, was approved by the FDA in 1998 for the treatment of metastatic melanoma.[11] IL-2 is a glycoprotein that stimulates T-cell and natural killer cell proliferation. It is given as an intravenous infusion with varied dosing parameters.[10] In an analysis of 270 patients with metastatic melanoma treated with Il-2, the overall response rate was 16%.[11] A complete response was seen in 6% of patients, and the median OS rate was 11.4 months.[11] Among the small percentage of patients who had a complete response, the response duration was between 24 and 106 months for 10 of the 17 patients.[1] AEs with IL-2 can be severe and occur secondary to capillary leak syndrome and lymphoid infiltration of many organs.[12] They include fever, chills, hypotension, tachycardia, nausea, vomiting, diarrhea, shortness of breath, pulmonary edema, oliguria, erythema, pruritus, confusion, psychosis, thrombocytopenia, bilirubinemia, and increased creatinine level (**Table 2**).[11] Hypotension and tachycardia are the most common AEs, typically develop within the first 2 hours of treatment, and are treated initially with intravenous fluids.[12] There are currently several trials on combination therapy with IL-2 and immune checkpoint inhibitors and small molecule targeted therapy for metastatic melanoma.

SMALL MOLECULE TARGETED THERAPY
BRAF Inhibitors

BRAF, a component of the mitogen-activated protein kinase (MAPK) signaling pathway, is the most commonly mutated oncogene in human tumors.[13,14] Around 40% to 60% of metastatic cutaneous melanomas have mutations in BRAF. The most common mutation occurs at codon V600E with a substitution of glutamic acid for valine. Other mutations include BRAFV600K, BRAFV600D, and non-V600 BRAF mutations.[13,14]

Table 2
Adverse effects with interleukin-2 therapy

Mucocutaneous
- Morbilliform eruption

Extracutaneous
- Hypotension
- Fever
- Fatigue
- Chills
- Myalgia
- Arrhythmia
- Tachycardia
- Pulmonary edema
- Weight gain
- Peripheral edema
- Shortness of breath
- Acute respiratory distress syndrome
- Increased creatinine level
- Oliguria
- Hallucinations
- Confusion
- Delirium
- Neutropenia
- Thrombocytopenia
- Nausea
- Vomiting
- Diarrhea
- Hyperbilirubinemia
- Transaminitis
- Metabolic acidosis
- Hypocalcemia
- Hypomagnesemia
- Hypophosphatemia

Targeted treatment of this mutation has led to the development of 3 BRAF inhibitors: vemurafenib, dabrafenib, and encorafenib (see **Table 1**). Vemurafenib was the first BRAFV600E inhibitor approved by the FDA, in August 2011, for the treatment of metastatic melanoma with BRAFV600E mutations.[14,15] The standard dosage is 960 mg twice daily by mouth. In phase I to III trials, vemurafenib showed rapid tumor shrinkage and improved survival rates compared with DTIC (**Table 3**).[14,15] In phase III trial BRIM-3, PFS was 6.9 months with vemurafenib compared with 1.6 months with DTIC. Median OS was 13.6 months with vemurafenib compared with 9.7 months with DTIC.[14,15] Dabrafenib was approved by the FDA in 2013 for treatment of metastatic melanoma with BRAFV600E mutations.[16] The standard dosage is 150 mg twice daily by mouth. In phase III trial BREAK-3, the response rate was 50% with dabrafenib compared with 6% with DTIC. PFS was 5.1 months with dabrafenib compared with 2.7 months with DTIC.[17] Encorafenib has been approved in combination with binimetinib for metastatic melanoma in 2018. This combination has shown improved PFS and OS in BRAF mutant melanoma compared with vemurafenib monotherapy.[18]

Malignant melanoma cells develop resistance to BRAF inhibitor monotherapy within 5 to 7 months of treatment.[14,15,17] Resistance occurs either through MAPK pathway–dependent or MAPK pathway–independent mutations (**Box 1**).[19–24] MAPK pathway–dependent mutations occur by paradoxic reactivation of the MAPK pathway via new NRAS or MEK mutations, or overexpression of COT. MAPK-independent resistance bypasses the MAPK pathway entirely, usually by signaling via the phosphatidylinositol 3 kinase (PI3K) pathway. This process occurs through upregulation of platelet-derived growth factor receptor, upregulation of insulinlike growth factor receptor, and genomic loss of phosphatase and tensin homolog (PTEN).[19–24] Because of the rapid resistance seen with BRAF monotherapy, BRAF inhibitors are combined with MEK

Table 3
Efficacy of BRAF and MEK inhibitor monotherapy

Studies	Treatment	Response Rate (%)	PFS (mo)	Median OS (mo)
Chapman et al,[14] 2011; Chapman et al,[15] 2017 (BRIM-3)	Group 1 (n = 337): Vemurafenib 960 mg BID Group 2: (n = 338) dacarbazine IV 1000 mg/m² every 3 wk	Group 1: 48 Group 2: 5	Group 1: 6.9 Group 2: 1.6	Group 1: 13.6 Group 2: 9.7
Hauschild et al,[16] 2012 (BREAK-3)	Group 1: (n = 187) Dabrafenib 150 mg BID Group 2: (n = 63) Dacarbazine IV 1000 mg/m² every 3 wk	Group 1: 50 Group 2: 6	Group 1: 5.1 Group 2: 2.7	Group 1: NA Group 2: NA
Flaherty et al,[16] 2012 (METRIC)	Group 1: (n = 214) Trametinib 2 mg daily Group 2: (n = 108) Dacarbazine IV 1000 mg/m² every 3 wk	Group 1: 22 Group 2: 8	Group 1: 4.8 Group 2: 1.5	Group 1: 81% at 6 mo Group 2: 67% at 6 mo

Abbreviations: BID, twice a day; IV, intravenous; NA, not available.

Box 1
Mechanisms of resistance to BRAF inhibitors

MAPK-dependent mutations:

- NRAS mutations[19,24]
- MEK mutations[23,24]
- COT overexpression[20]

MAPK-independent mutations via phosphatidylinositol 3 kinase/protein kinase B pathway alterations[23]

- Upregulated platelet-derived growth factor receptor
- Upregulated insulinlike growth factor receptor
- Loss of phosphatase and tensin homolog[20–24]

inhibitors for the treatment of melanoma with BRAF mutations.

The most common AEs with BRAF inhibitors are skin toxicities, pyrexia, fatigue, headache, arthralgia, and gastrointestinal events (**Table 4**).[14,15,17,25–30] Most AEs are similar across BRAF inhibitors except for 2 notable differences. Photosensitivity and increased liver enzyme levels occur more frequently with vemurafenib, whereas pyrexia is worse with dabrafenib.[14,15,17,27] Epidermal neoplasms including verrucal keratoses, plantar hyperkeratosis, actinic keratoses, keratoacanthomas (KAs), and squamous cell carcinomas (SCCs) are the most common cutaneous effects and develop because of paradoxic activation of the MAPK pathway.[26–28,31] Verrucal keratoses are the most common of the epidermal neoplasms.[27] They occurred in 66.4% of patients on dabrafenib and 72.2% on vemurafenib monotherapy in one study. These lesions develop as early as 1 week into therapy and can be removed with cryotherapy.[27] SCCs and KAs develop within the first 3 months of therapy.[31] Therapeutic options include excision, electrodessication and fulguration, systemic retinoids, intralesional fluorouracil injections, and photodynamic therapy (**Table 5**).[28,29,32–35] Grover disease is seen in up to 42.9% of patients on dabrafenib and 38.9% of patients on vemurafenib.[27] Other BRAF inhibitor–induced rashes include morbilliform exanthem, folliculocentric eruption, drug rash with eosinophilia and systemic symptoms (DRESS), Stevens-Johnson syndrome (SJS), and toxic epidermal necrolysis (TEN).[25,36–39] Additional cutaneous side effects include erythema nodosum–like lesions, Sweet syndrome,

Table 4
Adverse effects with BRAF inhibitor therapy

Mucocutaneous

- Morbilliform exanthem
- Folliculocentric eruption
- Acneiform eruption
- Keratosis pilaris–like Eruption
- Seborrheic dermatitis–like Eruption
- Hyperkeratotic hand-foot reaction
- Stevens-Johnson syndrome/toxic epidermolysis necrosis
- DRESS
- Granuloma annulare
- Neutrophilic eccrine hidradenitis
- Erythema nodosum–like panniculitis
- Sweet syndrome
- Pyoderma gangrenosum
- Sarcoidal-like reaction
- Granulomatous eruption
- Pruritus
- Xerosis

- Photosensitivity
- Seborrheic keratosis
- Hyperkeratosis
- Verrucal keratosis
- Skin papillomas
- Actinic keratosis
- Keratoacanthoma
- Squamous cell carcinoma
- Eruptive/changing nevi
- Plantar hyperkeratosis
- Vitiligo
- Curly, brittle hair
- Onycholysis
- Paronychia
- Brittle nails
- Alopecia
- Grover disease
- Radiation recall
- New melanoma

Extracutaneous

- Constitutional: fatigue, arthralgia, myalgia, fever, weight loss
- Neurologic: headache, neuropathy, encephalopathy
- Cardiovascular: prolonged QT, peripheral edema, hypertension
- Pulmonary: cough
- Gastrointestinal: nausea, vomiting, constipation, diarrhea, increased bilirubin level, increased LFTs, granulomatous hepatitis
- Hematologic: neutropenia, anemia, thrombocytopenia
- Ophthalmologic: uveitis, central retinal vein occlusion
- Other: increased cholesterol level, dysgeusia

Abbreviations: DRESS, drug rash with eosinophilia and systemic symptoms; LFTs, liver function tests.

pyoderma gangrenosum, granulomatous reactions, vitiligo, melanocytic nevi, neutrophilic eccrine hidradenitis, and radiation recall.[25–51] New primary melanomas have been reported with BRAF inhibitor monotherapy.[27] Management recommendations for cutaneous side effects from BRAF inhibitors are listed in **Table 5**.[26,28,29,32,34,35,40,41]

Table 5
Management of cutaneous adverse effects from BRAF inhibitors

SCCs and KAs	• Excision • Electrodessication and fulguration • Systemic retinoids • Pulse dynamic therapy • Topical chemotherapy • Cryotherapy • Intralesional 5-fluoruracil injections
Verrucal Keratosis	• Treatment: cryotherapy • Prevention: systemic retinoids (acitretin)
Grover Disease	• Emollients • Topical steroids • Topical keratolytics (urea and salicylic acid) • Systemic antihistamines • Systemic steroids • Systemic retinoids
Eruptive and Changing Melanocytic Nevi	• Frequent monitoring: baseline skin examination then every month for first 6 mo then every 8 wk while on therapy • Biopsy all suspicious lesions
Morbilliform Eruption	• Consider stopping or decreasing dose of BRAF inhibitor • Topical steroids • Systemic steroids
Panniculitis	• NSAIDs • Systemic steroids
Alopecia	• Concealment measures • Topical 5% minoxidil until 6 mo posttherapy
Photosensitivity	• Strict sun protection and sun avoidance • Broad-spectrum sunscreen • Topical steroids • Systemic steroids • Systemic antihistamines
Hyperkeratotic Hand-Foot Reaction	• Emollients Keratolytic agents (urea and salicylic acid) • Topical steroids (class I/II) • NSAIDs • Antiseptic soaks • Gabapentin and pregabalin • Stop treatment

Abbreviation: NSAIDs, nonsteroidal antiinflammatory drugs.
Data from Refs.[26,28–30,32–35,40,41]

BRAF inhibitors cross the placenta in pregnant monkeys and are associated with an increased risk of miscarriage, stillbirth, premature birth, neonatal death, and urogenital tract malformations.[52] There are 2 reports of pregnant women with metastatic melanoma taking vemurafenib.[53,54] The first patient developed toxic epidermolysis necrosis from vemurafenib and the second patient delivered a baby with intrauterine growth restriction, likely caused by the vemurafenib.[53,54]

MEK Inhibitors

The 3 MEK inhibitors approved by the FDA are trametinib, binimetinib, and cobimetinib (see **Table 1**). Trametinib was the first, approved in 2013 for metastatic or unresectable melanoma with BRAF V600E or V600K mutations. The standard dosage is 2 mg daily. In the METRIC trial, PFS was 4.8 months with trametinib compared with 1.5 months with DTIC[16] OS was 81% at 6 months for trametinib compared with 67% for DTIC.[16] Binimetinib and cobimetinib have been approved for advanced melanoma in combination with encorafenib and vemurafenib, respectively.[55,56] Cobimetinib is also approved for NRAS-positive melanoma.[55] In phase III NEMO trial, binimetinib had longer PFS compared with DTIC in patients with NRAS-positive melanoma.[57]

AEs of MEK inhibitors include cutaneous reactions, fatigue, myalgia, cardiovascular toxicities (peripheral edema, decreased ejection fraction, hypertension), gastrointestinal distress, blurred vision, and chorioretinopathy (**Tables 6** and **7**).[55–57] Cutaneous AEs include acneiform eruption, morbilliform eruption, pruritus, xerosis, pyoderma gangrenosum, alopecia, paronychia, hyperpigmentation, hair depigmentation, trichomegaly, hypertrichosis, telangiectasias, stomatitis, and angular cheilitis.[26,28,30,32–35,40,41] Prophylactic tetracycline antibiotics, including doxycycline 100 mg twice daily or minocycline 100 mg twice daily, may help in the treatment of acneiform eruptions with MEK inhibitors. More severe cases may require treatment with systemic steroids or systemic retinoids.[28,58]

BRAF and MEK Inhibitor Combination Therapy

Three different combinations of BRAF and MEK inhibitor therapy have been approved by the FDA for use in metastatic melanoma with BRAF V600E or V600K mutation. They are dabrafenib with trametinib, vemurafenib with cobimetinib, and encorafenib with binimetinib (see **Table 1**). In phase III trials COMBI-d and COMBI-v, dabrafenib with trametinib had improved PFS and OS compared with dabrafenib and vemurafenib monotherapy.[59,60] In

Table 6
Adverse effects with MEK inhibitors

Mucocutaneous

- Acneiform eruption
- Morbilliform eruption
- Hyperpigmentation
- Alopecia
- Pyoderma gangrenosum
- Stomatitis
- Angular cheilitis
- Panniculitis
- Paronychia
- Pruritus
- Xerosis
- Trichomegaly
- Hair depigmentation
- Telangiectasia
- Hypertrichosis

Extracutaneous

- Constitutional: fatigue, fever, chills, myalgia
- Neurologic: dropped head syndrome
- Cardiovascular: decreased ejection fraction, cardiomyopathy, hypertension, peripheral edema
- Gastrointestinal: nausea, vomiting, diarrhea
- Ophthalmologic: decreased visual acuity, halo spots, central serous retinopathy, retinal vein occlusion
- Other: osteopenia, increased creatinine kinase level

Data from Refs.[28,55–62]

the phase III trial COLUMBUS, encorafenib with binimetinib had higher PFS of 14.9 months compared with 9.6 and 7.3 months with encorafenib and vemurafenib monotherapy, respectively.[55] OS was 33.6 months with encorafenib with binimetinib compared with 23.5 and 16.9 months with encorafenib and vemurafenib monotherapy.[55] In the phase III trial CoBrim, vemurafenib with cobimetinib had PFS of 12.3 months compared with 7.2 months with vemurafenib monotherapy.[56] All 3 approved combination therapies have improved survival rates compared with BRAF and MEK inhibitor monotherapy.[55,56,59,61] Combination small molecule targeted therapy is currently under investigation for use as neoadjuvant and adjuvant therapy for stage III melanoma.

AEs with combination therapy are similar to BRAF inhibitor and MEK inhibitor monotherapies. The most frequent side effects include pyrexia, chills, fatigue, hypertension, gastrointestinal issues (nausea, vomiting, diarrhea, constipation), central serous retinopathy, increased creatinine kinase level, and increased aminotransferase level.[16,55–58,61] Epidermal neoplasms, acneiform eruption, alopecia, pruritus, and palmoplantar erythrodysesthesia syndrome were seen less frequently with combination therapy compared with single-agent BRAF inhibitor or MEK inhibitor.[16,56,57,60,61]

IMMUNE CHECKPOINT INHIBITORS
Cytotoxic T Lymphocyte–associated Antigen-4 Inhibitors

Cytotoxic T lymphocyte–associated antigen-4 (CTLA-4) is a glycoprotein expressed on the surface of T cells. By binding to CD80/86 on antigen-presenting cells, CTLA-4 inhibits activation of T cells, thereby serving as an essential mechanism preventing autoimmune disease.[62] It also allows malignant cells to evade the immune system. Three anti–CTLA-4 monoclonal antibodies were developed, but only ipilimumab has been FDA approved for use in metastatic melanoma in adults and pediatric patients (12 years and older).[62,63] Ipilimumab is a fully human, immunoglobulin (Ig) G1 monoclonal antibody that blocks CTLA-4. In one phase III trial, median OS was 10 months with ipilimumab compared with 6.4 months with the melanoma vaccine gp100 only (**Tables 8** and **9**).[62] In another phase III trial, OS with ipilimumab was 11.2 months compared with 9.1 months with DTIC.[63] Dosing for ipilimumab has varied in clinical trials with regimens ranging from 3 mg/kg to 10 mg/kg. Although ipilimumab is FDA approved at 3 mg/kg, OS is highest with 10 mg/kg dosing, although higher doses are associated with a more unfavorable side effect profile.[64] Ipilimumab is also approved for adjuvant therapy in stage III melanoma after a phase III trial showed prolonged recurrence-free survival compared with placebo.[65]

Anti–Programmed Cell Death-1 Therapy

Programmed cell death-1 (PD-1) is an immune checkpoint receptor expressed on activated effector T cells.[66] It binds programmed death ligand (PDL)-1 (B7H1) and PDL-2 (B7DC) on antigen-presenting cells, resulting in downstream signaling that inhibits T-cell proliferation. Nivolumab and pembrolizumab are both fully human, monoclonal IgG4 PD-1 receptor antibodies approved for treatment of metastatic melanoma. Although one study found similar PFS and OS with nivolumab compared with DTIC, another showed improved PFS of 5.1 months with nivolumab compared with 2.2 months with DTIC.[66,67] Nivolumab showed superior PFS (6.9 vs 2.9 months) and OS (36.9 vs 19.9 months) compared with ipilimumab.[68] Pembrolizumab also showed prolonged PFS of 5.6 months compared with 2.8 months with ipilimumab.[69] The best outcomes were seen with combination treatment with nivolumab and ipilimumab, with PFS of 11.5 months compared with 6.9 months with nivolumab monotherapy and 2.9 months

Table 7
Efficacy of combination BRAF and MEK inhibitor therapy

Author	Treatment	Response Rate (%)	PFS (mo)	Median OS (mo)
Long et al,[59] 2014 (COMBI-d)	Group 1: (n = 211) Dabrafenib 150 mg BID + trametinib 2 mg daily Group 2: (n = 212) Dabrafenib 150 mg BID	Group 1: 67% Group 2: 51%	Group 1: 9.3 Group 2: 8.8	Group 1: 93% at 5 mo Group 2: 85% at 5 mo
Robert et al,[60] 2015 (COMBI-v)	Group 1: (n = 352) Dabrafenib 150 mg BID + trametinib 2 mg daily Group 2: (n = 352) Vemurafenib 960 mg BID	Group 1: 64% Group 2: 51%	Group 1: 11.4 Group 2: 7.3	Group 1: 72% at 12 mo Group 2: 65% at 12 mo
Larkin et al,[57] 2014 (CoBRIM)	Group 1: (n = 247) Vemurafenib 960 mg BID + cobimetinib 60 mg daily Group 2: (n = 248) Vemurafenib 960 mg BID	Group 1: 70% Group 2: 50%	Group 1: 12.3 Group 2: 7.2	Group 1: 22.5 Group 2: 17.4
Dummer et al,[51] 2018 (COLUMBUS)	Group 1: (n = 192) Encorafenib 450 mg daily + binimetinib 45 mg BID Group 2: (n = 194) Encorafenib 300 mg once daily Group 3: (n = 191) Vemurafenib 960 mg BID	Group 1: 65% Group 2: 52% Group 3: 49%	Group 1: 14.9 Group 2: 9.6 Group 3: 7.3	Group 1: 33.6 Group 2: 23.5 Group 3: 16.9

Table 8
Efficacy of ipilimumab for metastatic melanoma

Author	Treatment	Response Rate (%)	PFS (mo)	Median OS (mo)
Hodi et al,[63] 2010	Group 1: (n = 403) ipilimumab 3 mg/kg + gp100 peptide vaccine Group 2: (n = 137) ipilimumab 3 mg/kg Group 3: (n = 136) gp100 peptide vaccine	Group 1: 5.7 (best overall response) Group 2: 10.9 Group 3: 1.5	Group 1: 2.76 Group 2: 2.86 Group 3: 2.76	Group 1: 10 Group 2: 10.1 Group 3: 6.4
Robert et al,[64] 2011	Group 1: (n = 250) ipilimumab 10 mg/kg + DTIC 250 mg/m^2 Group 2: (n = 252) DTIC 250 mg/m^2	Group 1: 33.2% Group 2: 30.2%	Reported as the same between the 2 groups	Group 1: 11.2 Group 2: 9.1
Ascierto et al,[65] 2017	Group 1: (n = 365) ipilimumab 10 mg/kg Group 2: (n = 362) Ipilimumab 3 mg/kg	Group 1: 15% Group 2: 12%	Group 1: 2.8 Group 2: 2.8	Group 1: 15.7 Group 2: 11.5

Table 9
Efficacy of anti–cytotoxic T lymphocyte–associated antigen-4 therapy for metastatic melanoma

Author	Drug	Response Rate (%)	PFS (mo)	Median OS (mo)
Larkin et al,[70] 2018 (Checkmate 037)	Group 1: (n = 272) Nivolumab 3 mg/kg every 2 wk Group 2: (n = 102) DTIC 1000 mg/m^2 every 3 wk or carboplatin paclitaxel	Group 1: 27 Group 2: 10	Group 1: 3.1 Group 2: 3.7	Group 1: 15.7 Group 2: 14.4
Robert et al,[67] 2015 (CheckMate 066)	Group 1: (n = 210) Nivolumab 3 mg/kg Group 2: (n = 208) DTIC 1000 mg/m^2	Group 1: 40 Group 2: 13.9	Group 1: 5.1 Group 2: 2.2	Group 1: Not reached Group 2: 10.8
Larkin et al,[68] 2015; Hodi et al,[69] 2018 (CheckMate 067)	Group 1: (n = 316) Nivolumab 3 mg/kg Group 2: (n = 314) Nivolumab 1 mg/ kg + ipilimumab 3 mg/kg every 3 wk for 4 doses, then nivolumab 3 mg/kg every 2 wk Group 3: (n = 315) Ipilimumab 3 mg/kg every 3 wk for 4 doses	Group 1: 43.7 Group 2: 57.6 Group 3: 19	Group 1: 6.9 Group 2: 11.5 Group 3: 2.9	Group 1: 36.9 Group 2: Not reached Group 3: 19.9
Schachter et al,[71] 2017 (KEYNOTE-006)	Group 1: (n = 279) Pembrolizumab 0 mg/kg every 2 wk Group 2: (n = 277) Pembrolizumab 10 mg/kg every 3 wk Group 3: (n = 278) Ipilimumab 3 mg/kg every 3 wk	Group 1: 37 Group 2: 36 Group 3: 13	Group 1: 5.6 Group 2: 4.1 Group 3: 2.8	Group 1: Not reached Group 2: Not reached Group 3: 16

with ipilimumab monotherapy.[68,70] Based on these results, the FDA has approved combination nivolumab and ipilimumab as the first-line treatment of advanced BRAF-negative melanoma.[68,70] Nivolumab is also approved for use as an adjuvant treatment of high-risk melanoma that has been surgically resected. In the phase III trial Checkmate-238, nivolumab had significantly fewer relapses and adverse events compared with ipilimumab.[71]

ADVERSE EFFECTS WITH IMMUNE CHECKPOINT INHIBITORS

Ipilimumab and PD-1 inhibitors share a similar side effect profile (**Table 10**). In general, ipilimumab has a higher incidence of AEs compared with both PD-1 inhibitors.[62,64,66,68,70] The most common AE is rash, which presents as an erythematous morbilliform or reticular eruption on the trunk and extremities.[72] It develops within the first 2 weeks of therapy. Management options include supportive care, topical corticosteroids, systemic antihistamines, and systemic corticosteroids.[72,73] Other cutaneous AEs include an eczematous dermatitis, lichenoid eruption, pruritus, SJS/TEN, DRESS, acute generalized exanthematous pustulosis (AGEP), alopecia areata, drug-induced subacute cutaneous lupus erythematosus, vasculitis, psoriasis, sarcoidal reaction, panniculitis, neutrophilic dermatoses, bullous pemphigoid, dermatomyositis, vitiligolike lesions, photosensitivity, radiation recall, and mucositis.[72–87] Vitiligolike lesions and lichenoid eruptions are more common with PD-1 agents than with ipilimumab.[76] Vitiligolike lesions usually develop after 3 weeks of therapy and may indicate a favorable treatment response.[72,87] Management of cutaneous side effects is reviewed in **Table 11**.[76]

Other immune-related AEs with ipilimumab and PD-1 inhibitors include gastrointestinal

Table 10
Adverse effects with immune checkpoint inhibitors

Mucocutaneous

- Morbilliform eruption
- Eczematous dermatitis
- Psoriasiform dermatitis
- Acute generalized exanthematous pustulosis
- SJS/TEN
- Erythema multiforme
- DRESS
- Lichenoid eruption
- Lichen planus pemphigoid
- Bullous pemphigoid
- Dermatomyositis
- Subacute lupus erythematosus
- Vasculitis
- Repigmentation of gray hair
- Sarcoidosis and sarcoidlike lesions, including subcutaneous
- Panniculitis
- Radiation recall
- Sweet syndrome
- Neutrophilic dermatoses
- Psoriasis
- Eruptive KAs
- Oral ulcers
- Alopecia areata
- Vitiligolike lesions
- Vogt-Koyanagia-Harada–like syndrome
- Pruritus

Extracutaneous

- Constitutional: fatigue, myalgia, headache, pyrexia, chills
- Neurologic: Guillain-Barré syndrome, posterior reversible encephalopathy syndrome
- Cardiovascular: myocarditis
- Pulmonary: pneumonitis, sarcoidosis
- Gastrointestinal: enteritis/colitis, diarrhea, nausea, vomiting, hepatitis, pancreatitis
- Hematological: leukopenia, anemia, thrombocytopenia
- Endocrine: autoimmune thyroiditis, hypothyroidism, hyperthyroidism, hypophysitis, hypopituitarism, adrenal insufficiency, adrenal crisis, type 1 diabetes
- Pulmonary: pneumonitis, sarcoidosis
- Renal: nephritis, hyperkalemia
- Neurologic: Guillain-Barré syndrome, posterior reversible encephalopathy syndrome
- Ophthalmologic: uveitis, episcleritis
- Hematological: leukopenia, anemia, thrombocytopenia
- Other: vasculitis

Data from Refs[63–65,68–87].

(diarrhea, colitis), autoimmune hepatitis, pneumonitis, endocrinopathies (hypophysitis, hypothyroidism, adrenal insufficiency, and adrenal crisis), pancreatitis, and hematological abnormalities.[62–72] Diarrhea and autoimmune hepatitis are more severe with ipilimumab than with anti-

PD-1 agents.[68,70,72] Of note, AEs are more common and more severe with combined PD-1 and CTLA-4 inhibitor therapy compared with monotherapy, with severe AEs seen in 55% of patients in the phase III trial on combination therapy.[68,70]

ONCOLYTIC VIRAL THERAPY

In 2015, talimogene laherparepvec (T-VEC) was approved by the FDA for treatment of metastatic melanoma.[87–89] T-VEC is a modified herpes simplex virus-1 oncolytic virus that is injected directly into cutaneous metastases. In a phase III trial of 436 patients with stage III and IV melanoma, the response rate was 26%, with a complete response seen in 11% of patients.[88] No improvement in OS was seen. Common AEs include fever, chills, injection site pain, nausea, fatigue, and cellulitis (**Box 2**, **Table 12**).[90] Cellulitis was the most severe side effect in clinical trials.[90] There are ongoing phase I and II clinical trials investigating T-VEC in combination with ipilimumab, PD-1 inhibitors, BRAF inhibitors, and MEK inhibitors. Other oncolytic viruses are also under investigation as therapies for metastatic melanoma.[91]

INTERFERON ALFA

Interferon alfa (IFN-α) is an immune regulatory protein that is antiangiogenic, antiproliferative, and proapoptotic.[92] IFN-α promotes a shift from T helper (Th) 2 to Th1 in host immunity, which enhances cell-mediated cytotoxicity against tumor cells.[92] IFN-α was the first adjuvant treatment approved by the FDA for high-risk, surgically resected melanoma including stages IIB and stage III.[92] The recommended dosing regimen consists of a high-dose intravenous phase 5 times per week for a total of 4 weeks followed by a maintenance subcutaneous dose 3 times per week for at least 1 year.[93] In one phase III trial, E1684, IFN-α had higher median relapse-free survival (RFS) of 20.6 months compared with 11.8 months in the observation group after surgical removal of melanoma.[93] Another phase III trial, E1690, had improved median RFS but found no survival benefit. This trial differed from the previous in that regional lymph node removal was not required, which is thought to have contributed to lack of survival benefit.[94] A third phase III trial, E1694, showed improved RFS and OS with IFN-α therapy compared with ganglioside Gm2/keyhole limpet hemocyanin (GMK) vaccine.[95] The most common AEs with IFN-α are fatigue, neutropenia, increased liver enzyme levels, and

Table 11
Management of cutaneous adverse effects from anti–cytotoxic T lymphocyte–associated antigen-4 and anti–programmed cell death-1 inhibitors

Lichenoid Reaction	• Topical steroids • Systemic steroids • Systemic antihistamines • Systemic retinoids • Consider stopping treatment
Morbilliform Reaction	• Emollients • Topical steroids • Topical calcineurin inhibitors • Systemic antihistamines • Systemic steroids
Psoriasiform Dermatitis	• Topical steroids • Topical vitamin D analogues • Systemic steroids • Systemic retinoids
Bullous Dermatoses (Bullous Pemphigoid, Bullous Lichenoid Reactions, Bullous Lichen Planus–like Reactions)	• Topical steroids • Systemic steroids • Methotrexate • Rituximab • Systemic retinoids • Consider stopping treatment
DRESS	• Topical steroids • Systemic steroids • Systemic immunosuppressants including cyclosporine, IV immunoglobulin, cyclophosphamide, mycophenolate mofetil, rituximab, interferon, muromonab-CD3
AGEP	• Stop therapy • Systemic steroids
SJS/TEN	• Stop therapy • Recommend burn care/special supportive unit • Systemic steroids • Intravenous immunoglobulin • Cyclosporine • Cyclophosphamide • Anti–tumor necrosis factor alpha agents
Neutrophilic Dermatosis (Sweet syndrome, Pyoderma Gangrenosum)	• Systemic steroids • Aggressive wound care
Pruritus	• Emollients • Topical antipruritics (menthol 0.5%, doxepin 5%, pramoxine hydrochloride 1%, camphor 0.5%) • Topical steroids • Systemic agents: gabapentin, pregabalin, mirtazapine, doxepin
Vitiligolike Lesions	• Sun protection • Camouflage
Eruptive or Changing Melanocytic Lesions	• Regular skin checks • Biopsy if suspicious

headache. These side effects can be severe, and 10% to 26% of patients discontinued IFN-α because of the AEs.[93–95]

Pegylated IFN-α (Peg-IFN) is IFN-α with a covalently attached polyethylene glycol.[96] Peg-IFN has a longer half-life and increased absorption compared with IFN-α. Peg-IFN was FDA approved in 2011 for adjuvant therapy in high-risk melanoma with lymph node metastases. A phase III trial showed improved RFS of

---

Box 2
Adverse effects with talimogene laherparepvec therapy

Mucocutaneous

- Pruritus
- Cellulitis
- Injection-site erythema and pruritus
- Vitiligo

Extracutaneous

- Constitutional: fever, chills, fatigue pyrexia, headache, myalgia, arthralgia
- Gastrointestinal: nausea, vomiting, diarrhea, constipation
- Pulmonary: cough, dyspnea
- Other: peripheral edema

---

36 months compared with 26.4 months with Peg-IFN, but no survival benefit was found.[96] Side effects include fatigue, increased liver enzyme levels, pyrexia, headache, myalgia, and depression. The most severe AEs were fatigue, increased liver enzyme levels, and depression, and 37% of patients discontinued treatment because of the severity.[96] At present, there are trials evaluating use of IFN-α and Peg-IFN in combination with immune checkpoint inhibitors and small molecule targeted therapy for adjuvant and neoadjuvant therapy in high-risk melanoma.

DISCUSSION

The treatment of advanced or unresectable melanoma is extremely challenging. The last several decades have witnessed a breakthrough in therapeutic options with the development of immune checkpoint inhibitors, small molecule targeted therapy, and oncolytic viral therapy. The prognosis for advanced melanoma is poor, with a median survival of less than 1 year for patients with distant metastases; however, the development of newer systemic therapies for melanoma have provided improvement in PFS and OS. With increased use of novel combination systemic therapies, dermatologists should be aware of the potential cutaneous AEs listed earlier and help their oncology colleagues manage these side effects.

Table 12
Efficacy of interferon alfa and pegylated interferon as adjuvant therapy in high-risk melanoma

Author	Treatment	Median RFS (mo)	OS (%)
Kirkwood et al,[93] 1996 (E1684)	Group 1: (n = 143) IFN-α2b 20 MU/m² IV 5 d/wk × 4 wk; then 10 MU/m² TIW × 48 wk Group 2: (n = 137) Observation	Group 1: 20.64 Group 2: 11.76	Group 1: 46% at 5 y Group 2: 37% at 5 y
Kirkwood et al,[94] 2000 (E1690)	Group 1: (n = 215) IFN-α2b 20 MU/m² IV 5 d/wk × 4 wk; then 10 MU/m² TIW × 48 wk Group 2: (n = 215) IFN-α2b 3 MU/m² TIW × 2 y Group 3: (n = 212) Observation	Group 1: 44% 5-y RFS Group 2: 40% 5 y RFS Group 3: 35% 5 y RFS	Group 1: 52% at 5 y Group 2: 53% at 5 y Group 3: 55% at 5 y
Kirkwood et al,[95] 2001 (E1694)	Group 1: (n = 389) GMK vaccine on days 1, 8, 15, 22, then every 12 wk Group 2: (n = 385) IFN-α2b 20 MU/m² IV 5 d/wk × 4 wk; then 10 MU/m² TIW × 48 wk	Group 1: 22.5 Group 2: not reached	Group 1: 73% at 2 y Group 2: 78% at 2 y
Eggermont et al,[96] 2011	Group 1: (n = 627) pIFN-α 6 µg/kg/wk × 8 wk; then 3, 2, or 1 µg/kg/wk × 5 y Group 2: (n = 629) Observation	Group 1: 36 Group 2: 26.4	Group 1: 47.8% at 7 y Group 2: 46.4% at 7 y

Abbreviations: IFN, interferon; pIFN, pegylated interferon; TIW, 3 times a week.

REFERENCES

1. Torres-Collado AX, Knott J, Jazirehi AR. Reversal of resistance in targeted therapy of metastatic melanoma: lessons learned from vemurafenib (BRAF^{V600E}-Specific Inhibitor). Cancer 2018; 24(10):6.

2. Long GV, Hauschild A, Santinami M, et al. Adjuvant dabrafenib plus trametinib in stage III BRAF-Mutated melanoma. N Engl J Med 2017;377(19): 1813–23.

3. Sam D, Gresham G, Adbel-Rahmnan O, et al. Generalizability of clinical trials of advanced melanoma in the real-world, population-based settings. Med Oncol 2018;35(7):110.

4. Chapman PB, Hauschild A, Robert C, et al. Improved survival with vemurafenib in melanoma. N Engl J Med 2005;353:2135–47.

5. Bhatia S, Tykodi SS, Thompson JA. Treatment of metastatic melanoma: an overview. Oncology 2009;23(6):488–96.

6. Patel PM, Suciu S, Mortier L, et al. Extended schedule, escalated dose temozolomide versus dacarbazine in stage IV melanoma: final results of a randomized phase III study (EORTC 18032). Eur J Cancer 2011;47(10):1476–83.

7. Lui P, Cashin R, Machado M, et al. Treatments for metastatic melanoma: Synthesis of evidence from randomized trials. Cancer Treat Rev 2007;33: 665–80.

8. Lattanzi SC, Tosteson T, Chertoff J, et al. Dacarbazine, cisplatin, carmustine, with or without tamoxifen, for metastatic melanoma: a 5-year follow-up. Melanoma Res 1995;5:365–9.

9. Chapman PB, Einhorn LH, Meyers ML, et al. Phase III multicenter randomized trial of the Dartmouth regimen versus dacarbazine in patients with metastatic melanoma. J Clin Oncol 1999; 17:2745–51.

10. Pasquali S, Hadjinicolaou AV, Chiarlion Sileni C, et al. Systemic treatments for metastatic cutaneous melanoma. Cochrane Database Syst Rev 2018;6:2.

11. Atkins MB, Lotze MT, Dutcher JP, et al. High-dose recombinant interleukin-2 therapy for patients with metastatic melanoma: analysis of 270 patients treated between 1985 and 1993. J Clin Oncol 1999;17(7):2105–16.

12. Schwartzentruber DJ. Guidelines for safe administration of high-dose interleukin-2. J Immunother 2001;24(4):287–93.

13. Sosman JA, Kim KB, Schuchter L, et al. Survival in BRAF 600E-mutant advanced melanoma treated with vemurafenib. N Engl J Med 2012;366:707–14.

14. Chapman PB, Hauschild A, Robert C, et al. Improved survival with vemurafenib in melanoma with BRAF V600E mutation. N Engl J Med 2011; 354(26):2507–16.

15. Chapman PB, Robert C, Larkin J, et al. Vemurafenib in patients with BRAFV600 mutation-positive metastatic melanoma: final overall survival results of the randomized BRIM-3 study. Ann Oncol 2017;28(10): 2581–7.

16. Flaherty KT, Robert C, Hersey P, et al. Improved survival with MEK inhibition in BRAF-mutated melanoma. N Engl J Med 2012;367(2):107–14.

17. Hauschild A, Grob JJ, Demidov L, et al. Dabrafenib in BRAF-mutated metastatic melanoma: a multicenter, open-label, phase 3 randomized controlled trial. Lancet 2012;380:358–65.

18. Graf NP, Koelblinger P, Galliker N, et al. The spectrum of cutaneous adverse events during Encorafenib and Binimetinib treatment in BRAF mutant advanced melanoma. J Eur Acad Dermatol Venereol 2018;33(4):686–92.

19. Nazarian R, Shi H, Qang Q, et al. Melanomas acquired resistance to B-RAF (V600E) inhibition by RTK or N-RAS upregulation. Nature 2010;468: 973–7.

20. Johannessen CM, Boem JS, Kim SY, et al. COT drives resistance to BRAF inhibition through MAP kinase pathway reactivation. Nature 2010;468: 968–72.

21. Paraiso KH, Xiang Y, Rebecca VW, et al. PTEN loss confers RAF inhibitor resistance to melanoma cells through suppression of BIM expression. Cancer Res 2011;71:2750–60.

22. Nathanson KI, Martin AM, Wubbenhorst B, et al. Tumor genetic analyses of patients with metastatic melanoma treated with BRAF inhibitor dabrafenib. Clin Cancer Res 2013;19:4868–78.

23. Villaneuva J, Vultur A, Lee JT, et al. Acquired resistance to BRAF inhibitors mediated by a RAF kinase switch in melanoma can be overcome by cotargeting MEK and IGF-1R/PI3K. Cancer Cell 2010;18(6): 683–95.

24. Trunzer K, Pavlick AC, Schuchter L, et al. Pharmacodynamic effects and mechanisms of resistance to vemurafenib in patients with metastatic melanoma. J Clin Oncol 2013;31(14):1767–74.

25. Lacouture ME, McArthur GA, Chapman PB, et al. PLX4032(RG7204), a selective mutant RAF inhibitor: Clinical and histological characteristics of therapy-associated cutaneous neoplasms in a phase I trial. J Clin Oncol 2010;28(suppl 15):8592.

26. Sinha R, Edmonds K, Newton-Bishop J, et al. Cutaneous adverse events associated with vemurafenib in patients with metastatic melanoma: Practical advice on diagnosis, prevention, and management of main treatment-related skin toxicities. Br J Dermatol 2012;167(5):987–94.

27. Anforth RM, Blumetti TC, Sharma R, et al. Cutaneous manifestations of dabrafenib(GSk2118436): a selective inhibitor of mutant BRAF in patients with metastatic melanoma. Br J Dermatol 2012;167:1153–60.

28. Macdonald JB, Macdonald B, Golitz LE, et al. Cutaneous adverse effects of targeted therapies. J Am Acad Dermatol 2015;72(2):221–36.

29. Tang N, Ratner D. Managing cutaneous side effects from targeted molecular inhibitors for melanoma and nonmelanoma skin cancer. Dermatol Surg 2016; 42(suppl 1):S40–8.

30. Sanlorenzo M, Choudry A, Vujic I, et al. Comparative profile of cutaneous adverse events: BRAF/MEK inhibitor combination therapy versus BRAF monotherapy in melanoma. J Am Acad Dermatol 2014;71(6): 1102–9.

31. Su F, Viros A, Milagre C, et al. Ras mutations in cutaneous squamous-cell carcinomas in patients treated with BRAF inhibitors. N Engl J Med 2012;366: 207–15.

32. Anforth R, Bluemetti TC, Mohd Affandi A, et al. Systemic retinoid therapy for chemoprevention of nonmelanoma skin cancer in a patient treated with vemurafenib. J Clin Oncol 2012;30:e165–7.

33. Alloo A, Garbiyan L, LeBoeuf N. Photodynamic therapy for multiple eruptive keratoacanthomas associated with vemurafenib treatment for metastatic melanoma. Arch Dermatol 2012;148(3): 363–6.

34. Sachse MM, Wagner G. Clearance of BRAF inhibitor-associated keratoacanthomas by systemic retinoids. Br J Dermatol 2014;170(2):475–7.

35. LaPresto L, Cranmer L, Morrison L, et al. A novel therapeutic combination approach for treating multiple vemurafenib-induced keratoacanthomas: systemic acitretin and intralesional fluorouracil. JAMA Dermatol 2013;149(3):279–81.

36. Munch M, Peuvrel L, Brocard A, et al. Early-onset vemurafenib-induced DRESS syndrome. Dermatology 2016;232(1):126–8.

37. Bellon T, Lerma V, Gonzalez-Valle O, et al. Vemurafenib-induced toxic epidermal necrolysis: possible cross-reactivity with other sulfonamide compounds. Br J Dermatol 2016;174(3):621–4.

38. Boyd KP, Vincent B, Andrea A, et al. Nonmalignant cutaneous findings associated with vemurafenib use in patients with metastatic melanoma. J Am Acad Dermatol 2012;67(6):1375–9.

39. Lacouture ME, Duvic M, Hauschild A, et al. Analysis of dermatologic events in vemurafenib-treated patients with melanoma. Oncologist 2013;18(3): 314–22.

40. Mossner R, Zimmer L, Berking C, et al. Erythema nodosum-like lesions during BRAF inhibitor therapy: report on 16 new cases and review of the literature. J Eur Acad Dermatol Venereol 2015;29(9): 1797–806.

41. Zimmer L, Livingstone E, Hillen U, et al. Panniculitis with arthralgia in patients with melanoma treated with selective BRAF inhibitors and its management. Arch Dermatol 2012;148:357–61.

42. Dummer R, Rinderknect J, Goldinger SM. Ultraviolet A and photosensitivity during vemurafenib therapy. N Engl J Med 2012;366:480–1.

43. Zimmer L, Hillen U, Livingstone E, et al. Atypical melanocytic proliferations and new primary melanomas in advanced melanoma patients undergoing selective BRAF inhibition. J Clin Oncol 2012;30: 2375–83.

44. Fusumae T, Kamiya K, Maekawa T, et al. Vogt-Koyanagi-Harada disease-like uveitis induced by vemurafenib for metastatic cutaneous malignant melanoma. J Dermatol 2018;45(6):e159–60.

45. Boussemart L, Boivin C, Claveau J, et al. Vemurafenib and radiosensitization. JAMA Dermatol 2013; 149:855–7.

46. Herms F, Frank N, Krankimel N, et al. Neutrophilic eccrine hidradenitis in two patients treated with BRAF inhibitors: a new cutaneous adverse event. Br J Dermatol 2017;176(6):1645–8.

47. Nasca MR, Lacarrubba F, Ferrau F, et al. Vitiligo of the face in a patient treated with vemurafenib for metastatic melanoma. J Drugs Dermatol 2016; 15(6):766–8.

48. Lee SB, Weide B, Ugurel S, et al. Vemurafenib-induced granuloma annulare. J Dtsch Dermatol Ges 2016;14(3):305–8.

49. Garrdio MC, Gutierrez C, Riveiro-Falkenbach E, et al. BRAF inhibitor-induced antitumoral granulomatous dermatitis eruption in advanced melanoma. Am J Dermatopathol 2015;37(10):795–8.

50. Lheure C, Kramkimel N, Franck N, et al. Sarcoidosis in patients treated with vemurafenib for metastatic melanoma: a paradoxical autoimmune activation. Dermatology 2015;231(4):378–84.

51. Silva Gde B, Mendes AP, de Macedo MP, et al. Vemurafenib and cutaneous adverse events-report of five cases. An Bras Dermatol 2015;90(suppl 1): 242–6.

52. Grunewald S, Jank A. New systemic agents in dermatology with respect to fertility, pregnancy, and lactation. J Dtsch Dermatol Ges 2015;13(4):277–89.

53. De Haan J, van Thienen JV, Casaer M, et al. Severe adverse reaction to vemurafenib in a pregnant woman with metastatic melanoma. Case Rep Oncol 2018;11(1):119–24.

54. Maleka A, Enblad G, Sjors G, et al. Treatment of metastatic malignant melanoma with vemurafenib during pregnancy. J Clin Oncol 2013;31(11):e192–3.

55. Dummer R, Ascierto PA, Gogas HJ, et al. Encorafenib plus binimetinib versus vemurafenib or encorafenib in patients with BRAF-mutant melanoma (COLUMBUS): a multicenter, open-label randomised phase 3 trial. Lancet Oncol 2018;19(5): 603–15.

56. Larkin J, Ascierto PA, Dreno B, et al. Combined vemurafenib and cobimetinib in BRAF-mutated melanoma. N Engl J Med 2014;371:1867–76.

57. Dummer R, Schadendorf D, Ascierto PA, et al. Bini-metinib versus dacarbazine in patients with advanced NRAS-mutant melanoma (NEMO): a multicentre, open-label, randomised, phase 3 trial. Lancet Oncol 2017;18(4):435–45.

58. Choi JN. Dermatologic adverse events to chemotherapeutic agents, Part 2: BRAF inhibitors, MEK inhibitors, and ipilimumab. Semin Cutan Med Surg 2014;33(1):40–8.

59. Robert C, Karaszewska B, Schachter J, et al. Improved overall survival in melanoma with combined dabrafenib and trametinib. N Engl J Med 2015;364(26):2507–16.

60. Carlos G, Anforth R, Clements A, et al. Cutaneous toxic effect of BRAF inhibitors alone and in combination with MEK inhibitors for metastatic melanoma. JAMA Dermatol 2015;151(10):1103–9.

61. Long GV, Stroyakovskiy D, Gogas H, et al. Combined BRAF and MEK inhibition versus BRAF inhibition alone in melanoma. N Engl J Med 2014;371(20):1877–88.

62. Hodi FS, O'DAY SJ, McDermott DF, et al. Improved survival with ipilimumab in patients with metastatic melanoma. N Engl J Med 2010;363(8):711–23.

63. Robert C, Thomas L, Bondarenko I, et al. Ipilimumab plus dacarbazine for previously untreated metastatic melanoma. N Engl J Med 2011;364(26):2517–26.

64. Ascierto PA, Del Vecchio M, Robert C, et al. Ipilimumab 10 mg/kg versus ipilimumab 3 mg/kg in patients with unresectable or metastatic melanoma: a randomised, double-blind, multicentre phase 3 trial. Lancet Oncol 2017;18(5):611–22.

65. Eggermont AM, Chiarion-Sileni V, Grobb JJ, et al. Adjuvant ipilimumab versus placebo after complete resection of high-risk stage III melanoma (EORTC 18071): a randomised, double blind, phase III trial. Lancet Oncol 2015;16(5):522–30.

66. Robert C, Long GV, Brady B, et al. Nivolumab in previously untreated melanoma without BRAF mutation. N Engl J Med 2015;372(4):320–30.

67. Larkin J, Minor D, D'Angelo S, et al. Overall survival in patients with advanced melanoma who received nivolumab versus investigator's choice chemotherapy in checkmate 037: a randomized, controlled, open-label phase III trial. J Clin Oncol 2018;36(4):383–90.

68. Larkin J, Chiarion-Silenei V, Gonzalez R, et al. Combined nivolumab and ipilimumab or monotherapy in untreated melanoma. N Engl J Med 2015;373(1):23–34.

69. Schachter J, Ribas A, Long GV, et al. Pembrolizumab versus ipilimumab for advanced melanoma: final overall survival results of a multicentre, randomised, open-label phase 3 study (KEYNOTE-006). Lancet 2017;390(10105):1853–62.

70. Hodi FS, Chiarion-Sileni V, Gonzalez R, et al. Nivolumab plus ipilimumab or nivolumab alone versus ipilimumab alone in advanced melanoma (Checkmate 067): 4-year outcomes of a multicentre, randomised, phase 3 trial. Lancet Oncol 2018;19(11):1490–2.

71. Weber J, Mandala M, Del Vecchio, et al. Adjuvant nivolumab versus ipilimumab in resected stage III or IV melanoma. N Engl J Med 2017;377(19):1824–35.

72. Friedman CF, Proverbs-Singh TA, Postow MA. Treatment of immune-related adverse effects of immune checkpoint inhibitors: a review. JAMA Oncol 2016;2(10):1346–53.

73. Hwang SJ, Carlos G, Wakade D, et al. Cutaneous adverse events (AEs) of anti-programmed cell death (PD)-1 therapy in patients with metastatic melanoma: a single institution cohort. J Am Acad Dermatol 2016;74(3):455–61.

74. Macdonald JB, Macdonald B, Golitz LE, et al. Cutaneous adverse effects of targeted therapies: part II: Inhibitors of intracellular molecular signaling pathways. J Am Acad Dermatol 2015;72(2):221–36.

75. Dika E, Ravaioli GM, Fanti PA, et al. Cutaneous adverse effects during ipilimumab treatment for metastatic melanoma: a prospective study. Eur J Dermatol 2017;27(3):266–70.

76. Liu RC, Consuegra G, Fernández-Peñas P. Management of the cutaneous adverse effects of antimelanoma therapy. Melanoma Manag 2017;4(4):187–202.

77. Ma C, Armstrong AW. Severe adverse events from the treatment of advanced melanoma: a systematic review of severe side effects associated with ipilimumab, vemurafenib, interferon alfa-2b, dacarbazine and interleukin-2. J Dermatolog Treat 2014;25(5):401–8.

78. Sheik Ali S, Goddard AL, Luke JJ, et al. Drug-associated dermatomyositis following ipilimumab therapy: a novel immune-mediated adverse event associated with cytotoxic T-lymphocyte antigen 4 blockade. JAMA Dermatol 2015;151(2):195–9.

79. Reule RB, North JP. Cutaneous and pulmonary sarcoidosis-like reaction associated with ipilimumab. J Am Acad Dermatol 2013;69(5):e272–3.

80. Pintova S, Sidhu H, Friedlander PA, et al. Sweet's syndrome in a patient with metastatic melanoma after ipilimumab therapy. Melanoma Res 2013;23(6):498–501.

81. Rambhia PH, Honda K, Arbesman J. Nivolumab induced inflammation of seborrheic keratosis: a novel cutaneous manifestation in a metastatic melanoma patient. Melanoma Res 2018;28(5):475–7.

82. Lopez AT, Khanna T, Antonov N, et al. A review of bullous pemphigoid associated with PD-1 and PD-L1 inhibitors. Int J Dermatol 2018;57(6):664–9.

83. Sundaresan S, Nguyen KT, Nelson KC, et al. Erythema multiforme major in a patient with metastatic melanoma treated with nivolumab. Dermatol Online J 2017;23(9) [pii:13030/qt2513974h].

84. Diaz-Perez JA, Beveridge MG, Victor TA, et al. Granulomatous and lichenoid dermatitis after IgG4 anti-PD-1 monoclonal antibody therapy for advanced cancer. J Cutan Pathol 2018;45(6):434–8.

85. Tetzlaff MT, Jazaeri AA, Torres-Cabala CA, et al. Erythema nodosum-like panniculitis mimicking disease recurrence: a novel toxicity from immune checkpoint blockade therapy-Report of 2 patients. J Cutan Pathol 2017;44(12):1080–6.

86. Reddy SB, Possick JD, Kluger HM, et al. Sarcoidosis following anti-PD-1 and anti-CTLA-4 therapy for metastatic melanoma. J Immunother 2017;40(8): 307–11.

87. Larsabal M, Marti A, Jacquemin C, et al. Vitiligo-like lesions occurring in patients receiving anti-programmed cell death-1 therapies are clinically and biologically distinct from vitiligo. J Am Acad Dermatol 2017;76(5):863–70.

88. Kaufman HL, Andtbacka RHI, Collichio FA, et al. Primary overall survival from OPTIM, a randomized phase III trial of talimogene laherparepvec (T-VEC) versus subcutaneous (SC) granulocyte-macrophage colony-stimulating factor (GM-CSF) for the treatment of unresected stage IIIB/C and IV melanoma. J Clin Oncol 2014;32:900a.

89. Elissa IR, Bustos-Billalobos I, Ichinose T, et al. The current status and future prospects of oncolytic viruses in clinical trials against melanoma, glioma, pancreatic and breast cancers. Cancers (Basel) 2018;10(10):356.

90. Andtbacka RH, Kaufman HI, Collichio F, et al. Talimogene Laherparepvec improves durable response rate in patients with advanced melanoma. J Clin Oncol 2015;33(25):2780–8.

91. Babiker HM, Riaz IB, Husnain M, et al. Oncolytic virotherapy including Rigvir and standard therapies in malignant melanoma. Oncolytic Virother 2017;9(6): 11–8.

92. Achkar T, Tarhini AA. The use of immunotherapy in the treatment of melanoma. J Hematol Oncol 2017; 10(1):88.

93. Kirkwood JM, Strawderman MH, Ernstoff MS, et al. Interferon alfa-2b adjuvant therapy of high-risk resected cutaneous melanoma: the Eastern Cooperative Oncology Group Trial EST 1684. J Clin Oncol 1996;14(1):7–17.

94. Kirkwood JM, Ibrahim JG, Sondak VK, et al. High- and low-dose interferon alfa-2b in high-risk melanoma: first analysis of intergroup trial E1690/ S9111/C9190. J Clin Oncol 2000;18:2444–58.

95. Kirkwood JM, Ibrahim JG, Sosman JA, et al. High-dose interferon alfa-2b significantly prolongs relapse-free and overall survival compared with the Gm2-KLH/QS-21 vaccine in patients with resected stage IIB-III melanoma: results of intergroup trial E1694/S9512/C509801. J Clin Oncol 2001;19: 2370–80.

96. Eggermont AM, Suciu S, Santinami M, et al. Long-term results of randomized phase III trial EORTC 18991 of adjuvant therapy with pegylated interferon-a2b versus observation in resected stage III melanoma. J Clin Oncol 2012;30(3):3810–8.

Review and Update on Evidence-Based Surgical Treatment Recommendations for Nonmelanoma Skin Cancer

Megan E. Shelton, MD, Adewole S. Adamson, MD, MPP*

KEYWORDS

- Nonmelanoma skin cancer • Surgical treatment • Basal cell carcinoma • Squamous cell carcinoma
- Mohs micrographic surgery • Excision • Destruction • Curettage and electrodessication

KEY POINTS

- Surgery, including electrodesiccation and curettage, standard excision, and Mohs micrographic surgery, is the gold standard for the treatment of nonmelanoma skin cancer.
- Studies directly comparing the effectiveness of surgical modalities are scarce, and recurrence rates among various surgical treatments are based on low-quality evidence.
- Additional large, prospective, comparative studies are needed to further inform clinical practice.
- Given low-level evidence, shared decision making is important in treatment decisions to balance tumor clearance with other factors, including patient preference, life expectancy, and cost of treatment.

INTRODUCTION

Basal cell carcinoma (BCC) and cutaneous squamous cell carcinoma (cSCC), are the most common malignancy in the United States, and their incidence continues to increase.[1] Together, these 2 malignancies are commonly referred to as nonmelanoma skin cancer (NMSC). Best estimates of NMSC incidence are obtained from US Medicare databases and US national survey data, with a recent multi-year study reporting an increase of 35% between 2006 and 2012, from 4,013,890 to 5,434,193 cases per year.[1] Given the sheer number and low case-fatality rate of NMSC, cancer registries in the US do not record the frequency of NMSC diagnoses unlike other malignancies (eg, breast, lung, prostate, colon, melanoma).

Although a variety of therapeutic modalities are available, surgery is generally considered the most effective treatment of NMSC. Surgical modalities commonly used in the treatment of NMSC include curettage and electrodesiccation (C&E), standard surgical excision (SE), and Mohs micrographic surgery (MMS). The main objectives of surgical treatment encompass complete removal of the tumor to prevent tumor recurrence, minimizing functional impairment following tumor removal, and optimizing cosmetic appearance. However, there are limited high-quality data available to provide clinicians with comprehensive evidence-based recommendations in determining the most appropriate intervention based on anatomic location, size, risk of recurrence, and cost-effectiveness.[2,3] The most recent guidelines for the management of BCC and cSCC, released

Disclosure Statement: The authors have nothing to disclose.
Division of Dermatology, Department of Internal Medicine, University of Texas at Austin, Dell Medical School, 1601 Trinity Street, Building B, Stop Z0900, Austin, TX 78712, USA
* Corresponding author.
E-mail address: adewole.adamson@austin.utexas.edu
; @AdeAdamson (A.S.A.)

Dermatol Clin 37 (2019) 425–433
https://doi.org/10.1016/j.det.2019.05.002

by the American Academy of Dermatology (AAD) in 2018, were based on a combination of expert opinion and available data, most of which was observational and retrospective.[4,5]

In addition to an overall paucity of prospective randomized controlled trials (RCTs), direct comparison studies of NMSC recurrence rates between different surgical modalities are scarce. Surgical treatment outcomes are often difficult to compare between studies because inclusion criteria, treatment protocols (including body site and tumor histology), and definition of recurrence vary. Further complicating recommendations regarding surgical treatments is the matter of financial cost. This is an increasingly relevant consideration given substantial overall expense to the health care system, and particularly germane when discussing treatment of NMSC among older adults with limited life expectancy.[6,7] Because numerous factors have an impact on the appropriateness of each surgical procedure for an individual patient's tumor, dermatologists must reconcile the uncertainty and science of medicine in their decision-making process.

This article aims to help clinicians make evidence-based decisions by reviewing the various surgical modalities and discussing the available data to support the use of these procedures in the treatment of BCC and cSCC.

SURGICAL MODALITIES
Curettage and Electrodesiccation

Tumor destruction with C&E is a commonly used and effective treatment modality for NMSC. There is wide variability in the technique performed among providers, but conventional practice involves removing the tumor by scraping it away with a curette, followed by denaturing the tissue with electrodessication until normal dermis is identified. One to 3 cycles of curettage and electrodessication are typically performed, but evidence to support this particular method, including treatment margins around the clinical tumor, are lacking.[8–10] An alternate technique involves curettage without electrodesiccation, because some report increased hypopigmentation and scarring after electrodesiccation, without an increased benefit of reduced tumor recurrence.[11,12] C&E is not recommended on terminal hair-bearing skin, such as the scalp or beard area in men, because of the potential risk of follicular extension of the tumor and subsequently increased recurrence rate.[13,14] However, limited data to support this practice are available.

C&E is most often used to treat superficial and nodular BCC and cSCC in situ. The main

advantages of C&E are time efficiency and cost-effectiveness. Most dermatologists perform C&E during a normally scheduled office visit with no follow-up visit necessary for suture removal. Studies examining treatment cost consistently identify significantly decreased cost of C&E compared with MMS and SE.[15] However, a notable drawback of C&E is the lack of histologic confirmation of tumor clearance, in contrast to SE and MMS. Thus, uncertainty surrounding treatment of clinically and histologically aggressive tumors (such as morpheaform BCCs or invasive cSCC) using C&E remains.

Remarkably, much of the data cited regarding the efficacy of C&E in treating NMSC originate from studies performed more than 40 years ago.[10,16,17] For example, the commonly cited 7.7% BCC 5-year recurrence rate after C&E is based on a retrospective review of studies published from 1950 to 1985.[18] Although more informative data now exist, current evidence to support C&E in the treatment of NMSC is derived from observational studies, and there are no RCTs comparing C&E with MMS or SE.[2,3]

Among more recent data, 257 primary nonmorpheaform BCCs on high- and medium-risk facial sites had a best case 5-year nonrecurrence rate of 98.80% (95% confidence interval [CI], 97.4%–100%).[19] A 2013 prospective cohort study of 1585 patients with BCC and cSCC reported an overall recurrence rate of 4.9% after C&E over 7.4 years, which was nonsignificant compared with MMS and SE.[20] In the subanalysis of high-risk tumors defined according to the National Comprehensive Cancer Network (NCCN) guidelines, recurrence was more likely after destruction of invasive tumors or those located in the H zone of the face. In addition, a 2013 systematic review and pooled analysis of observational studies investigating primary cSCC found low recurrence rates (4.5% in 109 patients; 95% CI, 1.4%–9.0%) after C&E, but the analysis included just 2 studies and was based on small, low-risk tumors.[21] Most recently, the results of a 2018 network meta-analysis support the effectiveness of C&E for low-risk BCC.[22]

Although C&E is effective, the least time intensive, and requires the least postoperative lifestyle modifications among the surgical treatments, how it affects skin-related quality of life is important. Chren and colleagues[23] found patients treated with C&E did not experience improvements in tumor-related quality of life (specifically, bother from the treatment site, including its unsatisfactory appearance), in contrast to both MMS and SE for which quality of life scores improved. Although not specifically investigated in this study, the investigators hypothesized that this could be explained by larger post-C&E scars than the initial tumor, which may be cosmetically unacceptable or symptomatic. Rigorous study of patient satisfaction regarding cosmesis after C&E or in comparison with other surgical modalities has not been performed.

Overall, C&E is an important intervention for the treatment of NMSC, offering low cost and a high cure rate, although trials comparing it head to head with other surgical techniques are needed.

Standard Surgical Excision

Another surgical modality used in the treatment of NMSC is SE. This technique involves excising predetermined margins of clinically normal tissue around the tumor, followed by postoperative histologic examination of tissue with "bread loaf" permanent sectioning. Similar to C&E, SE offers relative time efficiency and cost-effectiveness and is easily performed in the office by most dermatologists. A commonly cited disadvantage of SE is the inability to examine the full peripheral and deep margins of the excised tissue with "bread loaf" permanent sectioning.

When considering the optimal margins for SE, the importance of tumor clearance must be balanced with unnecessary resection of normal tissue. Tumor recurrence is strongly associated with excision margin size and thus must carefully considered. Unfortunately, most studies reporting data on surgical margins and recurrence rates are observational. The NCCN and AAD currently recommend SE with 4-mm margins for BCC and 4- to 6-mm margins for cSCC.[4,5] These guidelines are primarily based on single-center studies performed by Wolf and Zitelli[24] and Brodland and Zitelli[25] whereby MMS was used to identify the extent of subclinical tumor extension. They reported a 95% tumor clearance rate for excision with 4-mm margins for BCC and cSCC less than 2 cm in diameter, and at least 6-mm margins for high-risk cSCC and NMSC larger than 2 cm in diameter. However, these studies did not specifically aim to define the cure rate, which necessitates long-term follow-up.

Although there are no RCTs examining outcomes after various excision margins, Smeets and colleagues[26] conducted an RCT comparing SE with 3-mm margins with MMS for facial primary BCC.[27,28] In this study, SE was noninferior to MMS for both recurrence rates and cosmesis over 10 years. A 2010 meta-analysis investigating surgical margins for BCC found the relative risk of recurrence increased with smaller surgical margins.[29] The data suggested that 3-mm surgical margins for nonmorpheaform BCCs less than 2 cm correspond to a 95% cure rate over 2 to 5 years.

The implication of a positive margin after SE is unclear. In clinical practice, a positive surgical margin for BCC does not unequivocally result in tumor recurrence, because pooled data from a meta-analysis suggest a positive pathologic margin has a mean recurrence rate of only 27%.[29] In addition, both facial BCC and cSCC have been found to have high rates of "no residual carcinoma" on SE specimens, ranging from 25% to 48%, indicating either wound healing may clear the residual carcinoma or the entire lesion is removed with the initial biopsy.[30]

Data on SE margins and recurrence rates for cSCC are limited, although an extensive systematic review of observational studies identified 12 studies investigating SE of cSCC.[21] An average local recurrence rate of 5.4% was reported among all studies (n = 1144; 95% CI, 2.5%–9.1%), with excision margins ranging from 2 to 10 mm. Studies included were mostly retrospective case series with variable quality and follow-up. In addition, Chren and colleagues[20] reported an overall recurrence rate of 3.5% (95% CI, 1.8%–5.2%) after SE with 3-mm margins in a prospective cohort study of 1585 patients with BCC and cSCC over a median follow-up of 7.4 years. A diagnosis of SCC did not significantly increase the risk of recurrence with SE, although subgroup analyses found histologically invasive NMSC and those located in the H zone of the face were more likely to recur compared with those tumors treated with MMS.

At present, optimal margins for SE have not been determined, and additional RCTs comparing SE to other surgical techniques are needed. However, current data suggest margins of at least 3 mm provide acceptable long-term outcomes for most tumors less than 2 cm. Assurance provided by histologic margin examination, as well as relative cost and time efficiency, indicate that SE is an effective treatment option for NMSC.

Mohs Micrographic Surgery

MMS was developed by a general surgeon, Dr. Frederic Mohs, in the 1930s to treat large or recurrent tumors, and the technique has evolved over time. Presently, a disc of tissue encompassing the tumor and a small margin of surrounding normal tissue is excised at a 45-degree angle. As opposed to vertical sectioning with SE, horizontal sectioning of the excised tissue is performed during MMS, thereby permitting histologic evaluation of the entire epidermal and subcutaneous margins.

MMS has become a cornerstone in the management of NMSC, particularly on the head and neck, given its efficacy of tumor clearance by way of complete histologic margin examination while also maximizing tissue conservation. Ideally, MMS results in smaller, shallower wounds, thus facilitating smaller, simpler repairs or healing by secondary intention. However, compared with C&E and SE, MMS is more time intensive for the patient, uses additional resources, and generally requires additional surgical training to perform adeptly.

Tumor recurrence is a critical consideration when evaluating treatment approaches, and MMS has demonstrated low recurrence rates in many uncontrolled studies.[18,31,32] In 1 of the most frequently cited studies published by Rowe and colleagues[18] in 1989, a retrospective review of 106 studies found primary BCC 5-year recurrence rates to be 1% for MMS, compared with 10.1% for SE and 7.7% for C&E. However, the heterogeneity of the studies included, along with variable procedural methods and definitions of recurrence, do not permit generalization of the recurrence rates. Subsequent prospective cohort studies have failed to identify a definitive benefit of MMS over SE, including a study that found similar recurrence rates for BCC and cSCC after SE and MMS, even after adjusting for conventional risk factors for recurrence.[20]

The first prospective RCT comparing MMS with SE for the treatment of facial BCC was published by Smeets and colleagues[26] in 2004, followed by the release of 5- and 10-year recurrence data.[27,28] Performed in the Netherlands, the study investigated 408 primary BCC (pBCC) and 204 recurrent BCC (rBCC) involving high-risk facial areas of at least 1 cm in size or those with an aggressive histologic subtype treated with either SE with 3-mm margins or MMS. Initial results indicated 18% pBCC and 32% rBCC treated with SE were not completely excised after the first attempt, especially BCC with aggressive histologic patterns.[26] At 5- and 10-year follow-up, recurrence rates for rBCC were significantly greater in tumors treated with SE compared with MMS, with 10-year recurrence rates of 13.5% and 3.9%, respectively ($P = .023$).[27,28] However, recurrence rates for pBCC were not statistically different at either time point.

Overall, the results of this RCT indicate that SE and MMS are both effective treatments for pBCC, but response has been critical.[33] Opponents of the study cite a higher number of histologically aggressive pBCCs were treated with MMS than SE after randomization. In addition, for tumors larger than 16 mm treated with SE, en-face sectioning was used for margin assessment, instead of vertical sectioning. Although an intention-to-treat analysis was correctly performed despite several cases of protocol deviation and MMS rescue, a per-protocol analysis was not reported. Finally, follow-up at 10 years was approximately 35%, which may have had an impact on the ability to detect differences in recurrence-free survival.

Compared with BCC, studies investigating the recurrence rates of cSCC after MMS are limited. To date, no RCTs comparing MMS with other surgical modalities for the treatment of cSCC have been performed. Furthermore, given the higher risk of cSCC regional and distant metastasis, data demonstrating subsequent decrease in metastatic disease among treatment options is needed to inform clinical practice. However, retrospective data support the use of MMS to treat cSCC, including high-risk cSCC.[34,35] In addition, prospective cohort studies by Leibovitch and colleagues[32] reported a 5-year cSCC recurrence rate of 3.9% (95% CI, 2.2%–6.4%).[20] Finally, a systematic review and pooled analysis of observational studies of MMS for primary cSCC, a local recurrence rate of 3% (n = 1572; 95% CI, 2.2%–3.9%; 10 studies) and regional recurrence of 4.2% (n = 1162; 95% CI, 2.3%–6.6%; 6 studies) were reported.[21] Further studies investigating cSCC-specific treatment outcomes are crucial, considering recent reports suggest an increase in the incident ratio of SCC to BCC.[1]

Appropriate Use Criteria

As of 2008, MMS was used to treat 1 in 4 skin cancers in the Medicare population.[7] From 1996 to 2008, the number of MMS procedures performed increased by 248%, a stark contrast compared with the rates of excision and destruction, which increased 20% and 37%, respectively.[7] Despite its frequent use in the treatment of NMSC, most of the data supporting the use of MMS are limited to low-quality retrospective studies yielding low-quality meta-analyses. With the exception of an RCT assessing MMS and SE, direct comparison studies of recurrence rates between different surgical modalities are scarce, and treatment modalities are difficult to compare because studies often use different inclusion criteria or treatment protocols, as mentioned previously.

In light of increasing use of MMS and scrutiny by the Centers for Medicare and Medicaid Services, the first appropriate use criteria (AUCs) were created for the application of MMS in 2012.[36] Following an initial review of available evidence, indications for MMS were developed based on a combination of size and histologic subtype of tumor, location, and patient-specific characteristics, including immunosuppression or genetic syndromes. Indications were then categorized as appropriate, inappropriate, or uncertain by a review panel in a modified Delphi exercise. Of 270 scenarios discussed, MMS was deemed appropriate in 200 (74.1%), inappropriate in 24 (8.9%), and uncertain in 46 (17.0%). Designation of inappropriate use of MMS included low-risk tumors on the trunk and extremities given less costly management options with acceptable recurrence data and cosmetic outcomes.

Although the AUCs were intended to present guidelines to better define clinical scenarios that are best treated by MMS based on available evidence and expert opinion, they were not meant to establish the standard of care, although they may be increasingly interpreted in this manner. In addition, the AUCs did not comment on the role of MMS compared with other treatment options. Perhaps more fundamentally problematic to the creation of the MMS AUCs, however, is that guidelines heavily relied on expert opinion, given the lack of prospective trial data. Only studies performed in the US were assessed, thus excluding the only published RCT by Smeets and colleagues.[26]

ADDITIONAL CONSIDERATIONS
Cost-Effectiveness Analysis of Surgery for Nonmelanoma Skin Cancer

When considering various surgical options, physicians must weigh therapeutic efficacy with treatment expense. Multiple cost analyses of surgical treatment approaches have been performed, although most have been modeling studies heavily reliant on assumptions regarding practice patterns. A cost analysis of various surgical modalities found MMS to be less expensive than excision with frozen sections in an ambulatory surgical facility.[37] MMS has similarly been shown to be less expensive than excision in an operating room.[38] Furthermore, when considering the likelihood of tumor recurrence, it has been asserted MMS is less costly than in-office SE with permanent sectioning,[37,39,40] which has been reinforced by others. However, in the initial MMS cost analysis published by Cook and Zitelli,[37] it was assumed that ~65% of SE would require repair with a flap or graft, and ~40% of MMS cases would heal by secondary intention. It is highly unlikely that this represents the practice of most dermatologists, thus making the conclusions uncertain.

In the only prospective cost analysis based on an RCT, Essers and colleagues[41] found MMS to be more expensive than SE of facial BCCs when considering resource utilization. However, the results are difficult to generalize given an 18- to 30-month follow-up limited the ability to detect long-term differences, as well as variations in cost allocation between surgical modalities (eg, pathology costs for MMS were higher than for SE, which is disparate from cost comparisons in the US). For the diagnosis, treatment, and 2-month follow-up of primary NMSC, Wilson and colleagues[15] found an average total unadjusted fee of $463 for tumors treated using ED&C, $1222 for SE, and $2085 for MMS based on 2007 Medicare-approved fee schedule payments. Adjusted models controlling for treatment selection bias found total MMS fees to be $857 more than for SE, mostly as a result of higher repair fees, although this study did not incorporate long-term cost estimates of recurrence.

The relative cost between surgical modalities is not insignificant, with MMS often cited as being the costliest. However, considering that clinically relevant long-term recurrence rates may not differ significantly, this may support an increased role of SE and C&E for more patients.

Surgery in Patients with Limited Life Expectancy

Given that most NMSC have exceeding low mortality rates, recent conversations within dermatologic surgery have focused on the impact of surgery among patients with limited life expectancy. Not only do these patients generally prefer less invasive treatment approaches but long-term benefit from more intensive and expensive treatments such as MMS may not be realized.[30,42] Thus, when considering both the lower cost of treatment and infrequent tumor recurrence with C&E and SE, there may be an increased role for these surgical procedures in patients with limited life expectancy. Clinical practice may evolve to treat even those tumors traditionally classified as higher risk in this patient population, and there are certainly retrospective data to support this, because a recurrence rate of 4.5% was found for BCC less than 6 mm in high-risk sites after C&E.[43] As previously noted, there are also high rates of "no residual carcinoma" on SE specimens, and even if a positive surgical margin was identified, such patients could simply be observed for recurrence after informed discussion.[30] Thus, shared decision making with consideration of life expectancy, patient preference, and risk of tumor recurrence is critical to ensure optimal individual patient outcomes.

Table 1
NMSC recurrence rates as reported in recent systematic reviews and meta-analyses

Reference, Year	Study Type	Total Number of Studies Included	NMSC Subtype	Outcome of Interest		Other Notes
Drucker et al,[22] 2018	Systematic review and network meta-analysis	45 total; 40 RCTs and 5 NRCS	Primary BCC	**Surgical Intervention** Surgical excision MMS Diathermy + curettage Curettage	**Mean Recurrence Rate, % (95% CI)** 3.3 (1.3–7.8) 3.8 (0.7–18.9) 5.9 (0.7–34.9) 15.4 (2.6–55.3)	
Lansbury et al,[21] 2013	Systematic review of observational studies	118 total; 106 noncomparative studies and 12 single case reports	Primary, invasive cSCC (nonmetastatic)	**Surgical Intervention** Surgical excision MMS C&E	**Recurrence Average** Local recurrence average, 5.4% (95% CI, 2.5%–9.1%; 12 studies, n = 1144) Local recurrence average, 3.0% (95% CI, 2.2%–3.9%; 10 studies, n = 1572) Unspecified recurrence average, 1.7% (95% CI, 0.5%–3.4%; 7 studies, n = 1131)	
Bath-Hextall et al,[44] 2007	Systematic review	27 RCTs	Primary BCC	**Treatment Intervention** Surgical, destructive, other (topical, intralesional, and chemotherapy)	**Result** Only 1 comparative RCT for surgical excision versus MMS identified (Smeets et al[26]): lower recurrence rates found after MMS than after surgery, but the difference was nonsignificant	No RCTs investigating C&E identified

				Surgical Intervention	Primary BCC, all histologic subtypes	Surgical Intervention	Mean Recurrence Rate (%)	Cumulative 5-y recurrence rate
Thissen et al,[45] 1999	Systematic review of prospective studies	18 prospective studies			Primary BCC, all histologic subtypes	Surgical excision MMS	Cumulative 5-y rate, 5.3 Strict 5-y recurrence rate, 1.1	Cumulative 5-y recurrence rate unavailable for MMS and C&E
Gulleth et al,[29] 2010	Meta-analysis	37 prospective and retrospective studies			Primary BCC, nonmorpheaform	**Surgical Excision Margins** 5 mm 4 mm 3 mm 2 mm	**Mean Recurrence Rate ± SD (%)** 0.39 ± 0.26 1.62 ± 1.8 2.56 ± 1.6 3.96 ± 1.9	27% recurrence rate for BCC with positive pathologic margins

Abbreviations: BCC, basal cell carcinoma; C&E, curettage and electrodesiccation; cSCC, cutaneous squamous cell carcinoma; MMS, Mohs micrographic surgery; NMSC, nonmelanoma skin cancer; NRCS, nonrandomized comparative study; RCT, randomized controlled trial.

SUMMARY

C&E, SE, and MMS are effective surgical techniques for the treatment of NMSC (**Table 1**). However, there are scarce high-quality data to create comprehensive, evidence-based recommendations that assist clinicians in selecting the most appropriate intervention. It is astonishing that in the most common cancer in man, NMSC, there are so few prospective RCTs to guide practice. Although guidelines for clinical practice and management of NMSC are certainly necessary, it is important to appreciate that current guidelines published by the AAD and NCCN are heavily reliant on expert opinion informed by low-quality evidence.

Ideally, a large, multisite RCT comparing MMS, SE, and C&E for treatment of both BCC and cSCC on different body sites with long-term follow-up is required to further delineate the role of each surgical treatment. Completion of such a study is vital for the specialty of dermatology and the patients it serve.

Many factors have an impact on the clinical decision making of dermatologists, and each patient requires an individualized treatment plan. Because the overall recurrence rate between surgical modalities is not radically different, the authors implore dermatologists to use shared decision making, taking into consideration the cost and long-term benefit to the patient, during selection of surgical treatment.

REFERENCES

1. Rogers HW, Weinstock MA, Feldman SR, et al. Incidence estimate of nonmelanoma skin cancer (keratinocyte carcinomas) in the U.S. population, 2012. JAMA Dermatol 2015;151(10):1081–6.
2. Bath-Hextall FJ, Perkins W, Bong J, et al. Interventions for basal cell carcinoma of the skin. Cochrane Database Syst Rev 2007;(1):CD003412.
3. Lansbury L, Leonardi-Bee J, Perkins W, et al. Interventions for non-metastatic squamous cell carcinoma of the skin. Cochrane Database Syst Rev 2010;(4):CD007869.
4. Kim JYS, Kozlow JH, Mittal B, et al. Guidelines of care for the management of basal cell carcinoma. J Am Acad Dermatol 2018;78(3):540–59.
5. Kim JYS, Kozlow JH, Mittal B, et al. Guidelines of care for the management of cutaneous squamous cell carcinoma. J Am Acad Dermatol 2018;78(3):560–78.
6. Guy GP, Machlin SR, Ekwueme DU, et al. Prevalence and costs of skin cancer treatment in the U.S., 2002-2006 and 2007-2011. Am J Prev Med 2015;48(2):183–7.
7. Rogers HW, Coldiron BM. Analysis of skin cancer treatment and costs in the United States Medicare population, 1996-2008. Dermatol Surg 2013;39(1 Pt 1):35–42.
8. Edens BL, Bartlow GA, Haghighi P, et al. Effectiveness of curettage and electrodesiccation in the removal of basal cell carcinoma. J Am Acad Dermatol 1983;9(3):383–8.
9. Salasche SJ. Curettage and electrodesiccation in the treatment of midfacial basal cell epithelioma. J Am Acad Dermatol 1983;8(4):496–503.
10. Spiller WF, Spiller RF. Treatment of basal cell epithelioma by curettage and electrodesiccation. J Am Acad Dermatol 1984;11(5 Pt 1):808–14.
11. Reymann F. 15 years' experience with treatment of basal cell carcinomas of the skin with curettage. Acta Derm Venereol Suppl (Stockh) 1985;120:56–9.
12. McDaniel WE. Therapy for basal cell epitheliomas by curettage only. Further study. Arch Dermatol 1983;119(11):901–3.
13. National Comprehensive Care Center. NCCN clinical practice guidelines in oncology; basal cell carcinoma (V1.2019. Available at: www.nccn.org. Accessed October 1, 2018.
14. National Comprehensive Care Center. NCCN Clinical practice guidelines in oncology; squamous cell skin cancer (V2.2019. 2018. Available at: www.nccn.org. Accessed October 1, 2018.
15. Wilson LS, Pregenzer M, Basu R, et al. Fee comparisons of treatments for nonmelanoma skin cancer in a private practice academic setting. Dermatol Surg 2012;38(4):570–84.
16. Knox JM, Lyles TW, Shapiro EM, et al. Curettage and electrodesiccation in the treatment of skin cancer. Arch Dermatol 1960;82:197–204.
17. Kopf AW, Bart RS, Schrager D, et al. Curettage-electrodesiccation treatment of basal cell carcinomas. Arch Dermatol 1977;113(4):439–43.
18. Rowe DE, Carroll RJ, Day CL. Long-term recurrence rates in previously untreated (primary) basal cell carcinoma: implications for patient follow-up. J Dermatol Surg Oncol 1989;15(3):315–28.
19. Rodriguez-Vigil T, Vázquez-López F, Perez-Oliva N. Recurrence rates of primary basal cell carcinoma in facial risk areas treated with curettage and electrodesiccation. J Am Acad Dermatol 2007;56(1):91–5.
20. Chren MM, Linos E, Torres JS, et al. Tumor recurrence 5 years after treatment of cutaneous basal cell carcinoma and squamous cell carcinoma. J Invest Dermatol 2013;133(5):1188–96.
21. Lansbury L, Bath-Hextall F, Perkins W, et al. Interventions for non-metastatic squamous cell carcinoma of the skin: systematic review and pooled analysis of observational studies. BMJ 2013;347:f6153.

22. Drucker AM, Adam GP, Rofeberg V, et al. Treatments of primary basal cell carcinoma of the skin: a systematic review and network meta-analysis. Ann Intern Med 2018;169(7):456–66.

23. Chren MM, Sahay AP, Bertenthal DS, et al. Quality-of-life outcomes of treatments for cutaneous basal cell carcinoma and squamous cell carcinoma. J Invest Dermatol 2007;127(6):1351–7.

24. Wolf DJ, Zitelli JA. Surgical margins for basal cell carcinoma. Arch Dermatol 1987;123(3):340–4.

25. Brodland DG, Zitelli JA. Surgical margins for excision of primary cutaneous squamous cell carcinoma. J Am Acad Dermatol 1992;27(2 Pt 1):241–8.

26. Smeets NW, Krekels GA, Ostertag JU, et al. Surgical excision vs Mohs' micrographic surgery for basal-cell carcinoma of the face: randomised controlled trial. Lancet 2004;364(9447):1766–72.

27. Mosterd K, Krekels GA, Nieman FH, et al. Surgical excision versus Mohs' micrographic surgery for primary and recurrent basal-cell carcinoma of the face: a prospective randomised controlled trial with 5-years' follow-up. Lancet Oncol 2008;9(12):1149–56.

28. van Loo E, Mosterd K, Krekels GA, et al. Surgical excision versus Mohs' micrographic surgery for basal cell carcinoma of the face: a randomised clinical trial with 10 year follow-up. Eur J Cancer 2014;50(17):3011–20.

29. Gulleth Y, Goldberg N, Silverman RP, et al. What is the best surgical margin for a basal cell carcinoma: a meta-analysis of the literature. Plast Reconstr Surg 2010;126(4):1222–31.

30. Chauhan R, Munger BN, Chu MW, et al. Age at diagnosis as a relative contraindication for intervention in facial nonmelanoma skin cancer. JAMA Surg 2018;153(4):390–2.

31. Leibovitch I, Huilgol SC, Selva D, et al. Basal cell carcinoma treated with Mohs surgery in Australia I. Experience over 10 years. J Am Acad Dermatol 2005;53(3):445–51.

32. Leibovitch I, Huilgol SC, Selva D, et al. Cutaneous squamous cell carcinoma treated with Mohs micrographic surgery in Australia I. Experience over 10 years. J Am Acad Dermatol 2005;53(2):253–60.

33. Otley CC. Mohs' micrographic surgery for basal-cell carcinoma of the face. Lancet 2005;365(9466):1226–7 [author reply: 1227].

34. Rowe DE, Carroll RJ, Day CL. Prognostic factors for local recurrence, metastasis, and survival rates in squamous cell carcinoma of the skin, ear, and lip.

Implications for treatment modality selection. J Am Acad Dermatol 1992;26(6):976–90.

35. Pugliano-Mauro M, Goldman G. Mohs surgery is effective for high-risk cutaneous squamous cell carcinoma. Dermatol Surg 2010;36(10):1544–53.

36. Connolly SM, Baker DR, Coldiron BM, et al. AAD/ACMS/ASDSA/ASMS 2012 appropriate use criteria for Mohs micrographic surgery: a report of the American Academy of Dermatology, American College of Mohs Surgery, American Society for Dermatologic Surgery Association, and the American Society for Mohs Surgery. J Am Acad Dermatol 2012;67(4):531–50.

37. Cook J, Zitelli JA. Mohs micrographic surgery: a cost analysis. J Am Acad Dermatol 1998;39(5 Pt 1):698–703.

38. Johnson RP, Butala N, Alam M, et al. A retrospective case-matched cost comparison of surgical treatment of melanoma and nonmelanoma skin cancer in the outpatient versus operating room setting. Dermatol Surg 2017;43(7):897–901.

39. Ravitskiy L, Brodland DG, Zitelli JA. Cost analysis: Mohs micrographic surgery. Dermatol Surg 2012;38(4):585–94.

40. Seidler AM, Bramlette TB, Washington CV, et al. Mohs versus traditional surgical excision for facial and auricular nonmelanoma skin cancer: an analysis of cost-effectiveness. Dermatol Surg 2009;35(11):1776–87.

41. Essers BA, Dirksen CD, Nieman FH, et al. Cost-effectiveness of Mohs micrographic surgery vs surgical excision for basal cell carcinoma of the face. Arch Dermatol 2006;142(2):187–94.

42. Linos E, Chren MM, Stijacic Cenzer I, et al. Skin cancer in U.S. elderly adults: does life expectancy play a role in treatment decisions? J Am Geriatr Soc 2016;64(8):1610–5.

43. Silverman MK, Kopf AW, Grin CM, et al. Recurrence rates of treated basal cell carcinomas. Part 2: curettage-electrodesiccation. J Dermatol Surg Oncol 1991;17(9):720–6.

44. Bath-Hextall FJ, Perkins W, Bong J, et al. Interventions for basal cell carcinoma of the skin. Cochrane Database Syst Rev 2007;1:CD003412.

45. Thissen MR, Neumann MH, Schouten LJ. A systematic review of treatment modalities for primary basal cell carcinomas. Arch Dermatol 1999;135(10):1177–83.

Nonsurgical Treatments for Nonmelanoma Skin Cancer

Alexandra Collins, BS[a], Jessica Savas, MD[a,b], Laura Doerfler, MD[a,b],*

KEYWORDS

- Nonmelanoma skin cancer (NMSC) • Basal cell carcinoma (BCC)
- Cutaneous squamous cell carcinoma (SCC) • Nonsurgical • Photodynamic therapy
- Radiation therapy • Cryosurgery

KEY POINTS

- Although surgical intervention remains the standard of care for nonmelanoma skin cancer, other treatment modalities have been studied and used.
- Nonsurgical treatment methods include cryotherapy, topical medications, photodynamic therapy, radiation, Hedgehog pathway inhibitors, programmed cell death protein 1 inhibitors, and active nonintervention.
- Despite the favorable efficacy of surgical treatment methods, many factors, including but not limited to patient age, comorbidities, patient preference, and severity of disease, must be taken into consideration when choosing the most appropriate, patient-centered treatment approach.

INTRODUCTION

More than 3 million Americans are affected by nonmelanoma skin cancer (NMSC) each year, making NMSC the most common malignancy in the United States.[1] NMSC comprises roughly 80% basal cell carcinoma (BCC) and 20% squamous cell carcinoma (SCC), whereas Merkel cell carcinoma and adnexal tumors make up less than 1% of NMSC cases.[2] Most NMSC occurs in patients more than 60 years of age, with incidence increasing as age increases.[3] Selecting the appropriate treatment of NMSC requires consideration of cure rates, preservation of function, potential adverse effects, and cost. Among the elderly population, general health condition, life expectancy, and patient preference regarding surgical intervention should also be considered.[4,5]

Surgical intervention is the most effective treatment modality for NMSC, with a cure rate of greater than 90%.[6–8] However, other treatments have been used for NMSC and must be considered in certain clinical contexts. Nonsurgical treatment methods, including cryotherapy, topical medications, photodynamic therapy (PDT), radiation therapy, Hedgehog pathway inhibitors, programmed cell death protein 1 (PD-1) inhibitors, and active nonintervention are reviewed.

CRYOSURGERY

Cryosurgery (also known as cryotherapy) is a rapid, cost-effective, in-office treatment that uses subzero temperatures for tumor cell destruction.[9–11] The fast freeze–slow thaw protocol reaches skin temperatures of −50°C to −60°C by freezing the lesion for 40 to 90 seconds, depending on tumor size and thickness. The ice ball should extend 3 to 10 mm beyond the gross tumor.[11–14] Typically, 2 fast freeze–slow thaw cycles

Disclosure: None.
[a] Wake Forest School of Medicine, Winston-Salem, NC, USA; [b] Department of Dermatology, Wake Forest Baptist Hospital, 4618 Country Club Road, Winston-Salem, NC 27104, USA
* Corresponding author. Department of Dermatology, Wake Forest Baptist Hospital, 4618 Country Club Road, Winston-Salem, NC 27104.
E-mail address: ldoerfle@wakehealth.edu

Dermatol Clin 37 (2019) 435–441
https://doi.org/10.1016/j.det.2019.05.003

are completed with at least 90 seconds of total thaw time between each freeze cycle.[14] The extended thaw period allows for sufficient accumulation of toxic electrolytes. Decreased thaw times have been associated with incomplete eradication of the tumor.[14]

The data supporting the efficacy of cryotherapy derive mostly from studies performed in the 1980s, with cure rates reported as high as 94% to 99%.[15,16] The techniques used in these studies varied greatly from lesion to lesion, with some techniques not representative of how clinicians now typically practice (ie, curettage before treatment with cryotherapy).[15] Cryosurgery should be primarily considered in low-risk lesions because of the lack of histologic margin control provided by this modality.[17,18] Low-risk lesions most amenable to cryotherapy include primary, small lesions (<20 mm), with well-defined borders. Lesions on the perialar crease, nasolabial fold, anterior to the tragus of the ear, retroauricular folds, and hair-bearing scalp should not be treated with cryotherapy.[16]

Common local reactions to cryosurgery include:

- Pain
- Blistering
- Delayed wound healing
- Alopecia
- Permanent hypopigmentation

Less common adverse effects include hypertrophic scarring, tissue distortion, and severe painful hemorrhagic bullae, which can often be seen in more aggressive cryotherapy treatments.[15,16]

Topical Therapies

Topical therapies are often used in the treatment of NMSC. Because of limited penetration, topical treatments should be restricted to the treatment of superficial lesions. 5-Fluorouracil and imiquimod are US Food and Drug Administration (FDA)–approved topical agents for the treatment of superficial BCC. Ingenol mebutate and diclofenac are topical treatments currently being used off label for the treatment of thin NMSC.

5-Fluorouracil

5-Fluorouracil is a pyrimidine analogue that acts as an antimetabolite by inducing cell cycle arrest and apoptosis. Topical 5-fluorouracil is FDA approved in the treatment of superficial BCC. 5-Fluorouracil can be applied by either the patient or a caregiver, thus mitigating the need for multiple office visits and allowing the patients to complete the treatment at their convenience. The 5% cream or solution is administered once to twice daily for 2 weeks or more.[19]

The data supporting the efficacy of topical 5-fluorouracil treatments show cure rates ranging from 27% to 90%.[19–21] The wide variability in cure rates correlates with the many different application methods: occlusion versus nonocclusion, once-daily application versus twice-daily application, 2-week duration versus 16-week duration. Gross and colleagues[19] report a cure rate of 90% for superficial BCCs using twice-daily application for an average of 11 weeks. Cure rates for SCC in situ treated with topical 5-fluorouracil are lower than those of superficial BCC, ranging from 54% to 85% with twice-daily application for 6 to 8 weeks.[20]

Common local reactions include pain, crusting, erythema, dermatitis, and pruritus. These associated adverse events can affect patient adherence and thus treatment outcomes.[19–21]

Imiquimod

Imiquimod is a toll-like receptor 7 agonist that stimulates the innate immune response, causing a release of proinflammatory cytokines that contribute to tumor destruction. Imiquimod is FDA approved for the treatment of superficial BCC less than 2 cm and is also used in the off-label treatment of SCC in situ. It is available as a 3.75% or 5% cream. The cream is applied between once and twice daily, up to 5 days a week, for a 6-week to 16-week duration.

Topical imiquimod is most efficacious in the treatment of superficial BCC. Studies with varying regimens ranging from twice-weekly to twice-daily application report cure rates for superficial BCC ranging from 43% to 94%.[22–34] Topical imiquimod use for nodular BCC as well as for SCC show lower cure rates. For nodular BCC, topical imiquimod has clearance rates of 50% to 65%.[22–34] For SCC in situ, topical imiquimod showed clearance rates of 57% to 80%.[21–23]

Local reactions with topical imiquimod are similar to those with 5-fluorouracil, including pain, erythema, edema, weeping, pruritus, scaling, and permanent hypopigmentation.[22–34] Although systemic toxicity is rare with topical 5-fluorouracil, topical imiquimod frequently causes systemic symptoms, including flulike symptoms, dizziness, and headaches. Because of the extended duration of topical imiquimod and potential for systemic symptoms, patient adherence must be considered. Imiquimod is also commonly used as an adjuvant treatment of incompletely resected tumors or in combination with photodynamic therapy or cryosurgery.[35]

Ingenol Mebutate

Ingenol mebutate is a plant extract that has multiple mechanisms of action, including necrosis of cancer cells and subsequent activation of protein C kinase. The activation of protein C kinase contributes to the destruction of malignant cells and prevention of relapse.[36–38] Ingenol mebutate comes in a 0.05% gel formulation and is FDA approved for the treatment of actinic keratoses. Ingenol mebutate can be used off label for the treatment of superficial BCC. A previous study showed superficial BCC histologic clearance in 63% of patients.[38] Application of the gel to superficial BCC is recommended for 2 to 7 consecutive days. Compared with other topical agents, ingenol mebutate has a short application course, potentially lending itself to improved adherence rates. Adverse reactions may include erythema, pain, and edema that typically resolve within 2 weeks.[36–38]

Diclofenac

Diclofenac is a cyclooxygenase-2 inhibitor that exerts antitumor effects via interference of the sonic hedgehog gene and canonical wingless signaling.[5] This pathway interference results in cancer cell death. Its approved treatment of actinic keratosis consists of twice-daily application for 60 to 90 days. There are few reports of off-label use for treatment of superficial BCC and SCC in situ. Histologic clearance of superficial BCC with diclofenac alone and with diclofenac in combination with calcitriol was 64.3%.[39] Two case series have reported clearance of SCC in situ in 7 patients treated with diclofenac.[40,41] Side effects are common with application and may include erythema, erosion, and pruritus.[39] Similar to other topical treatments for BCC, the advantage of diclofenac is at-home application. The twice-daily application for an 8-week duration may result in poor patient adherence.

PHOTODYNAMIC THERAPY

PDT is a light-based therapy that is FDA approved for the treatment of actinic keratoses but is used off label for the treatment of thin NMSC. PDT requires a 2-step process that consists of application of a photosensitizer, methyl aminolevulinate or 5-aminolevulinic acid (ALA), and subsequent activation by a light source. The procedure requires waiting for several hours following the application of the photosensitizers to produce sufficient porphyrin IX levels. Once porphyrin IX has accumulated, a light source from the blue (404–20 nm) or red (635 nm) spectrum must be applied. The red light is primarily used in the treatment of cutaneous cancers because of deeper tissue penetration. The illumination generates reactive oxygen species, which leads to cell death.[42]

PDT is used in superficial and nodular BCC with clearance rates from 70% to 90%.[43–46] Higher clearance rates are associated with superficial lesions compared with nodular lesions.[45,46] However, nodular BCC clearance has shown improvement when preceded by debulking via curettage.[5] The use of PDT for SCC in situ shows marked variation in complete clearance ranging from 52% to 98%.[47–49] This range of clearance rates may be explained by the variation in PDT regimens. In small, randomized trials, PDT has shown a greater complete clearance rate in SCC in situ than other topical therapies.[47–49] PDT is not recommended for invasive squamous cell carcinoma. One study of 35 superficially invasive SCCs treated with ALA-PDT showed a clearance rate of 54%; however, the projected disease-free rate at 36 months after treatment was only 8%.[43]

Although surgical intervention provides superior clearance rates (96% vs 76%), cosmetic outcomes are superior with PDT (33% vs 82%).[46] Disadvantages include pain during treatment, erythema, mild edema, and superficial erosions. To reduce pain and thus prevent discontinuation of PDT before a therapeutic benefit can be obtained, analgesics, anesthetics, or forced cold air can be administered during treatment.[6] To improve treatment outcomes, PDT can also be used in combination with radiation therapy (RT), curettage, diclofenac, 5-fluorouracil, and imiquimod.[35]

RADIATION THERAPY

Radiation therapy for the treatment of NMSC includes megavoltage electron beam RT, orthovoltage RT, superficial x-ray therapy (SXRT), and electronic brachytherapy. Megavoltage electron beam RT and orthovoltage RT are used by radiation oncologists in the hospital setting. SXRT and electronic brachytherapy are used by dermatologists in the outpatient setting.

Megavoltage and orthovoltage RT are often used for nonsurgical candidates, including large lesions for which surgical intervention poses the risk of functional deficits (ie, loss of sense, facial palsy, drooling) and as adjuvant therapy for aggressive or incompletely resected tumors. Fractionated radiation is applied, 3 to 5 Gy, 3 to 5 times a week, to the total dose of 50 to 80 Gy.[50] Treatment protocols can be modified for patients who need fewer in-office visits, such as the elderly.

The reported 5-year clearance rates for NMSC treatment with megavoltage and orthovoltage RT are 92% for BCC and 80% for SCC.[50] Clearance rates are higher in primary NMSC versus recurrent NMSC.[50] Compared with BCC, SCC has a different response to radiation therapy, including an increased risk of failure, earlier recurrence, and a higher proportion of death after RT.[5]

Adverse events associated with RT include acute skin toxicity, changes to underlying structures, alopecia, cartilage necrosis, skin pigment changes, and secondary malignancy. However, radiation-related tumors occur 10 to 20 years following radiation treatment.[18,50,51] Most patients who are not surgical candidates using radiation therapy are more than 60 years of age, making the risk of radiation-related tumorigenesis minimal. RT also requires a lengthy treatment course of several fractions over the course of several weeks, making this option cumbersome logistically.

Brachytherapy is a form of radiation that is growing in popularity for well-circumscribed, thin tumors. In brachytherapy, the radioactive source is applied on the surface mold versus external beam RT, in which the radiation source is at a distance from the patient and aimed at the site to be treated. It provides minimal dose delivery to surrounding healthy tissue, thus enabling good functional and cosmetic results.[52]

HEDGEHOG INHIBITORS

There are now 2 oral treatments for advanced BCC: vismodegib (Erivedge, Genentech) and sonidegib (Odomzo, Sun Pharma). These systemic therapies are indicated for large or difficult-to-treat BCCs that are not candidates for surgical resection or radiation. The drugs are often used to shrink tumors before surgical intervention or used as long-term management to control tumor growth.

Both drugs interfere with the Hedgehog signaling pathway via selective inhibition of the smoothened protein receptor and are similar in efficacy, showing local disease control rates of approximately 80%.[53–55] The sonic hedgehog pathway is involved in the pathogenesis of sporadic BCC and nevoid BCC syndrome through somatic mutations in the smoothened protein and the patched gene.[53]

In addition to its FDA approval for locally advanced BCC, vismodegib is also approved to treat metastatic BCC. Based on a 21-month follow-up from the ERIVANCE BCC trial, objective response was reported in 43% of locally advanced and 30% of metastatic cases, with median duration of response of 7.6 months for both.[55]

Long-term treatment with these systemic medications is often limited given their adverse event profile. Adverse events include muscle spasms, alopecia, dysgeusia, and weight loss. In patients with advanced BCC treated with vismodegib, 22.1% discontinued treatment because of an adverse event.[56] Alternative dosing regimens, including drug holidays of 1 to 3 weeks, have been reported showing clinical improvement and less toxicity.[57]

PROGRAMMED CELL DEATH PROTEIN 1 INHIBITOR

There is a 5% risk of metastasis of SCC, with a heightened risk in immunosuppressed populations.[50,51] Chemotherapeutics, including cisplatin, carboplatin, 5-fluorouracil, and epidermal growth factor receptor inhibitors (cetuximab), have been used for treatment of regional and distant metastatic SCC, with inconsistent results.[58–62] In September of 2018, the FDA approved a new intravenously infused drug called cemiplimab-rwlc (Libtayo, Regeneron and Sanofi) for the treatment of patients with metastatic SCC or locally advanced cutaneous SCC who are not candidates for curative surgery or curative radiation. This agent is the first to be approved by FDA specifically for advanced SCC.

Cemiplimab is a fully human monoclonal antibody targeting the immune checkpoint receptor PD-1. Blockade of the PD-1 pathway prevents tumor cell immune evasion and allows immune system detection and response to malignant cells.[58] SCC may be responsive to immune therapy given the high mutation burden and its strong association with immunosuppression.[63] Efficacy results from a multicenter phase 2 study and a multicenter phase 1 study, with a combined 108 patients, showed promising results, with a 47% response rate for metastatic SCC and 50% response rate for locally advanced SCC.[64]

OBSERVATION

Observation, or active nonintervention, is a strategy that can be used to manage elderly patients with BCC because of slow tumor growth and a low risk for progression to metastatic disease. Elderly patients with a significantly decreased life expectancy can potentially be placed under surveillance with regular 3-month follow-ups to track tumor progression.

SUMMARY

As a result of modern technological advancements and improvements in medical care, life expectancy has been prolonged. As a sustained growth is seen in the elder population, there will be a continued increase in the incidence of NMSC. Although surgical intervention remains the standard of care for NMSCs, many factors, including but not limited to patient age, preference, and severity of disease, must be taken into consideration when choosing the most appropriate, patient-centered treatment approach. The patient and provider should find a treatment modality that aligns with the patient's expectations and maintenance of quality of life.

REFERENCES

1. Guy GP, Machlin S, Ekwueme DU, et al. Prevalence and costs of skin cancer treatment in the US, 2002–2006 and 2007–2011. Am J Prev Med 2015;48:183–7.
2. Eisemann N, Waldman A, Geller AC, et al. Non-melanoma skin cancer incidence and impact of skin cancer screening on incidence. J Invest Dermatol 2014;134:43–50.
3. Diffey BL, Langtry JAA. Skin cancer incidence and the ageing population. Br J Dermatol 2005;153:679–80.
4. Chren MM, Sahay AP, Bertenthal DS, et al. Quality of life outcomes of treatments for cutaneous basal cell carcinoma and squamous cell carcinoma. J Invest Dermatol 2007;127(6):1351–7.
5. Čeović R, Petković M, Mokos ZB, et al. Nonsurgical treatment of nonmelanoma skin cancer in the mature patient. Clin Dermatol 2018;36(2):177–87.
6. Lanoue J, Goldenberg G. Basal cell carcinoma: a comprehensive review of existing and emerging nonsurgical therapies. J Clin Aesthet Dermatol 2016;9:26–36.
7. Bahner JD, Bordeaux JS. Non-melanoma skin cancers: photodynamic therapy, cryotherapy, 5-fluorouracil, imiquimod, diclofenac, or what? Facts and controversies. Clin Dermatol 2013;31:792–8.
8. Lewin JM, Carucci JA. Advances in the management of basal cell carcinoma. F1000Prime Rep 2015;7:53.
9. Kauvar ANB, Arpey CJ, Hruza G, et al. Consensus for nonmelanoma skin cancer treatment. Part II: squamous cell carcinoma, including a cost analysis of treatment methods. Dermatol Surg 2015;41:1214–40.
10. Kauvar ANB, Cronin T, Roenigk R, et al. Consensus for nonmelanoma skin cancer treatment: basal cell carcinoma, including a cost analysis of treatment methods. Dermatol Surg 2015;41:550–71.
11. Kuflik EG. Cryosurgery for cutaneous malignancy: an update. Dermatol Surg 1997;23:1081–7.
12. Kuflik EG. Cryosurgery for skin cancer: 30-year experience and cure rates. Dermatol Surg 2004;30:297–300.
13. Mallon E, Dawber R. Cryosurgery in the treatment of basal cell carcinoma. Dermatol Surg 1996;22:854–8.
14. Zimmerman EE, Crawford P. Cutaneous cryosurgery. Am Fam Physician 2012;86(12):1118–24.
15. Holt PJ. Cryotherapy for skin cancer: results over a 5-year period using liquid nitrogen spray cryosurgery. Br J Dermatol 1988;119:231–40.
16. Kufik EG, Gage AA. The five-year cure rate achieved by cryosurgery for skin cancer. J Am Acad Dermatol 1991;24:1002–4.
17. Bichakjian C, Armstrong A, Baum C, et al. Guidelines of care for the management of basal cell carcinoma. J Am Acad Dermatol 2018;78(3):540–59.
18. Rowe DE, Carroll RJ, Day CL Jr. Prognostic factors for local recurrence, metastasis, and survival rates in squamous cell carcinoma of the skin, ear, and lip. Implications for treatment modality selection. J Am Acad Dermatol 1992;26(6):976–90.
19. Gross K, Kircik L, Kricorian G. 5% 5-fluorouracil cream for the treatment of small superficial basal cell carcinoma: efficacy, tolerability, cosmetic outcome, and patient satisfaction. Dermatol Surg 2007;33:433–9.
20. Bargman H, Hochman J. Topical treatment of Bowen's disease with 5-fluorouracil. J Cutan Med Surg 2003;7:101–5.
21. Love WE, Bernhard JD, Bordeux JS. Topical imiquimod or fluorouracil therapy for basal and squamous cell carcinoma: a systematic review. Arch Dermatol 2009;15:1431–8.
22. Warshauer E, Warshauer BL. Clearance of basal cell and superficial squamous cell carcinomas after imiquimod therapy. J Drugs Dermatol 2008;7(5):447–51.
23. Peris K, Micantonio T, Fargnoli MC, et al. Imiquimod 5% cream in the treatment of Bowen's disease and invasive squamous cell carcinoma. J Am Acad Dermatol 2006;55(2):324–7.
24. Schulze HJ, Cribier B, Requena L, et al. Imiquimod 5% cream for the treatment of superficial basal cell carcinoma: results from a randomized vehicle-controlled phase III study in Europe. Br J Dermatol 2005;152:939–47.
25. Vun Y, Siller G. Use of 5% imiquimod cream in the treatment of facial basal cell carcinoma: a 3-year retrospective follow-up study. Australas J Dermatol 2006;47:169–71.
26. Schiessl C, Wolber C, Tauber M, et al. Treatment of all basal cell carcinoma variants including large and high-risk lesions with 5% imiquimod cream: histological and clinical changes, outcome, and follow-up. J Drugs Dermatol 2007;6:507–13.
27. Gollnick H, Barona CG, Frank RG, et al. Recurrence rate of superficial basal cell carcinoma following treatment with imiquimod 5% cream: conclusion of a 5-year long-term follow-up study in Europe. Eur J Dermatol 2008;18:677–82.

28. Ezughah FI, Dawe RS, Ibbotson SH, et al. A randomized parallel study to assess the safety and efficacy of two different dosing regimens of 5% imiquimod in the treatment of superficial basal cell carcinoma. J Dermatolog Treat 2008; 19:111–7.

29. Marks R, Gebauer K, Shumack S, et al. Imiquimod 5% cream in the treatment of superficial basal cell carcinoma: results of a multicenter 6- week dose–response trial. J Am Acad Dermatol 2001;44: 807–13.

30. Alessi SS, Sanches JA, Oliveira WR, et al. Treatment of cutaneous tumors with topical 5% imiquimod cream. Clinics (Sao Paulo) 2009;64:961–6.

31. Ruiz-Villaverde R, Sanchez-Cano D, Burkhardt-Perez P. Superficial basal cell carcinoma treated with imiquimod 5% topical cream for a 4-week period: a case series. J Eur Acad Dermatol Venereol 2009;23:828–31.

32. Quirk C, Gebauer K, De'Ambrosis B, et al. Sustained clearance of superficial basal cell carcinomas treated with imiquimod cream 5%: results of a prospective 5-year study. Cutis 2010;85:318–24.

33. Geisse J, Caro I, Lindholm J, et al. Imiquimod 5% cream for the treatment of superficial basal cell carcinoma: results from two phase III, randomized, vehicle-controlled studies. J Am Acad Dermatol 2004;50:722–33.

34. Sterry W, Ruzicka T, Herrera E, et al. Imiquimod 5% cream for the treatment of superficial and nodular basal cell carcinoma: randomized studies comparing low-frequency dosing with and without occlusion. Br J Dermatol 2002;147:1227–36.

35. Lucena SR, Salazar N, Garcia-Cazanaa T, et al. Combined treatments with photodynamic for nonmelanoma skin cancer. Int J Mol Sci 2015;16: 25912–33.

36. Cantisani C, Paolino G, Cantoresi F, et al. Superficial basal cell carcinoma successfully treated with ingenol mebutate gel 0.05%. Dermatol Ther 2014;27: 352–4.

37. Bettencourt MS. Treatment of superficial basal cell carcinoma with ingenol mebutate gel 0.05%. Clin Cosmet Investig Dermatol 2016;9:205–9.

38. Siller G, Rosen R, Freeman M, et al. PEP005 (ingenol mebutate) gel for the topical treatment of superficial basal cell carcinoma: results of a randomized control phase IIa trial. Australas J Dermatol 2010;51: 99–105.

39. Brinkhuizen T, Frencken KJ, Nelemans PJ, et al. The effect of topical diclofenac 3% and calcitriol 3 μg/g on superficial basal cell carcinoma (sBCC) and nodular basal cell carcinoma (nBCC): a phase II, randomized controlled trial. J Am Acad Dermatol 2016;75(1):126–34.

40. Dawe SA, Salisbury JR, Higgins E. Two cases of Bowen's disease successfully treated topically with 3% diclofenac in 2.5% hyaluronan gel. Clin Exp Dermatol 2005;30:712–3.

41. Patel MJ, Stockfleth E. Does progression from actinic keratosis and Bowen's disease end with treatment: diclofenac 3% gel, an old drug in a new environment? Br J Dermatol 2007;156(Suppl 3): 53–6.

42. Braathen LR, Szeimies R-M, Basset-Seguin N, et al. Guidelines on the use of photodynamic therapy for nonmelanoma skin cancer: an international consensus. J Am Acad Dermatol 2007;56:125–43.

43. Fink-Puches R, Soyer HP, Hofer A, et al. Long-term follow-up and histological changes of superficial nonmelanoma skin cancers treated with topical delta-aminolevulinic acid photodynamic therapy. Arch Dermatol 1998;134:821–6.

44. Cohen DK, Lee PK. Photodynamic therapy for nonmelanoma skin cancer. Cancer 2016;8:90.

45. Savoia P, Deboli T, Previgliano A, et al. Usefulness of photodynamic therapy as a possible therapeutic alternative in the treatment of basal cell carcinoma. Int J Mol Sci 2015;16(10):23300–17.

46. Rhodes LE, de rice MA, Lefifsdottir R, et al. Five-year follow-up of a randomized, prospective trial of topical methyl amino levulinate photodynamic therapy vs. surgery for nodular basal cell carcinoma. Arch Dermatol 2007;143:1131–6.

47. Salim A, Leman JA, McColl JH, et al. Randomized comparison of photodynamic therapy with topical 5-fluorouracil in Bowen's disease. Br J Dermatol 2003;148(3):539–43.

48. Cairnduff F, Stringer MR, Hudson EJ, et al. Superficial photodynamic therapy with topical 5-amino-laevulinic acid for superficial primary and secondary skin cancer. Br J Cancer 1994;69(3): 605–8.

49. Zaar O, Fougelberg J, Hermansson A, et al. Effectiveness of photodynamic therapy in Bowen's disease: a retrospective observational study in 423 lesions. J Eur Acad Dermatol Venereol 2017;31(8): 1289–94.

50. Locke J, Karimpour S, Young G, et al. Radiotherapy for epithelial skin cancer. Int J Radiat Oncol Biol Phys 2001;51:748–55.

51. Avril MF, Auperin A, Margulis A, et al. Basal cell carcinoma of the face: surgery or radiotherapy? Results of a randomized study. Br J Cancer 1997;76(1): 100–6.

52. Alam M, Nanda S, Mittal BB, et al. The use of brachytherapy in the treatment of nonmelanoma skin cancer: a review. J Am Acad Dermatol 2011; 65(2):377–88.

53. Otsuka A, Levesque MP, Dummer R, et al. Hedgehog signaling in basal cell carcinoma. J Dermatol Sci 2015;78:95–100.

54. Jain S, Song R, Xie J. Sonidegib: mechanism of action, pharmacology, and clinical utility for advanced

basal cell carcinomas. Onco Targets Ther 2017;10: 1645–53.

55. Sekulic A, Migden MR, Lewis K, et al. Pivotal ERIV-ANCE basal cell carcinoma (BCC) study: 12-month update of efficacy and safety of vismodegib in advanced BCC. J Am Acad Dermatol 2015;72(6): 1021–6.

56. Sekulic A, Migden MR, Basset-Seguin N, et al. Long-term safety and efficacy of vismodegib in patients with advanced basal cell carcinoma: final update (30-month) of the pivotal ERIVANCE BCC study. J Clin Oncol 2014;32(15):9013.

57. Becker LR, Aakhus AE, Reich HC, et al. A novel alternate dosing of vismodegib for treatment of patients with advanced basal cell carcinomas. JAMA Dermatol 2017;153(4):321–2.

58. Palyca P, Koshenkov VP, Mehnert JM. Developments in the treatment of locally advanced and metastatic squamous cell carcinoma of the skin: a rising unmet need. Am Soc Clin Oncol Educ Book 2014; e397–404.

59. Szturz P, Vermorken JB. Treatment of elderly patients with squamous cell carcinoma of the head and neck. Front Oncol 2016;6:199.

60. Lu SM, Lien WW. Concurrent Radiotherapy with cetuximab or platinum-based chemotherapy for locally advanced cutaneous squamous cell carcinoma of the head and neck. Am J Clin Oncol 2018;41(1):95–9.

61. Jarkowski A, Hare R, Loud P, et al. Systemic therapy in advanced cutaneous squamous cell Carcinoma (CSCC): the roswell park experience and a review of the literature. Am J Clin Oncol 2016;39(6):545–8.

62. Trodello C, Pepper JP, Wong M, et al. Cisplatin and cetuximab treatment for metastatic cutaneous squamous cell carcinoma: a systematic review. Dermatol Surg 2017;43(1):40–9.

63. Ritprajak P, Azuma M. Intrinsic and extrinsic control of expression of the immunoregulatory molecule PD-L1 in epithelial cells and squamous cell carcinoma. Oral Oncol 2015;51(3):221–8.

64. Migden M. PD-1 blockade with cemiplimab in advanced cutaneous squamous-cell carcinoma. N Engl J Med 2018;379:341–51.

Diagnosis and Management of Cutaneous B-Cell Lymphomas

Stephen J. Malachowski, MD, MS[a,1], James Sun, MD[b,1],
Pei-Ling Chen, MD, PhD[b], Lucia Seminario-Vidal, MD, PhD[a,b],*

KEYWORDS

- B-cell lymphoma • Cutaneous marginal zone lymphoma • Cutaneous follicle center lymphoma
- Cutaneous diffuse large B-cell lymphoma • Intravascular diffuse large B-cell lymphoma

KEY POINTS

- Primary cutaneous B-cell lymphomas (PCBCLs) are a group of rare diseases that have variable presentations, treatments, and prognoses.
- PCBCLs include indolent forms (ie, primary cutaneous marginal zone lymphoma and primary cutaneous follicle center lymphoma) and aggressive forms (ie, primary cutaneous diffuse large B-cell lymphoma, leg-type, and intravascular diffuse large B-cell lymphoma).
- A thorough work-up is necessary before diagnosing CBCL as a primary cutaneous malignancy and includes a thorough history and physical examination, histologic analysis of biopsies, molecular studies, laboratory studies, and imaging.

INTRODUCTION

Primary cutaneous lymphomas are uncommon diseases with an estimated incidence of 0.5 to 1 case per 100,000 people annually. Primary cutaneous B-cell lymphomas (PCBCLs) represent a relatively large proportion of cutaneous lymphomas, accounting for approximately 20% to 25% of all primary cutaneous lymphomas.[1–4] PCBCLs are classified into 3 major subtypes: cutaneous marginal zone lymphoma (PCMZL), cutaneous follicle center lymphoma (PCFCL), and cutaneous diffuse large B-cell lymphoma, leg-type (DLBCL-LT).[4] Intravascular diffuse large B-cell lymphoma (IVDLBCL) is a rare subtype that will be discussed further. The first 2 types are regarded as indolent, and the latter 2 types are relatively aggressive in terms of morbidity and mortality.[4]

Currently, the pathogenesis of PCBCL is poorly understood. There is some evidence that infection with *Borrelia burgdorferi* may play a role because of chronic inflammation from the infection, particularly in European cases. This is not a frequent finding, however, nor is it a geographically stable occurrence.[5–7]

By definition, PCBCLs are cutaneous manifestations of disease that are not secondary to extracutaneous spread. Therefore, a thorough work-up is necessary before diagnosing CBCL as a primary malignancy.[8] Diagnosis requires a thorough history and physical examination, tissue samples and analysis, laboratory studies and imaging for staging.[8–10] It is critical to mention that biopsy sampling must be done only with an incisional, excisional or punch biopsy to allow for adequate sampling.[8] In general, the National

---

Conflicts of interest: S.J. Malachowski, J. Sun, P.L Chen, and L. Seminario-Vidal have no conflicts to disclose.
[a] Department of Dermatology and Cutaneous Surgery, University of South Florida Morsani College of Medicine, 12901 Bruce B Downs Boulevard, Tampa, FL 33612, USA; [b] Department of Cutaneous Oncology, Moffitt Cancer Center, 10920 McKinley Drive, Tampa, FL 33612, USA
[1] These authors have equally contributed to this article.
* Corresponding author. Department of Dermatology and Cutaneous Surgery, University of South Florida, 12901 Bruce B. Downs Boulevard, MDC 79, Tampa, FL 33612.
E-mail address: luciasem@health.usf.edu

Dermatol Clin 37 (2019) 443–454
https://doi.org/10.1016/j.det.2019.05.004

Comprehensive Cancer Network (NCCN) recommends an initial immunohistochemistry (IHC) panel including CD3, CD5, CD10, CD20, BCL2, BCL6 and MUM1 for each case of suspected PCBCL. Additional items may include CD21, CD23, CD43, CyclinD1, Ki-67, surface immunoglobulins immunoglobulins (IgM) and IgD, and kappa/lambda light chain analysis.[8] Other studies include complete blood cell count with differential (CBC), comprehensive metabolic panel (CMP), lactate dehydrogenase (LDH), hepatitis B panel, serum protein electrophoresis (SPEP) and pregnancy testing in women of childbearing age prior to treatment.[4]

There are limited data for treatment recommendations for PCBCLs and a dearth of large randomized trials to guide therapy.[11] Generally, treatment modalities are determined by whether the disease is indolent or aggressive.[11] The following sections will discuss the epidemiologic details, clinical and histopathologic features, the key differential diagnoses and the work-up for each subtype, and conclude with current treatment options for patients afflicted with PCBCLs. **Table 1** summarizes the characteristics of each subtype of PCBCL.

PRIMARY CUTANEOUS MARGINAL ZONE LYMPHOMA
Epidemiology

Primary cutaneous marginal zone lymphoma (PCMZL) represents approximately 30% (range 24%–57%) of all cutaneous B-cell lymphomas,[4] and about 7% of all primary cutaneous B-cell lymphomas.[3,12,13] Patients tend to be young to middle aged, with a median age of 39 to 55 years.[3,14–16] PCMZL represents the majority of the rare cutaneous B-cell lymphomas in pediatric patients.[12] Some studies have found male predominance.[3,14–16] PCMZL also includes the diseases formerly known as immunocytoma and nonmyelomatous plasmacytomas.[4]

Clinical Presentation, Histopathological Findings, and Differential Diagnoses

PCMZL usually presents as asymptomatic solitary or multiple erythematous to brown-colored papules, nodules, or plaques (**Fig. 1**). Sometimes pruritus is noted, but ulceration and pain are not expected.[7,12,17] Lesions are distributed over the trunk and extremities with predominance in the upper extremity compared with the lower extremity. Constitutional symptoms such as fever, weight loss or night sweats are typically absent.[4,12] Rarely, PCMZL can transform into diffuse large B-cell lymphoma.[3] Dissemination is uncommon, and lesions have been reported to spontaneously

resolve with resultant atrophy at the original site. However, recurrence is common.[7,17–20] Overall, the prognosis is favorable, with 5-year overall survival cited at over 95%.[7,14,17,18,20,21]

Histopathologic examination reveals a nodular or diffuse dermal infiltrate of small, centrocyte-like B cells, lymphoplasmacytoid cells and plasma cells, with sparing of the epidermis and superficial papillary dermis. A reactive germinal center may have peripheral, small-to-intermediate sized B cells with copious cytoplasm and irregular nuclei.[4,22] Eosinophils, reactive T cells and relatively few centroblasts may be seen.[4,22] Periodic acid Schiff-positive immunoglobulin material may be identified in the nucleus of plasma cells (**Fig. 2**).[3]

The differential diagnosis includes primary cutaneous follicular zone lymphoma diffuse type, non-melanoma skin cancers, secondary cutaneous involvement of a systemic lymphoma such as CLL, mantle cell lymphoma, hypersensitivity or inflammatory reaction and reactive lymphoid hyperplasia.[2,4]

Work-Up

Diagnosis of PCMZL requires adequate tissue sampling that includes the infiltrates within the deeper dermis and subcutaneous tissues.[2,3,8] IHC of neoplastic cells is negative for bcl-6, CD5, and CD10 and is positive for bcl-2, CD20 and CD79a.[3,22] Plasma cells may express CD79a and CD138 without expression of CD20.[3,23] Cyclin D1 may be useful in differentiating PCMZL from mantle cell lymphoma, as the latter will be positive for CD5 and cyclin D1.[8,24] Fluorescent in situ hybridization (FISH) or cytogenetics may be useful in determining the presence of chromosomal translocations, as these translocations are less likely in PCMZL compared with systemic lymphomas; few cases of PCBCL have reported translocations involving the MLT and immunoglobulin heavy chain (IgH) genes on chromosomes 18 and 14, respectively.[25] Therefore, translocations should increase suspicion for systemic rather than primary cutaneous lymphoma. Neoplastic B cells typically express IgG in primary lesions, whereas secondary, extranodal disease tends to express IgM.[22]

Staging requires laboratory studies and imaging of the chest, abdomen, and pelvis with either positron emission tomography (PET) or computed tomography (CT) scans.[8] A bone marrow biopsy is not typically beneficial in PCMZL unless there is suspicion for extracutaneous disease (eg, unexplained cytopenias) in the setting of an indolent subtype.[9,10]

Table 1
Key features of primary cutaneous B-cell lymphomas

Subtype	Epidemiology	Clinical Features	Histology	Immunophenotype	Molecular	Prognosis
Marginal zone lymphoma	Median age: 55 y M = F/M > F	Solitary or multiple papules, plaques or nodules, predominantly of upper extremities and trunk	Patchy periadnexal or diffuse infiltrates of small B cells Lymphoplasmacytoid and plasma cells	CD20+, CD79a+, PAX5+, Bcl-2+, Bcl-6−[b], CD5−, CD10−, CD43+, MUM-1+, FOXP1−	IgH/MALT1 translocation t(14;18) (q32;21)	5-y survival: >95% Frequent relapse
Follicle center lymphoma	Median age: 60 y M = F	Solitary, grouped or multiple papules, plaques or nodules, predominantly of head, neck and trunk Most common CBCL	Follicular, nodular or diffuse infiltrates Centrocytes and centroblasts	CD20+, CD79a+, PAX5+, Bcl-2−, Bcl-6+, CD5−, CD10+[a], MUM-1−, FOXP1−, IgM−, p63−	Rarely: t(14:18)	5-y survival: >95%; if primary leg involvement, ~40%; if systemic involvement, 5%–10%
Diffuse large B-cell lymphoma, leg type	Median age: 76 y M < F	Solitary or multiple plaques and tumors, predominantly of the legs Frequent extracutaneous spread	Diffuse infiltrates to subcutaneous tissue Rare lymphocytes Centroblasts and immunoblasts	CD20+, CD79a+, PAX5+, Bcl-2+, Bcl-6 +/−, CD10−, CD5−, MUM-1+, FOXP1+, IgM+, p63+	IgH, myc, Bcl-6 translocations DNA amplification of 18q21.31-q21.33 CDKN2A and CDKN2B deletions	5-y survival: 60%
Intravascular	Median age: 67 y M = F	Diffuse or cutaneous subtype Solitary or multiple indurated patches/ plaques or diffuse telangiectasias Neurologic symptoms, most commonly AMS at diagnosis	Intravascular large atypical cells with scant cytoplasm and vesicular nuclei, prominent nucleoli	CD20+, CD79a+, PAX5+, Bcl-2+, Bcl-6−, CD5−, CD10−, MUM-1+		5-y survival: Systemic: 33% Cutaneous: 56%

[a] CD10 may show negativity in cases with diffuse growth pattern.
[b] Negative in the lesional cells but highlights the associated reactive germinal centers.

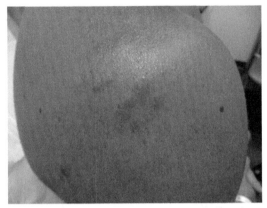

Fig. 1. Primary cutaneous marginal zone lymphoma. Grouped erythematous papules on the right shoulder.

Treatment: US Food and Drug Administration-Approved and Clinical Trials

Because of the association with *B burgdorferi* infection in European studies, the EORTC-CLG/ISCL consensus statement recommends antibiotic therapy prior to initiation of invasive therapy in antibody-positive cases.[11] In the United States, antibiotics are not recommended and are not mentioned in NCCN guidelines.[8,11] As PCMZL is largely an indolent disease, initial expectant management and observation are not unreasonable.

Should treatment be required, local therapies with radiation or surgical excision are first-line treatments.[4,8,11,26] There is some debate regarding the optimal dose of radiation therapy; doses from 24 Gy to 30 Gy have been effective. Ideally, the lowest effective dose should be used, with a margin of 1 to 1.5 cm of uninvolved skin included in the field of irradiation.[8,11,26] Parbhakar and Cin[27] performed a retrospective review comparing 6 patients treated with surgery to 7 patients treated with radiation. There were no recurrences in the surgery group, whereas one patient in the radiation group had recurrence. In addition, the patients treated with radiation also developed adverse effects such as erythema and edema. Based on this small retrospective review, surgery is an effective treatment without complications associated with radiation. However, radiation may be the more appropriate treatment for lesions in locations not amenable to surgery, such as facial or large lesions.

The NCCN guidelines also mention other topical therapies, including corticosteroids, topical nitrogen mustard and bexarotene, and intralesional steroid or rituximab injections.[8] All therapies have reportedly been effective to different degrees, but as stated previously, no randomized trial is available to systemically evaluate these treatments. Suárez and colleagues[11] report intralesional triamcinolone and cryotherapy in cosmetically sensitive areas such as the face where both radiotherapy and surgical excision would leave poor cosmetic results.

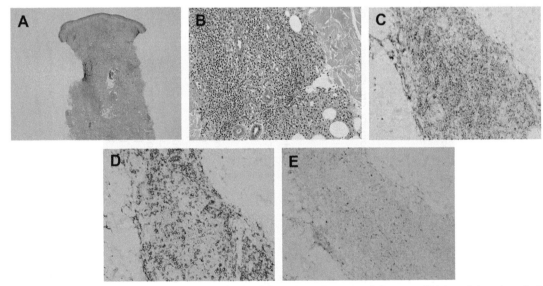

Fig. 2. Primary cutaneous marginal zone lymphoma. (*A*) Sections show a nodular, superficial, and deep lymphoid infiltrate composed of (*B*) small lymphocytes admixed with numerous plasma cells and rare larger atypical lymphocytes. Immunohistochemical staining reveals that the infiltrate is composed of nodular aggregates of (*C*) CD20-positive B-cells expressing Bcl-2, (*D*) surrounded by CD3, and (*E*) bcl-6 positive T cells. The plasma cells show lambda light chain restriction and are negative for kappa light chain. CD10 is negative.

For cases of multiple and symptomatic lesions not amenable to localized treatment, intralesional or systemic rituximab should be considered.[11,26] Rituximab is an anti-CD20 monoclonal antibody and is a logical choice, as both normal and malignant B cells express CD20 antigens. Morales and colleagues[28] and Valencak and colleagues[29] have reported small series of 10 and 11 patients, respectively, treated with systemic rituximab, that demonstrate near-complete overall response rates with low rates of relapse. A multicenter study conducted by the Spanish Working Group on Cutaneous Lymphoma indicated that intralesional rituximab induced complete response in 71% of patients with PCMZLs and PCFCLs, which is similar to the reported rate of complete response with systemic rituximab.[30] Unfortunately, there is no consensus on dosage or duration of treatment.

PCFCL rarely develops disseminated skin lesions or large tumors. In these rare cases, the first-line treatment is chemotherapy with R-CHOP (rituximab, cyclophosphamide, doxorubicin, oncovin/vincristine and prednisone).[11] Overall, recurrence is common, as high as 44% to 71% after primary treatment.[4]

Two notable experimental therapies are under investigation. The first is radioimmunotherapy with Yttrium-90 ibritumomab tiuxetan (Zevalin, V10XX02, Spectrum Pharmaceuticals, Henderson, Nevada), which is the first US Food and Drug Administration (FDA)-approved radioimmunotherapy approved for relapsed or refractory B-cell non-Hodgkin lymphoma and follicular lymphoma responsive to first-line chemotherapy. The monoclonal antibody binds to CD20, allowing the chelated radioisotope to apply radiation directly to CD20 expressing cells. The pilot study was reported in 2008 by Maza and colleagues,[31] with complete response in 100% of 10 patients treated with Yttrium-90 ibritumomab tiuxetan. Four patients achieved ongoing remission; however, median follow-up time was only 19 months. No further studies have built on initially promising results. The other therapy is adenovirus-interferon-γ (TG1042, now ASN-002). ASN-002 (Ascend Biopharmaceuticals, South Melbourne, Australia) is a genetically modified, nonreplicating adenovirus 5 containing human interferon-γ (IFN-γ) cDNA.[32] Intralesional injection leads to cytomegalovirus (CMV) promotor-driven expression of IFN-γ locally at the injection site.[33] In the Initial phase I/II, open label, multicenter, dose-escalation study conducted in 38 CTCL and CBCL patients, 5 patients had CBCL. Local response was observed in all CBCL patients (3 complete response, 2 partial response), and the treatment was well tolerated with mild-to-moderate injection site reactions and influenza-like symptoms.[32,33] Another multicenter phase II clinical trial was conducted by Dreno and colleagues,[34] examining TG1042/ASN-002 in relapsed primary CBCL. Thirteen patients received intralesional injections, and 11 patients had objective response (7 complete response, 4 partial response). The median time to disease progression in treated lesions was 23.5 months. Clinically, patients all demonstrated regression of their lesions. These studies demonstrate the effectiveness of immunotherapy for primary CBCL. Compared with existing therapies, TG1042/ASN-002 is safe, without the risk of serious infections associated with rituximab. Further research is required to directly compare TG1042 with current treatment modalities.

PRIMARY CUTANEOUS FOLLICLE CENTER LYMPHOMA
Epidemiology

PCFCL accounts for approximately 50% to 60% of PCBCLs.[3,13,35] It is also male predominant and tends to occur in middle-aged and older patients, with a median age in the 50s.[14–16] It rarely occurs in children, with only 3 previously reported pediatric cases.[35–38]

Clinical Presentation, Histopathological Findings, and Differential Diagnoses

Patients with PCFCL present with either single or multiple papules, plaques, or tumors with pink to purple coloration and may display peripheral erythema; surrounding plaques and papular lesions may also be seen (**Fig. 3**). The lesions tend to appear across the scalp and forehead, as well as the posterior torso, although any site can be affected.[2,3] Multiple lesions are often grouped, although widespread lesions may also be seen.[35] As both PCFCL and PCMZL are indolent subtypes, they share clinical features.[1–3] PCFCL that presents on the legs is associated with worse prognosis, with 5-year disease-specific survival reported at 41%.[2] Despite frequent recurrences up to 46.5%,[2] metastasis is rare and the overall prognosis is reassuring, as 5-year survival is near 95%[4,39] and 10-year survival is 88.8% in 1 large study.[2,14] If left untreated, the disease will slowly progress, with rare documented cases of spontaneous regression.[4]

Histologic examination reveals any combination of follicular, nodular, or diffuse patterns of malignant cells in the dermis and hypodermis with sparing of the epidermis (**Fig. 4**).[2,22,35] The growth patterns do not affect disease behavior or prognosis.[2] Familiar follicular architecture is present on

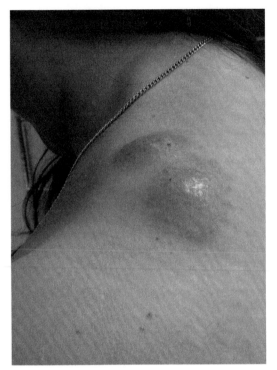

Fig. 3. Primary cutaneous follicle center lymphoma. Two erythematous tumors on the left shoulder.

a spectrum, with overt follicular patterns present in relatively fewer patients. In addition to degeneration of the usual mantle region, the follicle is missing signs of reactive processes such as tingible body macrophages and heterogeneity of the follicle's appearance. The infiltrate comprises large, multilobulated centrocytes and relatively fewer centroblasts with a varying number of interspersed eosinophils, reactive T cells, and histiocytes.[2,22] Earlier in the disease course, cells are more likely to display histologic features consistent with follicular architecture and familiar cell types such as follicular dendritic cells; these expected features are diminished as the lesion progresses.

Importantly, diffuse-patterned PCFCL may be confused with more aggressive large-cell lymphomas, but this represents a diagnostic challenge more than a clinical prognostic factor. Additional morphology such as spindle cells, which are also seen in sarcomas, also presents a diagnostic challenge.[40–42]

The differential diagnosis for PCFCL includes PCMZL with prominent follicular features, cutaneous lymphoma secondary to disseminated nodal disease, diffuse large B-cell lymphoma, reactive lymphoid hyperplasia, hypersensitivity reactions, and nonmelanoma skin cancer.[8,35]

Work-up

The standard work-up includes initial blood tests, staging imaging with PET and/or CT scan, bone marrow biopsy, and adequate tissue biopsy with IHC and FISH or cytogenetics for further classification.[8,35] Cells are positive for CD20, CD79a and bcl-6 and usually negative for CD5, CD43, bcl-2 and the MYD88 L265P mutation. On occasion, CD10 and bcl-2 will be positive; however, positive bcl-2 suggests a nodal lymphoma and CD10 may be negative in the diffuse pattern of PCFCL. Surface immunoglobulins will show monoclonal restriction to either kappa or lambda light chains. Additionally, IRF4, MUM1, and FOXP1 can be useful, as a negative result suggests PCFCL over primary cutaneous diffuse large B-cell lymphoma, leg-type.[23,25,40,41] Interestingly, a nontrivial percentage of PCFCL cases described tumor suppressor gene inactivation of p15 and p16.[43] As in PCMZL, chromosomal translocations are far less common than in systemic lymphoma; IgH, BCL-6, and MYC genes were not identified in a translocation.[44] An important feature to differentiate malignant proliferation is low Ki-67 staining (<50%), whereas reactive lymphoid hyperplasia expresses high mitotic activity and thus, a high Ki-67 index.[40,45]

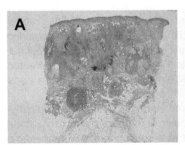
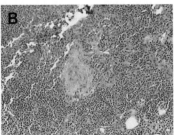
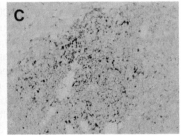

Fig. 4. Primary cutaneous follicle center lymphoma. (*A*) Sections show a nodular atypical lymphohistiocytic infiltrate in the dermis. (*B*) The atypical lymphocytes are small in size. Immunohistochemical studies reveal that the atypical lymphocytes are positive for CD20 and (*C*) bcl-6, but are negative for CD5, CD10, Bcl-2, CD23, and Bcl-1.

Treatment: US Food and Drug Administration-Approved and Clinical Trials

The treatment of PCFCL is essentially the same as for PCMZL.[8,26] However, there is less evidence for the benefit of rituximab for PCFCL.

PRIMARY CUTANEOUS DIFFUSE LARGE B-CELL LYMPHOMA, LEG TYPE
Epidemiology

Primary cutaneous diffuse large B-cell lymphoma, leg type (PCDLBCL-LT) is the least common variant of PCBCLs. This lymphoma accounts for 10% to 20% of all cutaneous B-cell lymphomas.[3,35] Elderly patients are more commonly affected, with a median age at presentation of 70 to 82. Some studies have described female preponderance, although this finding is not consistently reported.[35] The prototypic patient is a woman in her eighth decade of life.[8,46,47]

Clinical Presentation, Histopathological Findings, and differential Diagnoses

PCDLBCL-LT is classified as an aggressive PCBCL. Typically, there is rapid appearance of 1 or more red-brown to blue tumors on the lower extremity (Fig. 5). Lesions may be unilateral or bilateral, may exhibit ulceration and may be found in sites other than the lower extremity in roughly 20% of patients.[1,3,48–51] Erythematous, satellite papules may be seen near the larger tumors. The

5-year survival is roughly 30% to 70% and portends a poor prognosis, especially in the presence of a MYD88 L265P mutation.[52,53] However, a study by Grange and colleagues[49] suggests solitary lesions may have much higher survival, near 100%.

Tissue biopsy demonstrates a diffuse-patterned, dense infiltrate comprised of centroblasts and immunoblasts that extends from the papillary dermis to the hypodermis. Mitoses are common and reactive T cells are infrequently observed. Epidermal involvement may occur with large, neoplastic B cells, such that one may mistake this involvement for Pautrier microabscesses of cutaneous T-cell lymphoma (CTCL).[22,49,50]

Differential diagnoses for PCDLBCL-LT includes diffuse PCFCL, cutaneous manifestations of systemic lymphomas and leukemias and metastatic nonleukemic/lymphomatous disease.[3,35]

Work-up

As with the other subtypes, blood tests, staging imaging and tissue sampling are required. The malignant cells will be positive for CD20, CD79a, Bcl-2, Bcl-6, MUM1/IRF4 and FOX-P1 and negative for CD10; however, it is possible that the cells do not express Bcl-6 and do express CD10, although this is not the typical situation.[15,23,51,54–59] Analysis of IgM and IgD expression is useful for distinguishing PCDLBCL-LT from PCFCL when lesions are

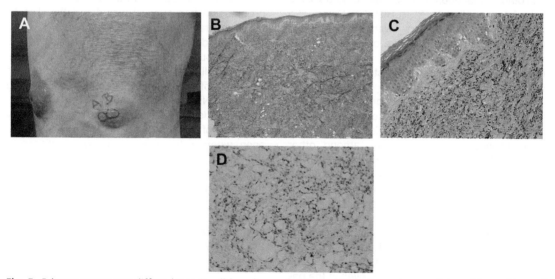

Fig. 5. Primary cutaneous diffuse large B-cell lymphoma, leg-type. (A) Erythematous nodules with markings of biopsy sites on the left knee. (B) A superficial and deep diffuse lymphoid infiltrate with a Grenz zone and no evidence of epidermal involvement is noted. (C) The lymphocytes are predominantly large cells with irregular nuclear contours, abundant cytoplasm, with frequent mitoses and associated nuclear debris; occasional smaller lymphocytes are scattered throughout. No germinal centers are seen. Immunohistochemical studies reveal that the large cells are positive for (D) Pax5 and CD10 and focally positive for CD20, while CD3, CD4, CD5, and CD8 highlight small, reactive-appearing T cells intervening.

not on the legs; these antibodies tend to be more strongly expressed in PCDLBCL-LT.[60] Further distinction for PCFCL may be gained by the presence of MYD88 L265P abnormalities and translocations of Bcl-6, IgH and MYC genes, which are more common in PCDLBCL-LT.[44] Overall, the classic lymphoma t(14;18) is again suggestive of a systemic disease.[44,52,53]

Treatment: US Food and Drug Administration-Approved and Clinical Trials

PCDLBCL-LT is classified as an aggressive lymphoma with many similarities to systemic diffuse large B-cell lymphoma.[11] As a result, the first-line treatment is multiagent chemotherapy with rituximab (R-CHOP; rituximab, doxorubicin, vincristine, cyclophosphamide, prednisone).[11] Grange and colleagues[61] published a large series with 115 patients demonstrating the efficacy of R-CHOP. Radiation therapy can be efficacious in combination with systemic therapy or as palliative monotherapy. Radiation monotherapy has good initial results; however most patients quickly recur.[26] Surgery also has a role to debulk large solitary lesions or lesions confined to a limited area.[26] Unfortunately, there are no further recommendations available for other treatment modalities. As with the other subtypes, there are no randomized clinical trials evaluating the available treatments. Upon review of current literature, many therapies for other cutaneous and systemic neoplasms have been applied to PCDLBCL-LT. Some, like isolated limb perfusion with hyperthermic melphalan[62] and ibrutinib[63] are only discussed in case reports with good results. Two treatments in particular have ongoing investigations and are worth discussion.

The first is pegylated liposomal doxorubicin (PLD; Doxil, Janssen Pharmaceuticals, Beerse, Belgium). Conventional doxorubicin is associated with significant cardiac toxicity, among other adverse effects. The liposomal pegylated formulation increases specificity and uptake by the skin.[64] PLD applied to PCBCL was first reported in a prospective phase II clinical trial of monotherapy.[65] Of the 5 patients in the trial, 1 patient was diagnosed with PCMZL and 4 patients had widespread PCDLBCL-LT. All 5 patients achieved complete response in this pilot study within a median time of 3 months, even in the patients previously treated with radiation and chemotherapy. Two patients relapsed. Upon follow-up at 69 months, 4 patients had continued complete response, defined as the absence of skin lesions, while 1 patient died from progressive disease. The treatment was well tolerated;

the only notable adverse effects were grade 1 neurotoxicity and grade 3 neutropenia, which were treatable. Based on the efficacy of rituximab, Fabbri and colleagues[64] performed a multicenter, single-arm, phase II clinical trial that studied the combination of rituximab and PLD (R-PLD) in 12 patients with refractory disease. Four of these patients had PCFCL; 5 patients had PCMZL and 3 patients had PCDLBCL-LT. Of the 3 patients with PCDLBCL-LT, 1 patient achieved complete response and 1 patient achieved partial response for an overall response rate of 66%. The last patient had progressive disease. The treatment was again well tolerated, with mild adverse effects. No dose interruptions or adjustments were made. Although the sample sizes are small, these 2 studies demonstrate that PLD is an effective treatment for all types of PCBCL and is well tolerated without significant adverse effects. Another experimental therapy is lenalidomide, an immunomodulatory drug that induces growth arrest and apoptosis in lymphoma cell lines[66] and increases natural killer cell expression, in turn enhancing the cytotoxic effect of rituximab.[67] Beylot-Barry and colleagues[68] conducted a prospective, multicenter, single-arm, phase II trial investigating the utility of lenalidomide in refractory or relapsing PCDLBCL-LT. Nineteen patients received therapy, of whom 4 patients demonstrated complete response and 1 patient had partial response. Two patients with initial CR relapsed within 12 months. Median progression-free survival was 4 months. The 6-month overall response rate was 26.3%. Overall, the study demonstrated modest efficacy in line with previous studies of lenalidomide for diffuse large B-cell lymphoma. There was also a high incidence of significant adverse effects, including 2 deaths. Nine patients required dose reduction, and 5 patients were discontinued on therapy because of adverse effects. It remains to be seen whether there is a role for lenalidomide therapy in relapsed disease. Overall, there are insufficient data supporting adoption of novel therapies for PCDLBCL-LT. There are limited therapeutic options in cases of relapsed disease. However, the number of medications under investigation is encouraging and will hopefully lead to new treatment options.

PRIMARY CUTANEOUS INTRAVASCULAR LARGE B-CELL LYMPHOMA
Epidemiology

Intravascular large B-cell lymphoma (IVBCL) is rare, diagnosed in less than 1 per million adults.

Median age of presentation is 67 years.[4] There is no gender predominance.[69]

Clinical Presentation, Histopathological Findings, and Differential Diagnoses

This subtype is an extranodal disease characterized by malignant lymphoid cells confined to the lumina of small- to medium-sized blood vessels. Two forms are identified, a cutaneous and systemic form. IVBCL presents with skin findings of livedo racemosa or panniculitis-like lesions, painful telangiectasias, or nodular lesions. The systemic form of the disease affects multiple organs, primarily, but not limited to, the small-to medium-sized vessels of the central nervous system and the skin. Clinically, patients present with skin findings and neurologic deficits. The cutaneous variant accounts for 25% of cases, with a better 5-year survival of 56%.[24,69] The systemic form is more aggressive, with a 5-year survival of 33%.[24]

Histopathologically, IVBCL is characterized by large, atypical cells with scant cytoplasm, vesicular nuclei and at least 1 prominent nucleoli; these cells are present within blood vessels.[35] These cells express pan-B cell antigens including CD20, CD79a with co-expression of CD5 in 38%, CD10 in 13% and Bcl-6 in 26% of cases.[70] Both MUM-1 and Bcl-2 are positive in most cases.[71] It is currently unknown why the neoplastic cells of IVBCL remain confined to the intravascular space. It is hypothesized that tumor cells express angiogenic factors or perhaps these cells lack adhesion molecules required for transendothelial migration.[24,35]

Differential diagnoses include reactive angioendotheliomatosis in the context of bacterial endocarditis and intralymphatic or intravascular histiocytosis in rheumatoid arthritis or following joint replacement surgery with metal implants.[24]

Treatment: US Food and Drug Administration-Approved and Clinical Trials

Intravascular large B-cell lymphoma is treated with multiagent chemotherapy in combination with rituximab (R-CHOP).[11,24,35] Again, there are no clinical trials available to guide therapy and the recommendation for R-CHOP is based on retrospective reviews and case reports.[69,72–74] No ongoing clinical trials have been identified.

DIFFERENTIATING PRIMARY CUTANEOUS B-CELL LYMPHOMA FROM SECONDARY CUTANEOUS B-CELL LYMPHOMA

Both nodal or systemic B-cell lymphomas can secondarily involve the skin. This typically signifies advanced disease and presents with multiple nodules. To differentiate these lesions from PCBCL, histology of the cutaneous lesions is examined, in addition to lymph node findings and/or bone marrow biopsy and radiological staging.[24] Ultimately, there is no reliable test to differentiate these diseases, so negative staging is required for a diagnosis of PCBCL.[4] Nodal follicular lymphomas are characterized by t(14:18) translocations and neoplastic cells are often Bcl-2 positive. PCBCL can exhibit both of these, but less commonly.[2]

Mantle cell lymphoma accounts for 10% of nodal B-cell non-Hodgkin lymphomas, with skin involvement in 2% to 6% of patients. This is usually the first sign of disseminated disease. The lesions have a predilection for the upper extremity and torso. Histologically, there are infiltrates of blastic or centrocytic tumor cells with cyclinD1 expression.[24]

Precursor B lymphoblastic lymphoma can present with secondary skin involvement in 20% of patients. This disease predominantly occurs in children. The skin lesions are purpuric plaques and red-blue nodules. Histologic examination reveals monomorphic infiltration by medium-sized B lymphoblasts with cobblestone growth pattern of neoplastic cells. These cells express CD10, CD79a, and TdT, but are CD20 negative.[24]

Finally, lymphomatoid granulomatosis is an Epstein-Barr virus (EBV)-associated systemic B-cell lymphoproliferative disorder with preferential extranodal involvement, especially of the lungs, skin, central nervous system and kidneys. Approximately 50% of patients have cutaneous involvement with multiple papules and subcutaneous ulcerated nodules and folliculitis-like lesions with facial edema. Histologically, angiocentric and angiodestructive infiltrates with necrosis are seen. Neoplastic cells express B-cell markers, and are EBV-RNA positive, embedded with reactive T cells.[24]

REFERENCES

1. Fink-Puches R, Zenahlik P, Bäck B, et al. Primary cutaneous lymphomas: applicability of current classification schemes (European Organization for Research and Treatment of Cancer, World Health Organization) based on clinicopathologic features observed in a large group of patients. Blood 2002; 99(3):800–5. Availble at: http://www.ncbi.nlm.nih.gov/pubmed/11806979. Accessed July 23, 2018.
2. Suárez AL, Pulitzer M, Horwitz S, et al. Primary cutaneous B-cell lymphomas: part I. Clinical features, diagnosis, and classification. J Am Acad Dermatol 2013;69(3):329.e1-13.

3. Willemze R, Jaffe ES, Burg G, et al. WHO-EORTC classification for cutaneous lymphomas. Blood 2005;105(10):3768–85.

4. Hope CB, Pincus LB. Primary cutaneous B-cell lymphomas. Clin Lab Med 2017;37(3):547–74.

5. Wood GS, Kamath NV, Guitart J, et al. Absence of *Borrelia burgdorferi* DNA in cutaneous B-cell lymphomas from the United States. J Cutan Pathol 2001; 28(10):502–7. Available at: http://www.ncbi.nlm.nih.gov/pubmed/11737518. Accessed July 23, 2018.

6. Goodlad JR, Davidson MM, Hollowood K, et al. Primary cutaneous B-cell lymphoma and Borrelia burgdorferi infection in patients from the Highlands of Scotland. Am J Surg Pathol 2000;24(9):1279–85. Available at: http://www.ncbi.nlm.nih.gov/pubmed/10976703. Accessed July 23, 2018.

7. Cerroni L, Signoretti S, Höfler G, et al. Primary cutaneous marginal zone B-cell lymphoma: a recently described entity of low-grade malignant cutaneous B-cell lymphoma. Am J Surg Pathol 1997;21(11): 1307–15. Available at: http://www.ncbi.nlm.nih.gov/pubmed/9351568. Accessed July 23, 2018.

8. NCCN: National Comprehensive Cancer Network. Clinical practice guidelines in oncology, Primary Cutaneous B-cell Lymphomas version 2.2018. Fort Washington (PA): National Comprehensive Cancer Network; 2018.

9. Kim YH, Willemze R, Pimpinelli N, et al. TNM classification system for primary cutaneous lymphomas other than mycosis fungoides and Sezary syndrome: a proposal of the International Society for Cutaneous Lymphomas (ISCL) and the Cutaneous Lymphoma Task Force of the European Organization of Research and Treatment of Cancer (EORTC). Blood 2007;110(2):479–84.

10. Senff NJ, Kluin-Nelemans HC, Willemze R. Results of bone marrow examination in 275 patients with histological features that suggest an indolent type of cutaneous B-cell lymphoma. Br J Haematol 2008; 142(1):52–6.

11. Suárez AL, Querfeld C, Horwitz S, et al. Primary cutaneous B-cell lymphomas: part 2. Therapy and future directions. J Am Acad Dermatol 2013;69(3): 343.e1-11.

12. Swerdlow SH. Cutaneous marginal zone lymphomas. Semin Diagn Pathol 2017;34(1):76–84.

13. Bradford PT, Devesa SS, Anderson WF, et al. Cutaneous lymphoma incidence patterns in the United States: a population-based study of 3884 cases. Blood 2009;113(21):5064–73.

14. Zinzani PL, Quaglino P, Pimpinelli N, et al. Prognostic factors in primary cutaneous B-cell lymphoma: the italian study group for cutaneous lymphomas. J Clin Oncol 2006;24(9):1376–82.

15. Senff NJ, Hoefnagel JJ, Jansen PM, et al. Reclassification of 300 primary cutaneous B-cell lymphomas according to the new WHO-EORTC classification for cutaneous lymphomas: comparison with previous classifications and identification of prognostic markers. J Clin Oncol 2007;25(12):1581–7.

16. Haverkos B, Tyler K, Gru AA, et al. Primary cutaneous B-cell lymphoma: management and patterns of recurrence at the multimodality cutaneous lymphoma Clinic of The Ohio State University. Oncologist 2015;20(10):1161–6.

17. Li C, Inagaki H, Kuo T-T, et al. Primary cutaneous marginal zone B-cell lymphoma: a molecular and clinicopathologic study of 24 Asian cases. Am J Surg Pathol 2003;27(8):1061–9. Available at: http://www.ncbi.nlm.nih.gov/pubmed/12883238. Accessed July 23, 2018.

18. Bailey EM, Ferry JA, Harris NL, et al. Marginal zone lymphoma (low-grade B-cell lymphoma of mucosa-associated lymphoid tissue type) of skin and subcutaneous tissue: a study of 15 patients. Am J Surg Pathol 1996;20(8):1011–23. Available at: http://www.ncbi.nlm.nih.gov/pubmed/8712288. Accessed July 23, 2018.

19. Child FJ, Woollons A, Price ML, et al. Multiple cutaneous immunocytoma with secondary anetoderma: a report of two cases. Br J Dermatol 2000; 143(1):165–70. Available at: http://www.ncbi.nlm.nih.gov/pubmed/10886154. Accessed July 23, 2018.

20. Rijlaarsdam JU, van der Putte SC, Berti E, et al. Cutaneous immunocytomas: a clinicopathologic study of 26 cases. Histopathology 1993;23(2): 117–25. Available at: http://www.ncbi.nlm.nih.gov/pubmed/8406383. Accessed July 23, 2018.

21. Torne R, Su WP, Winkelmann RK, et al. Clinicopathologic study of cutaneous plasmacytoma. Int J Dermatol 1990;29(8):562–6. Available at: http://www.ncbi.nlm.nih.gov/pubmed/2242944. Accessed July 23, 2018.

22. Chen ST, Barnes J, Duncan L. Primary cutaneous B-cell lymphomas— clinical and histopathologic features, differential diagnosis, and treatment. Semin Cutan Med Surg 2018;37(1):49–55.

23. Hoefnagel JJ, Vermeer MH, Jansen PM, et al. Bcl-2, Bcl-6 and CD10 expression in cutaneous B-cell lymphoma: further support for a follicle centre cell origin and differential diagnostic significance. Br J Dermatol 2003;149(6):1183–91. Available at: http://www.ncbi.nlm.nih.gov/pubmed/14674895. Accessed July 23, 2018.

24. Kempf W, Denisjuk N, Kerl K, et al. Primary cutaneous B-cell lymphomas. J Dtsch Dermatol Ges 2012;10(1):12–23.

25. Child FJ, Russell-Jones R, Woolford AJ, et al. Absence of the t(14;18) chromosomal translocation in primary cutaneous B-cell lymphoma. Br J Dermatol 2001;144(4):735–44. Available at: http://www.ncbi.nlm.nih.gov/pubmed/11298531. Accessed July 23, 2018.

26. Nicolay JP, Wobser M. Cutaneous B-cell lymphomas - pathogenesis, diagnostic workup, and therapy. J Dtsch Dermatol Ges 2016;14(12):1207–24.

27. Parbhakar S, Cin AD. Primary cutaneous B-cell lymphoma: Role of surgery. Can J Plast Surg 2011; 19(2):e12–4. Available at: http://www.ncbi.nlm.nih.gov/pubmed/22654537. Accessed July 21, 2018.

28. Morales AV, Advani R, Horwitz SM, et al. Indolent primary cutaneous B-cell lymphoma: experience using systemic rituximab. J Am Acad Dermatol 2008; 59(6):953–7.

29. Valencak J, Weihsengruber F, Rappersberger K, et al. Rituximab monotherapy for primary cutaneous B-cell lymphoma: response and follow-up in 16 patients. Ann Oncol 2009;20(2):326–30.

30. Peñate Y, Hernández-Machín B, Pérez-Méndez LI, et al. Intralesional rituximab in the treatment of indolent primary cutaneous B-cell lymphomas: an epidemiological observational multicentre study. The Spanish Working Group on Cutaneous Lymphoma. Br J Dermatol 2012;167(1):174–9.

31. Maza S, Gellrich S, Assaf C, et al. Yttrium-90 ibritumomab tiuxetan radioimmunotherapy in primary cutaneous B-cell lymphomas: first results of a prospective, monocentre study. Leuk Lymphoma 2008;49(9):1702–9.

32. Dummer R, Eichmüller S, Gellrich S, et al. Phase II clinical trial of intratumoral application of TG1042 (adenovirus-interferon-gamma) in patients with advanced cutaneous T-cell lymphomas and multilesional cutaneous B-cell lymphomas. Mol Ther 2010; 18(6):1244–7.

33. Dummer R, Hassel JC, Fellenberg F, et al. Adenovirus-mediated intralesional interferon-gamma gene transfer induces tumor regressions in cutaneous lymphomas. Blood 2004;104(6):1631–8.

34. Dreno B, Urosevic-Maiwald M, Kim Y, et al. TG1042 (Adenovirus-interferon-γ) in primary cutaneous B-cell lymphomas: a phase II clinical trial. PLoS One 2014;9(2):e83670.

35. Hope CB, Pincus LB. Primary cutaneous B-cell lymphomas with large cell predominance-primary cutaneous follicle center lymphoma, diffuse large B-cell lymphoma, leg type and intravascular large B-cell lymphoma. Semin Diagn Pathol 2017;34(1):85–98.

36. Amitay-Laish I, Feinmesser M, Ben-Amitai D, et al. Juvenile onset of primary low-grade cutaneous B-cell lymphoma. Br J Dermatol 2009;161(1):140–7.

37. Fink-Puches R, Chott A, Ardigo M, et al. The spectrum of cutaneous lymphomas in patients less than 20 years of age. Pediatr Dermatol 2004;21(5): 525–33.

38. Ghislanzoni M, Gambini D, Perrone T, et al. Primary cutaneous follicular center cell lymphoma of the nose with maxillary sinus involvement in a pediatric patient. J Am Acad Dermatol 2005;52(5 Suppl 1): S73–5.

39. Park J-H, Shin H-T, Lee D-Y, et al. World Health Organization–European Organization for Research and Treatment of Cancer classification of cutaneous lymphoma in Korea: A retrospective study at a single tertiary institution. J Am Acad Dermatol 2012;67(6): 1200–9.

40. Cerroni L, Arzberger E, Pütz B, et al. Primary cutaneous follicle center cell lymphoma with follicular growth pattern. Blood 2000;95(12):3922–8. Available at: http://www.ncbi.nlm.nih.gov/pubmed/10845929. Accessed July 23, 2018.

41. Goodlad JR, Krajewski AS, Batstone PJ, et al. Primary cutaneous follicular lymphoma: a clinicopathologic and molecular study of 16 cases in support of a distinct entity. Am J Surg Pathol 2002;26(6): 733–41. Available at: http://www.ncbi.nlm.nih.gov/pubmed/12023577. Accessed July 23, 2018.

42. Santucci M, Pimpinelli N, Arganini L. Primary cutaneous B-cell lymphoma: a unique type of low-grade lymphoma. Clinicopathologic and immunologic study of 83 cases. Cancer 1991;67(9):2311–26. Available at: http://www.ncbi.nlm.nih.gov/pubmed/2013039. Accessed July 23, 2018.

43. Child FJ, Scarisbrick JJ, Russell-Jones R, et al. Inactivation of tumor suppressor genes p15INK4b and p16INK4a in primary cutaneous B cell lymphoma. J Invest Dermatol 2002;118(6):941–8.

44. Hallermann C, Kaune KM, Gesk S, et al. Molecular cytogenetic analysis of chromosomal breakpoints in the IGH, MYC, BCL6, and MALT1 gene loci in primary cutaneous B-cell lymphomas. J Invest Dermatol 2004;123(1):213–9.

45. Leinweber B, Colli C, Chott A, et al. Differential diagnosis of cutaneous infiltrates of B lymphocytes with follicular growth pattern. Am J Dermatopathol 2004;26(1):4–13. Available at: http://www.ncbi.nlm.nih.gov/pubmed/14726817. Accessed July 23, 2018.

46. Fujita A, Hamada T, Iwatsuki K. Retrospective analysis of 133 patients with cutaneous lymphomas from a single Japanese medical center between 1995 and 2008. J Dermatol 2011;38(6):524–30.

47. Wilson LD, Hinds GA, Yu JB. Age, race, sex, stage, and incidence of cutaneous lymphoma. Clin Lymphoma Myeloma Leuk 2012;12(5):291–6.

48. Goodlad JR, Krajewski AS, Batstone PJ, et al. Primary cutaneous diffuse large B-cell lymphoma: prognostic significance of clinicopathological subtypes. Am J Surg Pathol 2003;27(12):1538–45. Available at: http://www.ncbi.nlm.nih.gov/pubmed/14657713. Accessed July 23, 2018.

49. Grange F, Bekkenk MW, Wechsler J, et al. Prognostic factors in primary cutaneous large B-cell lymphomas: a European multicenter study. J Clin Oncol 2001;19(16):3602–10.

50. Vermeer MH, Geelen FA, van Haselen CW, et al. Primary cutaneous large B-cell lymphomas of

the legs. A distinct type of cutaneous B-cell lymphoma with an intermediate prognosis. Dutch Cutaneous Lymphoma Working Group. Arch Dermatol 1996;132(11):1304–8. Available at: http://www.ncbi.nlm.nih.gov/pubmed/8915307. Accessed July 23, 2018.

51. Kodama K, Massone C, Chott A, et al. Primary cutaneous large B-cell lymphomas: clinicopathologic features, classification, and prognostic factors in a large series of patients. Blood 2005;106(7):2491–7.

52. Menguy S, Gros A, Pham-Ledard A, et al. MYD88 somatic mutation is a diagnostic criterion in primary cutaneous large B-cell lymphoma. J Invest Dermatol 2016;136(8):1741–4.

53. Pham-Ledard A, Beylot-Barry M, Barbe C, et al. High frequency and clinical prognostic value of MYD88 L265P mutation in primary cutaneous diffuse large B-cell lymphoma, leg-type. JAMA Dermatol 2014;150(11):1173–9.

54. Hoefnagel JJ, Mulder MMS, Dreef E, et al. Expression of B-cell transcription factors in primary cutaneous B-cell lymphoma. Mod Pathol 2006;19(9):1270–6.

55. Pham-Ledard A, Cowppli-Bony A, Doussau A, et al. Diagnostic and prognostic value of BCL2 rearrangement in 53 patients with follicular lymphoma presenting as primary skin lesions. Am J Clin Pathol 2015;143(3):362–73.

56. Paulli M, Viglio A, Vivenza D, et al. Primary cutaneous large B-cell lymphoma of the leg: histogenetic analysis of a controversial clinicopathologic entity. Hum Pathol 2002;33(9):937–43. Available at: http://www.ncbi.nlm.nih.gov/pubmed/12378521. Accessed July 23, 2018.

57. Grange F, Petrella T, Beylot-Barry M, et al. Bcl-2 protein expression is the strongest independent prognostic factor of survival in primary cutaneous large B-cell lymphomas. Blood 2004;103(10):3662–8.

58. Hoefnagel JJ, Dijkman R, Basso K, et al. Distinct types of primary cutaneous large B-cell lymphoma identified by gene expression profiling. Blood 2005;105(9):3671–8.

59. Geelen FA, Vermeer MH, Meijer CJ, et al. bcl-2 protein expression in primary cutaneous large B-cell lymphoma is site-related. J Clin Oncol 1998;16(6):2080–5.

60. Koens L, Vermeer MH, Willemze R, et al. IgM expression on paraffin sections distinguishes primary cutaneous large B-cell lymphoma, leg type from primary cutaneous follicle center lymphoma. Am J Surg Pathol 2010;34(7):1043–8.

61. Grange F, Joly P, Barbe C, et al. Improvement of survival in patients with primary cutaneous diffuse large B-cell lymphoma, leg type, in France. JAMA Dermatol 2014;150(5):535.

62. Kobold S, Killic N, Lütkens T, et al. Isolated limb perfusion with melphalan for the treatment of intractable primary cutaneous diffuse large B-cell lymphoma leg type. Acta Haematol 2010;123(3):179–81.

63. Gupta E, Accurso J, Sluzevich J, et al. Excellent outcome of immunomodulation or Bruton's tyrosine kinase inhibition in highly refractory primary cutaneous diffuse large B-cell lymphoma, leg type. Rare Tumors 2015;7(4):6067.

64. Fabbri A, Cencini E, Alterini R, et al. Rituximab plus liposomal pegylated doxorubicin in the treatment of primary cutaneous B-cell lymphomas. Eur J Haematol 2014;93(2):129–36.

65. Pulini S, Rupoli S, Goteri G, et al. Efficacy and safety of pegylated liposomal doxorubicin in primary cutaneous B-cell lymphomas and comparison with the commonly used therapies. Eur J Haematol 2009;82(3):184–93.

66. Zhu D, Corral LG, Fleming YW, et al. Immunomodulatory drugs Revlimid® (lenalidomide) and CC-4047 induce apoptosis of both hematological and solid tumor cells through NK cell activation. Cancer Immunol Immunother 2008;57(12):1849–59.

67. Wu L, Adams M, Carter T, et al. Lenalidomide enhances natural killer cell and monocyte-mediated antibody-dependent cellular cytotoxicity of rituximab-treated CD20+ tumor cells. Clin Cancer Res 2008;14(14):4650–7.

68. Beylot-Barry M, Mermin D, Maillard A, et al. A single-arm phase II trial of lenalidomide in relapsing or refractory primary cutaneous large B-cell lymphoma, leg type. J Invest Dermatol 2018. https://doi.org/10.1016/j.jid.2018.03.1516.

69. Ferreri AJM, Campo E, Seymour JF, et al. Intravascular lymphoma: clinical presentation, natural history, management and prognostic factors in a series of 38 cases, with special emphasis on the 'cutaneous variant. Br J Haematol 2004;127(2):173–83.

70. Saurel CA, Personett DA, Edenfield BH, et al. Molecular analysis of intravascular large B-cell lymphoma with neoangiogenesis. Br J Haematol 2011;152(2):234–6.

71. Murase T, Yamaguchi M, Suzuki R, et al. Intravascular large B-cell lymphoma (IVLBCL): a clinicopathologic study of 96 cases with special reference to the immunophenotypic heterogeneity of CD5. Blood 2007;109(2):478–85.

72. Ferreri AJM, Dognini GP, Govi S, et al. Can rituximab change the usually dismal prognosis of patients with intravascular large B-cell lymphoma? J Clin Oncol 2008;26(31):5134–6 [author reply: 5136-7].

73. Ferreri AJM, Dognini GP, Bairey O, et al. The addition of rituximab to anthracycline-based chemotherapy significantly improves outcome in 'Western' patients with intravascular large B-cell lymphoma. Br J Haematol 2008;143(2):253–7.

74. Shimada K, Kosugi H, Narimatsu H, et al. Sustained remission after rituximab-containing chemotherapy for intravascular large B-cell lymphoma. J Clin Exp Hematop 2008;48(1):25–8.

Cutaneous T Cell Lymphoma
A Difficult Diagnosis Demystified

Erik Peterson, BA, BS[a], Jason Weed, MD[a], Kristen Lo Sicco, MD[a],
Jo-Ann Latkowski, MD[a,b],*

KEYWORDS

- Cutaneous T cell lymphoma • Mycosis fungoides • CTCL treatment • Overview • Histology
- Clinical correlations

KEY POINTS

- Cutaneous T cell lymphoma (CTCL) represents a heterogeneous group of extranodal non-Hodgkin lymphomas in which monoclonal T lymphocytes infiltrate the skin.
- This article provides an overview of CTCL epidemiology, pathogenesis, diagnosis, subtypes, and therapeutic approaches.
- A strong grasp of our current understanding of CTCL can enable dermatologists to correlate clinical presentation and clinical behavior with the spectrum of histologic, immunophenotypic, and genetic components of each CTCL subtype, thereby playing a key role in diagnosis and treatment.
- A wide variety of treatment modalities including topical, systemic, phototherapy, radiation, chemotherapy, photopheresis, and biologics are available for CTCL.
- Because of a relatively low incidence and significant chronicity of disease, as well as the high morbidity of some therapeutic regimens, further clinical trials are warranted to better define the ideal treatment option for each subtype of CTCL.

INTRODUCTION

Cutaneous T cell lymphoma (CTCL) represents a heterogeneous group of extranodal non-Hodgkin lymphomas in which monoclonal T lymphocytes infiltrate the skin.[1–3] CTCL demonstrates a high degree of variance in clinical presentation and course, histology, immunotyping, and prognosis.[4] Characterized by a wide variety of findings both clinical and histologic, CTCL often demonstrates skin localization, avoidance of bone marrow, and infiltration of perifollicular T cell zones of lymph nodes and the spleen. These specific findings reflect the migratory pathway of cutaneous T cells and underscore the importance of clonal T cell populations in the disease pathogenesis.[5] Subtypes of CTCL include mycosis fungoides (MF), Sézary syndrome, cutaneous γ/δ T cell lymphoma, and primary cutaneous peripheral T cell lymphoma not otherwise specified (PCTCL-NOS).[6] This article provides an overview of CTCL epidemiology, pathogenesis, diagnosis, subtypes, and management and treatment approaches.

The classification schema of CTCL arose from an understanding that many types of cutaneous B cell lymphoma (CBCL) and CTCL may present as primarily cutaneous processes without any evidence of extracutaneous involvement at initial

---

Disclosure Statement: No disclosures to be made.
[a] The Ronald O. Perelman Department of Dermatology, 240 East 38th Street, 11th Floor, New York, New York 10016, USA; [b] New York Harbor VA Healthcare System, Dermatology Residency Training Program
* Corresponding author.
E-mail address: Jo-Ann.Latkowski@nyulangone.org

Dermatol Clin 37 (2019) 455–469
https://doi.org/10.1016/j.det.2019.05.007

diagnosis. Such primary cutaneous lymphomas were found to present, progress, and respond to treatment in entirely different fashions than their nodal counterparts. Each entity's particular morphologic, immunologic, genetic, and clinical characteristics necessitated the delineation of different subtypes, resulting in the development of the European Organization for Research and Treatment of Cancer (EORTC) classification system, as well as that of the World Health Organization (WHO).[7] The development of these classification systems enabled dermatologists to correlate clinical presentation and clinical behavior with the unique histologic, immunophenotypic, and genetic components of each condition, thereby playing a key role in diagnosis and treatment.

EPIDEMIOLOGY

The annual incidence of CTCL is roughly 0.5 in 100,000, with a median age of 55 to 60 years and a male predominance of 2.0:1 to 1.6:1.[8] The frequency and typical course of each subtype of CTCL is presented in **Table 1**. The incidence of CTCL increased sharply between 1973 and 2002, representing 3.4% of all non-Hodgkin lymphomas.[9] Subsequently, incidence stabilized through 2013.[10] MF is the most common subtype of CTCL, constituting approximately 44% of all cutaneous lymphomas.[11]

PATHOGENESIS

Since the first description of MF more than 200 years ago, a wide range of processes have been investigated as potential drivers of CTCL; modern proposals have included chronic antigen stimulation, infectious processes such as endogenous or exogenous oncogenic viruses, reactivation of RAG1/RAG2 endonuclease activity instrumental in T cell receptor somatic V(D)J recombination, and ultraviolet (UV) irradiation.[12] Thus far no definitive cause has been identified, although recent studies have characterized the genetic and functional changes in malignant cells and their environment in greater detail than previously was possible.

Gene-sequencing studies have revealed a complex landscape of mutations with a preponderance of copy-number alterations in commonly affected genes, including canonical oncogenes and tumor suppressors, genes involved in chromatin structure and epigenetic modulation, and genes closely tied to T cell maturation and activation. UV-mutation signatures have also been identified among point mutations.[13]

Cell-transcriptional profiles have demonstrated dysregulation of factors in many central signaling pathways including BRAF, COX-2, FOXP2, GATA-3, IL2, JAK-3/STAT, MTAP, MAPK1, NFκB, PTEN, and many others.[14–19] A full list can be found in **Table 2**. Cytokine profiles have

Table 1
Cutaneous T cell lymphoma subtypes

WHO-EORTC Classification	No. of Cases	Frequency (%)	Typical Disease Course
Mycosis fungoides (MF)	800	54	Indolent
Sézary syndrome	52	4	Aggressive
Folliculotropic MF	86	6	Indolent
Pagetoid reticulosis	14	<1	Indolent
Granulomatous slack skin	4	<1	Indolent
Primary cutaneous anaplastic large cell lymphoma	146	10	Indolent
Lymphomatoid papulosis	236	16	Indolent
Subcutaneous panniculitis-like T cell lymphoma	18	1	Indolent
Primary cutaneous CD4+ small/medium pleomorphic T cell lymphoma	39	3	Indolent
Primary cutaneous natural killer (NK)/T cell lymphoma, nasal type	7	0	Aggressive
Primary cutaneous aggressive CD8+ T cell lymphoma	14	1	Aggressive
Primary cutaneous γ/δ T cell lymphoma	13	1	Aggressive
Primary cutaneous peripheral T cell lymphoma, unspecified	47	3	Aggressive

Adapted from Willemze, R., Jaffe, E. S., Burg, G., Cerroni, L., Berti, E., Swerdlow, S. H.,... & Grange, F. (2005). WHO-EORTC classification for cutaneous lymphomas. Blood, 105(10), 3768–85.

Table 2
Mutations and expression abnormalities in cutaneous T cell lymphoma

Frequently Mutated Genes[13,20,21]	Function
TP53, PTEN, BRAF, MYC, RB1, CDKN2A, FAS	Cell cycling, apoptosis
ARID1A, DNMT3A, CTCF, ATM	Chromatin modification, DNA repair
ZEB1, NFKB2, PLCG1, STAT3, CD28, JAK2	T cell development and function

Genes with Aberrant Expression Profiles[22,23]	Function
TOX, BCL11A, SATB1, CD40, GATA3, JUNB, STAT4	T cell differentiation
NFKB-2, FYB, LCK, KIR3DL2, PTPRCAP	T cell activation or signaling
CCR4, SATB1, EPHA4, DNM3, PLS3	Cell migration, homing
BCL2, MCL1, STAT3, TWIST1, FAS	Apoptosis evasion

demonstrated T helper cell type 2 (Th2) skewing, raising concern for decreased Th1-mediated antitumor immune activity. Surface expression profile studies have suggested that separate memory T cell subpopulations may develop into distinct subtypes of CTCL. In this paradigm, MF may be a neoplasm of skin resident memory cells (CCR4+, CLA+, L-selectin−, CD27−, CCR7−), whereas leukemic CTCL such as Sézary syndrome may arise from central memory T cells (CCR4+, CLA+/−, L-selectin+, CD27+, CCR7+).[24]

Studies focused on specific genetic and functional changes underscore the diverse spectrum of cellular mechanisms harnessed by malignant cells to survive and proliferate. Dysregulation of the JAK-3/STAT and NFκB pathways may lead to chronic activation of T cells driving a proliferative response. Dysfunction of the negative regulators of the JAK-3/STAT pathway, such as SOCS3 and protein tyrosine phosphatase SHP1, may also play a role in CTCL pathogenesis.[25] In tumor-stage MF, the antitumor agent interleukin (IL)-12 is downregulated whereas expression of IL-9, regulated by STAT3, is increased.[26] The NOTCH family of transmembrane receptors enable cell differentiation and proliferation, and these may contribute to the pathogenesis of Sézary syndrome.[16] Aberrant cytokine signaling, including IL-2, IL-4, IL-7, IL-15, and IL-21, may enable the development or further the progression of CTCL.[25] Upregulation of chemokine receptors, such as CCR6 and CCR7, is purported to contribute to malignant T cell infiltration of lymph nodes, peripheral blood vessels, and viscera.[15,27] The chemokine CXCL12 is expressed on the endothelial and stromal cells of many organs, and can act on most CD34+ progenitor cells and CD4+ T cells to induce chemotaxis, invasion, angiogenesis, and proliferation, contributing to the pathogenesis of MF specifically.[28] Across the subtypes of CTCL, dysfunction of the T cell receptor (TCR) pathway has been shown to contribute to resistance to tumor-suppressive mechanisms, such as the FAS cell-surface death receptor for apoptosis and growth suppression via transforming growth factor β.[20,29,30]

Multiple entities have been investigated for diagnostic and prognostic implications. The transcription factor TOX plays a role in the development of CD4+ T cells; overexpression of TOX and its products has been associated with more advanced disease in MF, progression of disease, and a poorer prognosis.[17] In Sézary syndrome, peripheral blood and cutaneous lesions also demonstrate aberrant TOX expression.[17] MicroRNA (miRNA) expression also has been investigated in CTCL; miR-21 and miR-155 correlate with a poor prognosis and aggressive disease course by decreasing apoptotic mechanisms and increasing malignant proliferation.[8] These miRNAs may be a result of dysfunctional JAK-3/STAT pathways.[25]

Certain exposures or chronic cutaneous inflammation have been associated with the subsequent development of CTCL. Although the exact mechanism is not fully understood, chronic stimulation of T lymphocytes may result in eventual T cell clonality and malignant transformation.[31] The possible role of viral infection in CTCL development remains poorly elucidated. Although infection with human T cell leukemia/lymphotropic virus type 1 (HTLV-1) is not associated with MF, it has been strongly associated with development of adult T cell leukemia/lymphoma, an aggressive noncutaneous T cell malignancy.[32,33]

DIAGNOSIS

The wide variety of clinical presentations and complex diagnostic criteria can make CTCL a challenging diagnosis, in many cases leading to a delay of years from onset until diagnosis.[8,34] Guidelines for the diagnosis of CTCL have been developed internationally by groups including the International Society for Cutaneous Lymphomas (ISCL), the cutaneous lymphoma task force of the EORTC, and the National Comprehensive Cancer Network (NCCN).

Clinical suspicion of a diagnosis of CTCL should be supported by characteristic skin findings on physical examination. MF typically presents as erythematous patches or plaques with fine scaling and wrinkling on non–sun-exposed areas including the buttocks, axillae, and trunk as well as the extremities. Further evaluation of suspected CTCL should be made through biopsy and analysis via dermatopathology, immunophenotyping, and TCR gene-rearrangement analysis.[4,35] If early patch stage MF is suspected, a broad shave biopsy from untreated skin lesion should be performed. For plaques or tumors, punch biopsy is preferred. Treatment with topical corticosteroids or phototherapy may alter the histology and delay accurate diagnosis.[4] However, even early initial biopsies may not provide a definitive diagnosis as several subtypes of CTCL can be preceded by cutaneous lesions that take years to progress to overt lymphoma on histologic examination. Likewise, morphologic and phenotypic characteristics of CTCL demonstrate high variability and may not be visible on any one biopsy alone. Thus, repeat biopsies over the course of treatment are justified and recommended.[36]

Typical laboratory analysis comprises flow cytometry and TCR studies of tissue or blood, as well as lactate dehydrogenase (LDH), complete blood count, and complete metabolic profile. Analysis of peripheral blood for the presence of malignant cells may assist in the diagnosis of Sézary syndrome, but has limited diagnostic utility because of low sensitivity.[37] LDH can provide valuable information regarding tumor burden because high values correlate with a poorer prognosis.[35]

The clinician may also use immunophenotyping to distinguish among cutaneous neoplasms and within CTCL subtypes. Levels of CD3 and markers of major T cell subtypes CD4 and CD8 strongly influence the differential. For MF, decreased levels of pan–T cell markers CD2, CD5, and CD7 may be seen.[38,39] CD30 expression is characteristically positive in multiple variants of CTCL including subtypes of lymphomatoid papulosis and primary cutaneous anaplastic large cell lymphoma, and may be positive in a subset of MF and other patients. A wide variety of specialized stains, including CD25, CD56, TIA1, and granzyme B, among others, are routinely used as evidence for or against specific subtypes.[40] For blood samples, flow-cytometric evidence of loss of CD7 and/or CD26 expression among CD4$^+$ T cells supporting specified thresholds of greater than 40% and 30%, respectively, is consistent with blood involvement, as is CD4/CD8 ratio $\geq$10.[41] Flow cytometry should not represent the sole diagnostic

tool for CTCL, although it can supplement clinical and histologic examination and aid evaluation of leukemic burden during treatment.[42]

TCR gene rearrangement likewise provides valuable diagnostic information regarding the clonality of possible lymphomas. Polymerase chain reaction analysis can identify clonality in many patients, and high-throughput TCR sequencing may provide higher specificity and sensitivity in detection. However, detection of clonal T cell populations is not sufficient to make a diagnosis. Although clonal populations may be found in the cutaneous lesions, lymph nodes, and peripheral blood of patients with CTCL, clonality is also common to many benign dermatoses, such as pityriasis lichenoides et varioliformis acuta, lichen planus, chronic pigmented purpura, lichen sclerosis, and pseudolymphomas.[43] Atypical T cell infiltrates may also be present in reactive conditions, such as lymphomatoid drug eruptions.[44] Thus, the presence of a clonal T cell population without consistent clinical and histopathologic findings cannot be used to make a definitive diagnosis of CTCL.

Further diagnostic utility can be gained via MRI or contrast-enhanced computed tomography (CT). These studies enable determination of systemic or lymph node involvement, while fluorine-18 fluorodeoxyglucose PET-CT provides higher sensitivity and specificity to locate cutaneous or extracutaneous disease manifestations.[45] Imaging is recommended in any patient with stage $\geq$T2 (patches and/or plaques covering $\geq$10% body surface area), large cell transformation, folliculotropic MF, adenopathy on examination, or abnormal laboratory evaluation.[46]

CUTANEOUS T CELL LYMPHOMA SUBTYPES: MANAGEMENT AND TREATMENT APPROACHES

A wide variety of treatments modalities including topical, systemic, phototherapy, radiation, chemotherapy, photopheresis, and biologics are available for CTCL (Table 3).[8] Treatment goals include symptom relief, induction of remission, and halting disease progression, while simultaneously balancing the numerous side effects of various treatment approaches. More aggressive systemic regimens in early-stage disease have not been shown to provide any greater survival benefit, but rather may be associated with higher complication rates and morbidity.[67]

Management of CTCL requires accurate staging to determine the best therapeutic option.[8,68] For disease involving less than 20% of body surface area or of stage IA to IIA, skin-directed therapies

Table 3
Clinical highlights for subtypes of cutaneous T cell lymphoma

WHO-EORTC Classification	Clinical	Pathology	Workup	Treatment	Prognosis
Mycosis fungoides (MF)	Patches, plaques, or tumors. Erythematous to hyperpigmented polymorphic patches with epidermal atrophy (wrinkling) in non–sun-exposed areas is classic	Superficial band-like or lichenoid infiltrates, atypical lymphocytes with cerebriform nuclei, Pautrier microabscesses, dermal infiltrates[4]	PE, sequential skin biopsies, CBC, CMP, LDH, serum chemistries. May require flow cytometry of peripheral blood, TCR, or PET-CT	Skin-targeted therapy (corticosteroids, cytotoxic agents, phototherapy, radiotherapy), systemic chemotherapy, biological response modifiers, targeted MAB therapies including alemtuzumab, brentuximab, mogamulizumab	Depends on stage. Limited patch/plaque stage has similar life expectancy as general population. Prognosis is poorer for patients with lymph nodes or visceral involvement, or large cell transformation
Sézary syndrome	Pruritic erythroderma with exfoliation, edema, and lichenification. Lymphadenopathy, alopecia, onychodystrophy, and palmoplantar hyperkeratosis[4,7] Difficult to clinically distinguish Sézary from non-neoplastic erythroderma	Frequently nonspecific skin biopsy findings; may show monotonous cellular infiltrations with epidermotropism. Lymph nodes with dense infiltrate of Sézary cells and effacement of lymph node architecture	PE, sequential skin biopsies, CBC, CMP, LDH, serum chemistries, flow cytometry of peripheral blood, TCR, or PET-CT	Skin-directed therapies are adjuvant. Necessitates systemic treatment, including oral bexarotene, extracorporeal photopheresis, HDAC inhibitors, targeted monoclonal antibodies, chemotherapy including CHOP, bone marrow transplant	Poor. Overall 5-y survival is 25%. Death from opportunistic infections in setting of immunosuppression

(continued on next page)

Table 3
(continued)

WHO-EORTC Classification	Clinical	Pathology	Workup	Treatment	Prognosis
Folliculotropic MF	Follicular papules, acneiform lesions, indurated plaques, most often in head/neck area. Infiltrated plaques in eyebrow region with alopecia is highly characteristic	Perivascular and periadnexal localization of dermal infiltrates. Infiltration of T cells with cerebriform nuclei and sparing of epidermis, follicular mucinosis	Clinicopathologic correlation to differentiate from other types of MF/CTCL. Regular monitoring to assess for advancement. 68% show severe pruritus, 71% show alopecia[47]	Because of perifollicular localization of infiltrates, this entity is less responsive to skin-targeted treatment. Use oral retinoids	Sustained remission rarely achieved. Overall survival is poor. Early-stage disease shows 10-y survival of 82%, 15-y survival of 41%[47]
Pagetoid reticulosis	Solitary psoriasiform or hyperkeratotic patch/plaque, typically on extremity, slowly progressive[7]	Hyperplastic epidermis with marked infiltration of atypical pagetoid cells, hyperchromatic and cerebriform nuclei. Superficial dermis with infiltrate of small lymphocytes	Clinicopathologic correlation to differentiate from other types of CTCL	Radiotherapy, surgical excision, topical steroids, nitrogen mustard, PUVA, NB-UVB[48]	Life expectancy similar to that of matched general population. Associated morbidities of superinfection, pain, and functional impairment[48]
Granulomatous slack skin	Pendulous lax skin in axillae and groin. Associated classic MF. Indolent clinical course	Dense granulomatous dermal infiltrates with atypical T cells with cerebriform nuclei. Destruction of elastic tissue. Epidermal infiltration[49]	Clinicopathologic correlation to differentiate from other types of CTCL. Development of bulky skin folds[49]	Radiotherapy or surgical excision. Possible response to mechlorethamine, but no definitive therapy has been established[50]	Rapid recurrence after excision. Sustained remission rarely achieved. Development of second lymphoid neoplasia in 48% of patients[51]

	Clinical features	Histopathology	Diagnosis	Treatment	Prognosis
Primary cutaneous anaplastic large cell lymphoma	Solitary or localized nodules, tumors, or thick plaques with ulceration. Frequent cutaneous relapse[7]	Diffuse nonepidermotropic infiltrates with sheets of anaplastic CD30+ tumor cells. Reactive lymphocytes at periphery of tumor	Clinicopathologic correlation to differentiate from other forms of CTCL or secondary cutaneous involvement by nodal Hodgkin lymphoma. Complete excision or 4-mm incisional biopsy for histologic evaluation[52]	Radiotherapy or surgical excision for solitary tumor, chemotherapy for multifocal disease.[52] No further treatment is necessary after surgical excision or spontaneous resolution	Favorable. 5-y survival rates between 76% and 96%.[53] 10-y survival rate >85%.[4] Involvement of regional lymph node not associated with worse prognosis.[54] 39% with skin-limited relapse and 13% with extracutaneous spread[55]
Subcutaneous panniculitis-like T cell lymphoma	Self-healing subcutaneous nodules and plaques on extremities more often than trunk, typically indolent course. May be associated with serosal effusions, hemophagocytosis syndrome, and pancytopenia.[56] Rare dissemination to extracutaneous sites	Panniculitis-like subcutaneous infiltrate, with neoplastic T cells and macrophages. Epidermis and dermis not involved. Necrosis, karyorrhexis, and cytophagocytosis are common[4]	Clinicopathologic correlation to differentiate from other types of CTCL. Differential includes angiocentric T cell lymphoma[56]	Systemic chemotherapy or radiotherapy[56]	Favorable prognosis. 5-y survival rate is approximately 80%[4]
Primary cutaneous CD4+ small/medium pleomorphic T cell lymphoma	Solitary plaque or tumor, on face, neck, or upper trunk[57]	Dense, diffuse, or nodular dermal and subcutis infiltrates. Focal epidermotropism. Reactive lymphocytes and histiocytes observed	Differentiation from MF and reactive granulomatous conditions based on clinical course and presentation.[58] Demonstration of T cell clone and loss of pan–T cell antigens[59]	Surgical excision or radiotherapy for solitary skin lesions. Cyclophosphamide or IFN-α for generalized disease	Favorable prognosis, especially with solitary tumor or lesions localized to skin[4]

(continued on next page)

Table 3
(continued)

WHO-EORTC Classification	Clinical	Pathology	Workup	Treatment	Prognosis
Primary cutaneous NK/T cell lymphoma, nasal type	Multiple plaques or tumors on trunk and extremities. For nasal type, patients have midfacial destructive tumor, commonly ulcerated.[60] Aggressive clinical course	EBV-positive lymphoma with NK cell dense infiltrates of dermis, fat, and deeper tissues. Angiocentricity and angiodestruction	Clinicopathologic correlation to differentiate from other types of CTCL	Systemic chemotherapy. Pursue aggressive therapy at an early stage of disease. Anthracycline- or doxorubicin-based chemotherapy is ineffective as primary treatment[60]	Poor prognosis. Low treatment efficacy. Progression is common. Poor predictive factors age >60, advanced stage, presence of constitutional symptoms, bone marrow involvement[60]
Primary cutaneous aggressive CD8+ T cell lymphoma	Localized or disseminated eruptive papules, nodules, and tumors with central ulceration and necrosis. Preponderance for elderly male patients[61]	Epidermotropic infiltrates of T cells. Acanthotic or atrophic epidermis with necrotic keratinocytes, spongiosis, and ulceration. Adnexal structure destruction. Angiocentricity and angioinvasion[61]	Differentiation from other subtypes based on clinical course and presentation. Unlike MF, does not typically progress from patch to plaque to tumor[61]	Multiagent systemic chemotherapy. Skin-directed therapies or radiotherapy is usually ineffective.[62] Allogenic or autologous stem cell transplantation may be considered[63]	Aggressive clinical course. Poor prognosis. Average 5-y survival of 18%[61]

	Clinical features	Histology	Differentiation	Treatment	Prognosis
Primary cutaneous γ/δ T cell lymphoma	Disseminated plaques or ulceronecrotic nodules on the extremities. Mucosa and extranodal sites commonly involved, whereas lymph nodes, spleen, and bone marrow usually spared[64]	Epidermotropism and subcutaneous involvement. Medium to large neoplastic cells with clumped chromatin. Angiocentricity and angiodestruction are common[4,64]	Differentiation from MF or pagetoid reticulosis based on clinical course and presentation. Differentiate from subcutaneous panniculitis-like T cell lymphoma based on expression of TCR α/β^+ phenotype[64]	Few treatment options. Poor response to multiagent chemotherapy. Consider hematopoietic stem cell transplantation[64]	Aggressive and rapidly fatal disease. Resistant to multiagent chemotherapy. Subcutaneous fat involvement suggests poorer prognosis. 5-y survival rate of 33%, median survival of 15 mo[64]
Primary cutaneous peripheral T cell lymphoma, unspecified	Describes types of CTCL not consistent with previously described subtypes. Patients present with solitary or localized nodules or tumors, no specific sites of predilection[7,46]	Nodular or diffuse infiltrates with pleomorphic or immunoblast-like T cells. Little to no epidermotropism[65]	Differentiation from MF based on clinical course and presentation	Systemic chemotherapy, for example, doxorubicin-based multiagent therapy[65]	Poor prognosis, disease specific 5-y survival rate 16%[7,65]

Abbreviations: CBC, complete blood count; CHOP, cyclophosphamide, doxorubicin, vincristine, and prednisone; CMP, complete metabolic panel; EBV, Epstein-Barr virus; HDAC, histone deacetylase; IFN, interferon; LDH, lactate dehydrogenase; MAB, monoclonal antibody; MF, mycosis fungoides; NB-UVB, narrow-band ultraviolet B; PE, physical examination; PUVA, psoralen plus ultraviolet A; TCR, T cell receptor.
Data from Refs.[4,6,7,66]

are often optimal. For cases with advanced stages or refractory cases in early stages, systemic therapies should be used.[4]

Because of the high risk of infection in CTCL patients with poor skin-barrier function, caution should be exercised with multidrug regimens.[69] Use of emollients can decrease transepidermal water loss at the stratum corneum and minimize disruption of the skin barrier. Glycerin is a humectant that can decrease corneocyte loss from superficial epidermis and maintain the lipid profile to improve skin-barrier repair and minimize symptoms of pruritus and scale.[70]

Both topical and systemic corticosteroids have shown high efficacy in treatment, yet often ultimately result in relapse of disease.[8,71] Corticosteroids function as anti-inflammatory and antiproliferative agents by activating intracytoplasmic glucocorticoid receptors and decreasing production of interleukins, interferon (IFN)-γ, tumor necrosis factor (TNF), and granulocyte-monocyte colony-stimulating factor.[72] Such effects reduce mitotic activity and promote apoptosis of malignant cell populations.[73] However, these agents are accompanied by significant side effects, including atrophy, hypopigmentation, striae, acneiform eruptions, and purpura.[72,74] Topical clobetasol 0.05% is typically recommended for early-stage CTCL lesions.

Retinoids have also demonstrated therapeutic utility via the antiproliferative and proapoptotic effects of the retinoic acid receptor β2 tumor-suppressor gene.[75] The retinoid bexarotene (Targretin) is approved by the Food and Drug Administration (FDA) for the treatment of MF. Its functions include activating caspase-3, promoting apoptosis, and activating p53, a tumor-suppressor protein.[76,77] Other effects include decreased production of matrix metalloproteinases and vascular endothelial and epidermal growth factors, and increased production of gap junctions, which are typically lost in malignant transformation.[77,78] Ultimately, both topical and systemic retinoids function in CTCL treatment to promote normal cellular differentiation across the epithelium and decrease rates of carcinogenesis.[79] A 1% bexarotene gel applied up to 4 times per day can be used for early CTCL.[71] Reversible, dose-dependent side effects of oral bexarotene include severe mixed hyperlipidemia and central hypothyroidism.[80] Retinoids such as acitretin, isotretinoin, and tazarotene may also be used.[66]

Topical chemotherapeutic agents such as mechlorethamine can be effective therapies against early-stage CTCL while imposing significant side-effect profiles and offering dubious efficacy for advanced cases.[81] Mechlorethamine is an alkylating agent that inhibits proliferating cells and modulates the interactions between T cells and keratinocytes. In addition to typical chemotherapeutic side effects, patients may experience increased risk of nonmelanoma skin cancers when treated concurrently with phototherapy, radiation, or immunosuppressive chemotherapy.[81]

The toll-like receptor 7 (TLR7) agonist imiquimod is an effective treatment option for MF, and is recommended by the NCCN guidelines. Imiquimod functions via the production of IFN-α, TNF-α, IL-1α, IL-6, and IL-8, and leads to cellular apoptosis. Side effects include predominantly cutaneous reactions of erythema, pruritus, dysesthesias, ulceration, and bleeding.[71]

Various phototherapies and laser therapies such as narrow-band ultraviolet B (NB-UVB) and excimer laser are efficacious in inducing remission or halting progression of MF.[31,66] Studies demonstrate that NB-UVB is an effective first-line treatment for early-stage MF, with a minimal side-effect profile.[31,82] Clinical response rates are found to be 54% to 75% for NB-UVB in patients with MF, and although this effect can be prolonged with maintenance therapy every 2 to 4 weeks, many patients relapse after cessation of therapy.[83,84] More advanced-stage disease often necessitates the combination of UV therapy with other biological response modifiers such as IFN-α to achieve a more favorable patient outcome.[4] Although the mechanism of action of NB-UVB has not been clearly elucidated, therapy with UVB decreases the antigen-presenting capacity of Langerhans cells and increases production of IL-2, IL-6, and TNF-α, thereby suppressing functionality of neoplastic T cells in the skin and upregulating immune response.[84]

A variety of systemic therapies exist, within which are a range of mechanistic modalities. For refractory early-stage or more advanced MF, initial systemic treatment options to add to skin-directed therapy include extracorporeal photopheresis, methotrexate, or an oral retinoid such as bexarotene.

Biological response modifiers, such as the cytokine IFN-α, can be used in MF as well,[68] but are not advised in the setting of primary cutaneous peripheral T cell lymphoma not otherwise specified (PCTCL-NOS).[85] These therapies potentiate the host immune response to neoplastic T cells.[4] IFN-α is administered as 3 to 9 million units 3 times per week, and induces flu-like symptoms, hair loss, nausea, and bone marrow suppression.[4] Monotherapy with IFN-α can achieve response rates of 50% and complete remission rates of 17%.[86] Recombinant IL-12 can also induce cellular immunity and increase the responsiveness of cytotoxic T cells as a means to treat CTCL.[87]

Histone deacetylase inhibitors (HDACIs) are antineoplastic agents that preferentially target transformed cells over normal cells.[81] By promoting expression of proapoptotic genes, altering the structural integrity of chromatin, increasing the production of reactive oxygen species, and decreasing the stability of the mitochondrial membrane, HDACIs provide a novel therapy for CTCL management.[81] FDA-approved agents for progressive or recurrent CTCLs include vorinostat and romidepsin.[88] Response rates range from 30% to 35% as monotherapy, but complete remission has only been observed in 2% to 6% of cases.[81] HDACIs are fairly well tolerated but fatigue, gastrointestinal discomfort, neutropenia, anemia, and dehydration have all been reported.[8]

Traditional chemotherapeutic regimens such as CHOP (cyclophosphamide, doxorubicin, vincristine, and prednisone) have demonstrated variable efficacy in advanced CTCL.[69] Because of its high associated morbidity, systemic chemotherapeutic regimens such as CHOP should be reserved only for patients with lymph node or visceral involvement, or those with progressive skin-based diseases refractory to other treatment modalities.

Radiotherapy and electron-beam therapy for local lesions or the entire body surface area (total skin electron-beam irradiation) represents an appropriate treatment modality for advanced cases, especially those with skin-limited MF.[8,69] Response rates for CTCL cutaneous plaques can be as high as 98.3%, whereas the response rates of CTCL tumors are only 36%.[89] Side effects are relatively mild, including erythema and scale, with transient loss of hair, nails, and sweat-gland function.[4] The addition of aminolevulinic acid to photodynamic therapy aids in the expression of apoptotic receptors, such as FAS, to induce cell death. The combination of methotrexate with this treatment modality increases the overall efficacy by inhibiting the inactivation of the FAS promoter.[90]

Allogeneic stem cell transplantation has been shown to be highly efficacious for the treatment of CTCL, providing a sustained immune-mediated graft-versus-lymphoma effect.[11] Although morbidity and mortality after this therapy is relatively high, possibly given the advanced age of CTCL patients and the immunosuppression typical of the disease and its treatment, stem cell transplantation can provide long-term remission in a subset of patients.[91] However, this effect may be limited in patients with a large burden of disease or refractory disease with multiple relapses.[11]

Finally, several targeted treatment modalities offer additional options. Brentuximab, a CD30-targeted monoclonal antibody (mAb), has demonstrated efficacy in CD30$^+$ CTCL.[92] Alemtuzumab, an anti-CD52 mAb, has shown efficacy for CTCL with blood involvement.[93] Mogamulizumab has activity against the CC chemokine receptor (CCR4) universally overexpressed in the lesions of CTCL. Further studies are investigating the potential role of checkpoint inhibitors and targeted small molecules such as Bcl-2 and BET inhibitors.

PROGNOSIS

Mortality rates for CTCL range from 10% to 15% up to 43%. Poorer outcomes are associated with more advanced stages of MF, whereas patients with stages IA to IIA have more favorable prognoses.[94] Progression of the disease can occur via malignant infiltration of T cells into lymph nodes, peripheral blood vessels, and viscera. The resultant tumor stage of the disease occurs in ~5% of CTCL cases.[8] **Box 1** lists prognostic factors for CTCL. Involvement of viscera has been associated with increased severity of skin lesions and a resulting increased risk of skin infection.[8] Cases of death caused by MF demonstrate malignant infiltration of the viscera in 70% to 90% of cases.[96,97]

Box 1
Prognostic factors in CTCL

Factors strongly associated with worse prognosis in advanced MF/Sézary syndrome[8,95]

Age greater than 60

Folliculotropism

WBC count

LDH

Large cell transformation

Stage

Blood involvement

Other possible prognostic factors[4,6,8]

DNA mutation profile

RNA expression profile

CD30 staining

Ki-67 staining

TOX staining

Data from Scarisbrick, J. J., Prince, H. M., Vermeer, M. H., Quaglino, P., Horwitz, S., Porcu, P.,... & Foss, F. (2015). Cutaneous Lymphoma International Consortium study of outcome in advanced stages of mycosis fungoides and Sézary syndrome: effect of specific prognostic markers on survival and development of a prognostic model. Journal of Clinical Oncology, 33(32), 3766.

In early stages of CTCL, such as limited patch/plaque, no difference in life expectancy from that of the general population has been shown. However, in progressed disease life expectancy decreases by 3.2 to 9.9 years.[8,96] Because CTCL displays a chronic course, most affected patients die from other causes, and 25% die from lymphoma.[31] Other causes of death include secondary malignancy, immunosuppression, and resulting opportunistic infections.[81]

SUMMARY

The great variety in clinical presentation and course, histologic appearance, immunogenetics, and therapeutic options makes CTCLs a challenging entity to diagnose and treat. While many subtypes exist, the grouping of these diseases under the unified heading of CTCL has enabled dermatologists to better select treatment modalities and improve patient outcomes. Although many treatments can successfully induce remission in a majority of patients, disease may recur after treatment cessation. Because of relatively low incidence and significant chronicity of disease, as well as the high morbidity of some therapeutic regimens, further clinical trials are warranted to better define the ideal treatment option for each subtype of CTCL.

REFERENCES

1. National Comprehensive Cancer Network. Primary cutaneous CD30+ T cell lymphoproliferative disorders (version 1.2015). Available at: http://www.nccn.org/professionals/physician_gls/pdf/bone.pdf. Accessed February 6, 2014.
2. Kaminetzky D, Hymes KB. Denileukin diftitox for the treatment of cutaneous T-cell lymphoma. Biologics 2008;2(4):717.
3. Duvic M, Evans M, Wang C. Mogamulizumab for the treatment of cutaneous T-cell lymphoma: recent advances and clinical potential. Ther Adv Hematol 2016;7(3):171–4.
4. Bolognia J, Cerroni L, Schaffer J. Dermatology. 4th edition. Philadelphia: Elsevier Saunders; 2018.
5. Edelson RL. Cutaneous T cell lymphoma. Ann N Y Acad Sci 2001;941(1):1–11.
6. Bagherani N, Smoller BR. An overview of cutaneous T cell lymphomas. F1000Res 2016;5. https://doi.org/10.12688/f1000research.8829.1.
7. Willemze R, Kerl H, Sterry W, et al. EORTC classification for primary cutaneous lymphomas. A proposal from the Cutaneous Lymphoma Study Group of the European Organization for Research and Treatment of Cancer (EORTC). Blood 2005; 105(10):3768–85.
8. Rodd AL, Ververis K, Karagiannis TC. Current and emerging therapeutics for cutaneous T-cell lymphoma: histone deacetylase inhibitors. Lymphoma 2012;2012:1–10.
9. Criscione VD, Weinstock MA. Incidence of cutaneous T-cell lymphoma in the United States, 1973-2002. Arch Dermatol 2007;143(7):854–9.
10. Korgavkar K, Xiong M, Weinstock M. Changing incidence trends of cutaneous T-cell lymphoma. JAMA Dermatol 2013;149(11):1295–9.
11. Lansigan F, Choi J, Foss FM. Cutaneous T-cell lymphoma. Hematol Oncol Clin North Am 2008;22(5):979–96.
12. Fava P, Bergallo M, Astrua C, et al. Human endogenous retrovirus expression in primary cutaneous T-cell lymphomas. Dermatology 2016;232(1):38–43.
13. McGirt LY, Jia P, Baerenwald DA, et al. Whole genome sequencing reveals oncogenic mutations in mycosis fungoides. Blood 2015;126(4):508–19.
14. Litvinov IV, Netchiporouk E, Cordeiro B, et al. Ectopic expression of embryonic stem cell and other developmental genes in cutaneous T-cell lymphoma. Oncoimmunology 2014;3(11):e970025.
15. Lauenborg B, Christensen L, Ralfkiaer U, et al. Malignant T cells express lymphotoxin α and drive endothelial activation in cutaneous T cell lymphoma. Oncotarget 2015;6(17):15235.
16. Hameetman L, van der Fits L, Zoutman WH, et al. EPHA4 is overexpressed but not functionally active in Sézary syndrome. Oncotarget 2015;6(31):31868–76.
17. Dulmage BO, Akilov O, Vu JR, et al. Dysregulation of the TOX-RUNX3 pathway in cutaneous T-cell lymphoma. Oncotarget 2015. https://doi.org/10.18632/oncotarget.5742.
18. Katona TM, Smoller BR, Webb AL, et al. Expression of PTEN in mycosis fungoides and correlation with loss of heterozygosity. Am J Dermatopathol 2013; 35(5):555–60.
19. Katona TM, O'malley DP, Cheng L, et al. Loss of heterozygosity analysis identifies genetic abnormalities in mycosis fungoides and specific loci associated with disease progression. Am J Surg Pathol 2007; 31(10):1552–6.
20. Choi J, Goh G, Walradt T, et al. Genomic landscape of cutaneous T cell lymphoma. Nat Genet 2015; 47(9):1011.
21. da Silva Almeida AC, Abate F, Khiabanian H, et al. The mutational landscape of cutaneous T cell lymphoma and Sézary syndrome. Nat Genet 2015; 47(12):1465.
22. Dulmage BO, Geskin LJ. Lessons learned from gene expression profiling of cutaneous T-cell lymphoma. Br J Dermatol 2013;169(6):1188–97.
23. Litvinov IV, Netchiporouk E, Cordeiro B, et al. The use of transcriptional profiling to improve personalized diagnosis and management of cutaneous

T-cell lymphoma (CTCL). Clin Cancer Res 2015; 21(12):2820–9.

24. Campbell JJ, Clark RA, Watanabe R, et al. Sezary syndrome and MF arise from distinct T cell subsets: a biologic rationale for their distinct clinical behaviors. Blood 2010;116(5):767–71.

25. Sibbesen NA, Kopp KL, Litvinov IV, et al. Jak3, STAT3, and STAT5 inhibit expression of miR-22, a novel tumor suppressor microRNA, in cutaneous T-Cell lymphoma. Oncotarget 2015;6(24):20555.

26. Vieyra-Garcia PA, Wei T, Naym DG, et al. STAT3/5 dependent IL-9 overexpression contributes to neoplastic cell survival in mycosis fungoides. Clin Cancer Res 2016;22(13):3328–39.

27. Ikeda S, Kitadate A, Ito M, et al. Disruption of CCL20-CCR6 interaction inhibits metastasis of advanced cutaneous T-cell lymphoma. Oncotarget 2016;7(12):13563.

28. Maj J, Jankowska-Konsur AM, Hałoń A, et al. Expression of CXCR4 and CXCL12 and their correlations to the cell proliferation and angiogenesis in mycosis fungoides. Postepy Dermatol Alergol 2015;32(6):437.

29. Lebas E, Libon F, Nikkels AF. Koebner phenomenon and mycosis fungoides. Case Rep Dermatol 2015; 7(3):287–91.

30. Willerslev-Olsen A, Krejsgaard T, Lindahl LM, et al. Staphylococcus aureus enterotoxin A (SEA) stimulates STAT3 activation and IL-17 expression in cutaneous T-cell lymphoma. Blood 2016;127(10): 1287–96.

31. Eklund Y, Aronsson A, Schmidtchen A, et al. Mycosis fungoides: a retrospective study of 44 Swedish cases. Acta Derm Venereol 2016;96(5): 669–74.

32. Nahidi Y, Meibodi NT, Ghazvini K, et al. Evaluation of the association between Epstein-Barr virus and mycosis fungoides. Indian J Dermatol 2015;60(3): 321.

33. Whittaker SJ, Luzzatto L. HTLV-1 provirus and mycosis fungoides. Science 1993;259(5100):1470.

34. Kirsch IR, Watanabe R, O'malley JT, et al. TCR sequencing facilitates diagnosis and identifies mature T cells as the cell of origin in CTCL. Sci Transl Med 2015;7(308):308ra158.

35. Benjamin Chase A, Markel K, Tawa MC. Optimizing care and compliance for the treatment of mycosis fungoides cutaneous T-cell lymphoma with mechlorethamine gel. Clin J Oncol Nurs 2015;19(6):E131–9.

36. Smoller BR, Bishop K, Glusac E, et al. Reassessment of histologic parameters in the diagnosis of mycosis fungoides. Am J Surg Pathol 1995;19(12): 1423–30.

37. Gibson JF, Huang J, Liu KJ, et al. Cutaneous T-cell lymphoma (CTCL): current practices in blood assessment and the utility of T-cell receptor (TCR)-

38. Ralfkiaer E. Controversies and discussion on early diagnosis of cutaneous T-cell lymphoma: phenotyping. Dermatol Clin 1994;12:329–34.

39. Moll M, Reinhold U, Kukel S, et al. CD7-negative helper T cells accumulate in inflammatory skin lesions. J Invest Dermatol 1994;102:328–32.

40. DiCaudo D. Chapter 24. Cutaneous T-cell lymphoma, NK-cell lymphoma, and myeloid leukemia. In: Elston D, editor. Dermatopathology. Philadelphia (PA): Elsevier; 2018.

41. National Comprehensive Care Network. NCCN clinical practice guidelines in oncology: non-Hodgkin's lymphomas 2015. Available at: https://www.clfoundation.org/sites/default/files/2017-08/NCCN Guidelinesmfss2015.pdf.

42. Aggarwal S, Topaloglu H, Kumar S. Systematic review of burden of cutaneous T-cell lymphoma. Value Health 2015;18(7):A438.

43. Lukowski A, Muche JM, Sterry W, et al. Detection of expanded T-cell clones in skin biopsy samples of patients with lichen sclerosus et atrophicus by T-cell receptor-gamma polymerase chain reaction assays. J Invest Dermatol 2000;115:254–9.

44. Rijlaarsdam JU, Scheffer E, Meijer CJLM, et al. Cutaneous pseudo-T-cell lymphomas. A clinicopathologic study of 20 patients. Cancer 1992;69:717–24.

45. Alanteri E, Usmani S, Marafi F, et al. The role of fluorine-18 fluorodeoxyglucose positron emission tomography in patients with mycosis fungoides. Indian J Nucl Med 2015;30(3):199.

46. Bekkenk MW, Vermeer MH, Jansen PM, et al. Peripheral T-cell lymphomas unspecified presenting in the skin: analysis of prognostic factors in a group of 82 patients. Blood 2003;102:2213–9.

47. Gerami P, Rosen S, Kuzel T, et al. Folliculotropic mycosis fungoides: an aggressive variant of cutaneous T-cell lymphoma. Arch Dermatol 2008; 144(6):738–46.

48. Lee J, Viakhireva N, Cesca C, et al. Clinicopathologic features and treatment outcomes in Woringer-Kolopp disease. J Am Acad Dermatol 2008;59(4): 706–12.

49. Kempf W, Ostheeren-Michaelis S, Paulli M, et al. Granulomatous mycosis fungoides and granulomatous slack skin: a multicenter study of the Cutaneous Lymphoma Histopathology Task Force Group of the European Organization For Research and Treatment of Cancer (EORTC). Arch Dermatol 2008;144(12): 1609–17.

50. Hultgren TL, Jones D, Duvic M. Topical nitrogen mustard for the treatment of granulomatous slack skin. Am J Clin Dermatol 2007;8(1):51–4.

51. Clarijs M, Poot F, Laka A, et al. Granulomatous slack skin: treatment with extensive surgery and review of the literature. Dermatology 2003;206(4):393–7.

38. Vβ chain restriction. J Am Acad Dermatol 2016; 74(5):870–7.

52. Kempf W, Pfaltz K, Vermeer MH, et al. EORTC, ISCL, and USCLC consensus recommendations for the treatment of primary cutaneous CD30-positive lymphoproliferative disorders: lymphomatoid papulosis and primary cutaneous anaplastic large-cell lymphoma. Blood 2011;118(15):4024–35.

53. Benner MF, Willemze R. Applicability and prognostic value of the new TNM classification system in 135 patients with primary cutaneous anaplastic large cell lymphoma. Arch Dermatol 2009;145(12): 1399–404.

54. Bekkenk MW, Geelen FA, van Voorst Vader PC, et al. Primary and secondary cutaneous CD30(+) lymphoproliferative disorders: a report from the Dutch Cutaneous Lymphoma Group on the long-term follow-up data of 219 patients and guidelines for diagnosis and treatment. Blood 2000;95(12):3653–61.

55. Liu HL, Hoppe RT, Kohler S, et al. CD30+ cutaneous lymphoproliferative disorders: the Stanford experience in lymphomatoid papulosis and primary cutaneous anaplastic large cell lymphoma. J Am Acad Dermatol 2003;49(6):1049–58.

56. Jaffe ES. Subcutaneous panniculitis-like T cell lymphoma. In: Mason DY, Harris NL, editors. Human lymphoma: clinical implications of the REAL classification. London: Springer; 1999. p. 197–200.

57. Çetinözman F, Jansen PM, Willemze R. Expression of programmed death-1 in primary cutaneous CD4-positive small/medium-sized pleomorphic T-cell lymphoma, cutaneous pseudo-T-cell lymphoma, and other types of cutaneous T-cell lymphoma. Am J Surg Pathol 2012;36(1):109–16.

58. Beltraminelli H, Leinweber B, Kerl H, et al. Primary cutaneous CD4+ small-/medium-sized pleomorphic T-cell lymphoma: a cutaneous nodular proliferation of pleomorphic T lymphocytes of undetermined significance? A study of 136 cases. Am J Dermatopathol 2009;31(4):317–22.

59. Bakels V, van Oostveen JW, van der Putte SC, et al. Immunophenotyping and gene rearrangement analysis provide additional criteria to differentiate between cutaneous T-cell lymphomas and pseudo-T-cell lymphomas. Am J Pathol 1997;150:1941–9.

60. Lee J, Kim WS, Park YH, et al. Nasal-type NK/T cell lymphoma: clinical features and treatment outcome. Br J Cancer 2005;92(7):1226.

61. Nofal A, Abdel-Mawla MY, Assaf M, et al. Primary cutaneous aggressive epidermotropic CD8+ T-cell lymphoma: proposed diagnostic criteria and therapeutic evaluation. J Am Acad Dermatol 2012;67(4): 748–59.

62. Gormley RH, Hess SD, Anand D, et al. Primary cutaneous aggressive epidermotropic CD8+ T-cell lymphoma. J Am Acad Dermatol 2010;62(2):300–7.

63. Kimby E. Management of advanced-stage peripheral T-cell lymphomas. Curr Hematol Malig Rep 2007;2(4):242–8.

64. Kempf W. Primary cutaneous γ/δ T-cell lymphoma. In: Rongioletti F, Margaritescu I, Smoller BR, editors. Rare malignant skin tumors. New York: Springer; 2015. p. 295–7.

65. Ryan AJA, Robson A, Hayes BD, et al. Primary cutaneous peripheral T-cell lymphoma, unspecified with an indolent clinical course: a distinct peripheral T-cell lymphoma? Clin Exp Dermatol Clin Dermatol 2010;35(8):892–6.

66. Olsen EA, Hodak E, Anderson T, et al. Guidelines for phototherapy of mycosis fungoides and Sézary syndrome: a consensus statement of the United States Cutaneous Lymphoma Consortium. J Am Acad Dermatol 2016;74(1):27–58.

67. Kaye FJ, Bunn PA, Steinberg SM, et al. A randomized trial comparing combination electron-beam radiation and chemotherapy with topical therapy in the initial treatment of mycosis fungoides. N Engl J Med 1989;321:1784–90.

68. Scarisbrick JJ, Prince HM, Vermeer MH, et al. Cutaneous Lymphoma International Consortium study of outcome in advanced stages of mycosis fungoides and Sézary syndrome: effect of specific prognostic markers on survival and development of a prognostic model. J Clin Oncol 2015;33(32):3766.

69. Chmielowska E, Studziński M, Giebel S, et al. Follow-up of patients with mycosis fungoides after interferon α2b treatment failure. Postepy Dermatol Alergol 2015;32(2):67.

70. Rawlings A, Harding C, Watkinson A, et al. The effect of glycerol and humidity on desmosome degradation in stratum corneum. Arch Dermatol Res 1995; 287:457–64.

71. Nguyen CV, Bohjanen KA. Skin-directed therapies in cutaneous T-cell lymphoma. Dermatol Clin 2015; 33(4):683–96.

72. Del Rosso JQ, Cash K. Topical corticosteroid application and the structural and functional integrity of the epidermal barrier. J Clin Aesthet Dermatol 2013;6(11):20.

73. Schwartzman RA, Cidlowski JA. Glucocorticoid-induced apoptosis of lymphoid cells. Int Arch Allergy Immunol 1994;105:347–54.

74. Zackheim HS. Treatment of patch-stage mycosis fungoides with topical corticosteroids. Dermatol Ther 2003;16(4):283–7.

75. Huen AO, Kim EJ. The role of systemic retinoids in the treatment of cutaneous T-cell lymphoma. Dermatol Clin 2015;33(4):715–29.

76. Marciano DP, Kuruvilla DS, Pascal BD, et al. Identification of Bexarotene as a PPAR Antagonist with HDX. PPAR Res 2015;2015:254560.

77. Burg G, Dummer R. Historical perspective on the use of retinoids in cutaneous T-cell lymphoma (CTCL). Clin Lymphoma 2000;1:S41–4.

78. Heller EH, Shiffman NJ. Synthetic retinoids in dermatology. Can Med Assoc J 1985;132:1129–36.

79. Lippman SM, Kavanagh JJ, Paredes-Espinoza M, et al. 13-cis-retinoic acid plus interferon-2a: highly active systemic therapy for squamous cell carcinoma of the cervix. J Natl Cancer Inst 1992;84: 241–5.

80. Suarez SR, Andreu EP, Grijalvo OM, et al. Thyroid and lipidic dysfunction associated with bexarotene in cutaneous T-cell lymphoma. Med Clin (Barc) 2016;146(3):117–20.

81. Moyal L, Feldbaum N, Goldfeiz N, et al. The therapeutic potential of AN-7, a novel histone deacetylase inhibitor, for treatment of mycosis fungoides/Sézary syndrome alone or with doxorubicin. PLoS One 2016;11(1):e0146115.

82. Gathers RC, Scherschun L, Malick F, et al. Narrowband UVB phototherapy for early-stage mycosis fungoides. J Am Acad Dermatol 2002;47(2):191–7.

83. Querfield C, Rosen ST, Kuzel TM, et al. Long-term follow-up of patients with early-stage cutaneous T-cell lymphoma who achieved complete remission with psoralen plus UV-A monotherapy. Arch Dermatol 2005;141:305–11.

84. Gökdemir G, Barutcuoğlu B, Sakız D, et al. Narrowband UVB phototherapy for early-stage mycosis fungoides: evaluation of clinical and histopathological changes. J Eur Acad Dermatol Venereol 2006; 20(7):804–9.

85. Aderhold K, Carpenter L, Brown K, et al. Primary cutaneous peripheral T-cell lymphoma not otherwise specified: a rapidly progressive variant of cutaneous T-cell lymphoma. Case Rep Oncol Med 2015;2015: 429068.

86. Olsen EA, Bunn PA. Interferon in the treatment of cutaneous T-cell lymphoma. Hematol Oncol Clin North Am 1995;9:1089–97.

87. Rook AH, Gelfand JM, Wysocka M. Topical resiquimod can induce disease regression and enhance T-cell effector functions in cutaneous T-cell lymphoma (vol 126, pg 1452, 2015). Blood 2015; 126(25):2765.

88. Zinzani PL, Bonthapally V, Huebner D, et al. Panoptic clinical review of the current and future treatment of relapsed/refractory T-cell lymphomas: cutaneous T-cell lymphomas. Crit Rev Oncol Hematol 2016;99:228–40.

89. Ahmed SK, Grams MP, Locher SE, et al. Adaptation of the Stanford technique for treatment of bulky cutaneous T-cell lymphoma of the head. Pract Radiat Oncol 2016;6(3):183–6.

90. Salva KA, Wood GS. Epigenetically Enhanced Photodynamic Therapy (ePDT) is superior to conventional photodynamic therapy for inducing apoptosis in cutaneous T-cell lymphoma. Photochem Photobiol 2015;91(6):1444–51.

91. Herbert KE, Spencer A, Grigg A, et al. Graft-versus-lymphoma effect in refractory cutaneous T-cell lymphoma after reduced-intensity HLA-matched sibling allogeneic stem cell transplantation. Bone Marrow Transplant 2004;34(6):521.

92. Duvic M, Tetzlaff MT, Gangar P, et al. Results of a phase II trial of brentuximab vedotin for CD30+ cutaneous T-cell lymphoma and lymphomatoid papulosis. J Clin Oncol 2015;33(32):3759.

93. de Masson A, Guitera P, Brice P, et al. Long-term efficacy and safety of alemtuzumab in advanced primary cutaneous T-cell lymphomas. Br J Dermatol 2014;170(3):720–4.

94. Zackheim HS, Amin S, Kashani-Sabet M, et al. Prognosis in cutaneous T-cell lymphoma by skin stage: long-term survival in 489 patients. J Am Acad Dermatol 1999;40:418–25.

95. Benton EC, Crichton S, Talpur R, et al. A cutaneous lymphoma international prognostic index (CLIPi) for mycosis fungoides and Sezary syndrome. Eur J Cancer 2013;49(13):2859–68.

96. Gomez Venegas AA, Vargas Rubio RD. Unusual involvement in mycosis fungoides: duodenal papilla. Rev Esp Enferm Dig 2015;10.

97. Tensen CP. PLCG1 gene mutations in cutaneous T-cell lymphomas revisited. J Invest Dermatol 2015;135(9):2153–4.

Lymphomatoid Papulosis and Other Lymphoma-Like Diseases

Adrian Moy, MS[a,1], James Sun, MD[b,1], Sophia Ma, MD[a], Lucia Seminario-Vidal, MD, PhD[a,*]

KEYWORDS

- Pityriasis lichenoides et varioliformis acuta • Pityriasis lichenoides chronica
- CD30 lymphoproliferative disorder • Lymphomatoid papulosis • Anaplastic large cell lymphoma

KEY POINTS

- Pityriasis lichenoides is represented by 2 subtypes, pityriasis lichenoides et varioliformis acuta and pityriasis lichenoides chronica, representing the acute and chronic presentations of the disease. They can be distinguished based on morphology and histopathology, but treatment options share many similarities.
- Lymphomatoid papulosis is characterized by crops of papulonodular lesions and currently has no known 100% effective treatment.
- Primary cutaneous anaplastic large cell lymphoma needs to be differentiated from systemic anaplastic large cell lymphoma, and is best treated by surgical excision or radiation therapy.

PITYRIASIS LICHENOIDES

Epidemiology

Pityriasis lichenoides (PL) is an inflammatory dermatitis first described in 1894 by Neisser and Jadassohn.[1] It was initially categorized as a parapsoriasis, but it is currently recognized as its own disorder, typically classified into 2 main variants.[1] The acute variant of PL is known as pityriasis lichenoides et varioliformis acuta (PLEVA), and the chronic variant is known as pityriasis lichenoides chronica (PLC) (Fig. 1). Many dermatologists consider PL a spectrum, with PLEVA on 1 end and PLC on the opposite. Both PLEVA and PLC are difficult to diagnose and categorize, and are sometimes indistinguishable between each other.[2] To date, no prevalence or incidence rate has been reported for the general population. No predispositions have been published, and cases have been reported in many ethnic groups across geographic boundaries without discrimination.[3–6] PLC is relatively more common than PLEVA and is more likely to affect children.[2,7] Zang and colleagues[8] found that black patients are more likely to be affected by PLC (53%) than PLEVA (9%), whereas Caucasian patients are more likely be have PLEVA (71% to 25%).

PLEVA is most commonly seen in patients in the second or third decade of life, but both children and adults can be affected by the disorder. Reported cases have an age range from as young as 1 year old and up to 90 years old.[3,9,10] It is considered a benign disease and will generally resolve on its own, but the timeline can vary

Conflicts of Interest: The authors have no conflicts to disclose.
[a] Department of Dermatology and Cutaneous Surgery, University of South Florida Morsani College of Medicine, 12901 Bruce B. Downs Boulevard, Tampa, FL 33612, USA; [b] Department of Cutaneous Oncology, Moffitt Cancer Center, 10920 McKinley Drive, Tampa, FL 33612, USA
[1] These authors contributed equally to this work.
* Corresponding author.
E-mail address: luciasem@health.usf.edu

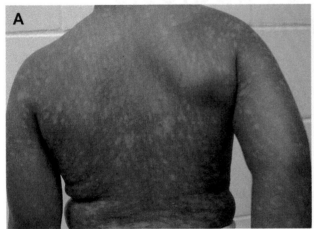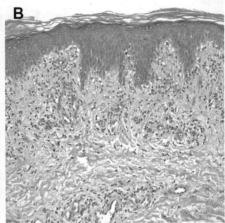

Fig. 1. Pityriasis lichenoides chronica. (*A*) Scaly hypopigmented macules on trunk. (*B*) Epidermal parakeratosis, lichenoid inflammation with necrotic keratinocytes, along with dermal edema and lymphohistiocytic perivascular inflammatory infiltrate (hematoxylin and eosin, magnification 200X).

between weeks and years. A more severe subtype of PLEVA known as febrile ulceronecrotic Mucha-Habermann disease (FUMHD) has had 11 reported fatalities, with only 1 of the reported cases occurring in a child.[11,12]

Pathophysiology

The pathogenesis of PL is not fully understood, and there are 3 major pathogenic theories. The first theory points to an antigenic etiologic trigger. Epstein-Barr virus (EBV), toxoplasma gondii, and human immunodeficiency virus (HIV) have all been associated with cases of PLEVA.[3] In these cases, patients generally present with the initial infection, followed by acute onset of PLEVA. The list of reported antigenic triggers continues to grow, with cases of PLEVA reportedly being induced by the measles, mumps, and rubella (MMR) vaccine; the influenza vaccine; and human herpesviruses.[13–17] The exact relationship between these antigenic agents and PLEVA is not known, and there is speculation that it may actually be PLEVA-induced immune dysregulation that raises susceptibility to these infections.[2] In addition to the reported infectious agents that may cause PLEVA, drugs have been associated with PLC.[18]

The second theory is a T-cell dyscrasia causing an inflammatory response. The combined work of Wood and colleagues[19,20] and Magro and colleagues[21,22] suggests that the lesions of PLEVA and PLC fall under the lymphoproliferative disorders regardless of detectable atypical clonal T cells, and the regression or progression of a case of PLEVA is attributed to the host immune response. PLC has been reported to evolve into mycosis fungoides,[23,24] supporting this theory.

The third theory describes an immune complex-mediated hypersensitivity vasculitis. Clayton and Haffenden[25] showed 16 patients with immunoglobulin depositions in lesion biopsies. Additionally, circulating immune complexes were detected in 8 patients; most were immunoglobulin M (IgM)-positive at either the dermo-epidermal junction or vessel wall. The authors suggest that the immune complex may deposit in the skin, leading to PL. Although other studies supporting this theory exist, not all investigators have been able to show a relationship between immune complexes and PL.

Recently, Karouni and colleagues[26] showed that plasmacytoid dendritic cells contribute to the inflammatory infiltrate in PL through the production of type I interferons, suggesting a new mechanism of pathogenesis. This was shown in both PLEVA and PLC, and is a process shared by other skin disorders that present with an interface dermatitis.

Clinicopathological Presentation and Differential Diagnoses

PLEVA and PLC are regarded as the 2 opposite ends of the PL spectrum. A patient with PL may present with both PLEVA-type and PLC-type lesions; thus, most clinical and pathologic findings apply to both conditions.[3] PLEVA is characterized by sudden onset of erythematous macules that progress into papules with a fine micaceous scale. The micaceous scale will thicken, often becoming unattached at the periphery. The papule commonly presents with a central vesiculopustular point, often with a hemorrhagic adherent crust and varioliform scars. The papule may become ulcerated and form a red-brown crust.[2,3,6] PLC may present synchronously or after PLEVA subsides.

PLC lesions can be distinguished from PLEVA by their slower development of small, dim, erythematous or brownish maculopapules with lack of epidermal necrosis.[6] Up to 90% of PLC patients may present with parakeratotic scales attached centrally, which leave a shiny pink or brown surface after removal.[3,8] Although rare, systemic symptoms such as pruritus and fever may occur in PL.[9]

Hyper- and hypopigmentation are common in both PLEVA and PLC.[27] The lesions are 2 to 3 mm in diameter and most commonly found on the trunk, extremities, and flexural areas, but they may present on any area of the skin. Lesions may stay in affected areas, as the eruptions often present at all stages of lesion development.[2,28]

Patients with PLEVA report burning and pruritus associated with the papules. Systemic symptoms are rare, but malaise, fever, lymphadenopathies, and arthritis have all been reported.[3]

Histologically, PL is characterized by a lichenoid inflammation with necrotic keratinocytes, epidermal parakeratosis, along with dermal edema and lymphohistiocytic perivascular inflammatory infiltrate. In PLEVA, the denser dermal infiltrates extend deep into the reticular dermis and are commonly wedge-shaped. Lymphocytes are usually CD8+, but may also be CD4+; the epidermis is predominantly CD8+.[3] Blood vessels may also become affected by the inflammatory cells, including perivascular neutrophils, resulting in leukocytoclastic vasculitis and fibrinoid necrosis.[2] Histology of PLC shows a more superficial and sparse CD4+ T-cell dominant lymphocytic perivascular infiltrate. Occasional keratinocytic dyskeratosis and basilar vacuolar change can be identified. Hemorrhage, neutrophilic infiltrate, spongiosis, and vesicle formation are rarely seen.[2]

The differential diagnosis is broad, and disorders such as varicella zoster, guttate psoriasis, Gianotti-Crosti syndrome, lichen planus, and pityriasis rosea can all present similarly to PL. It is also important to rule out generalized arthropod bite reaction, drug or viral exanthemas, polymorphous light reaction, cutaneous small-vessel vasculitis, secondary syphilis, and folliculitis.[2,3,29] The condition most commonly confused with PLEVA is lymphomatoid papulosis (LyP), a CD30+ lymphoproliferative disorder.[30] Although these 2 diseases have lesions that may share some characteristics, it is uncommon to find CD30+ atypical cells in PL.[28]

Work-Up

Clinical examination and a thorough history are the primary methods of diagnosing PL, and a full work-up is necessary to exclude other conditions.

Laboratory tests include complete blood cell count (CBC) and serology for HIV, EBV, cytomegalovirus, herpes simplex virus, and *Toxoplasmosis*.[2,3,28]

Treatment

Because of the unpredictable nature of the disease and the high rate of spontaneous remission, there are currently no standard guidelines for the treatment of PL. The disease course often resolves on its own within weeks but may persist for years. Many modalities have been employed to treat PL, and often multiple modalities are combined.[3]

Many consider oral antibiotics to be the first-line treatment. Tetracycline, erythromycin, and azithromycin have been shown to be effective in the treatment of PL, along with the antiviral acyclovir.[28] When treating PL with any of these antibiotics, it is important to gradually taper down the treatment to prevent recurrence. Topical corticosteroids may also be used as a first-line therapy, or in conjunction with oral antibiotics. They are most useful in relieving inflammation and pruritus and do not affect the disease course.[9] Simon and colleagues[31] reported a case in which PL resolved with topical tacrolimus, although insufficient evidence is available.

Phototherapy is also an effective therapy that is well tolerated.[3] UVB is safe for pediatric populations, and nb-UVB has been shown to have the lowest recurrence rate. Some studies have suggested that phototherapy is more effective for children with PLC than systemic treatments.[32] Fernandez-Guarino and colleagues[33] showed a positive outcome in patients with PLC treated with photodynamic therapy, but the mechanism behind its efficacy is unknown.

In severe cases of PL, methotrexate, acitretin, dapsone, or cyclosporine may be used.[34] FUMHD is potentially fatal, and thus its treatment differs slightly from that of PLEVA. Again, no consensus has been made on the most effective therapy. However, a review of cases by Nofal and colleagues[11] suggested that methotrexate is an effective therapy that limited immunosuppression, thus reducing the risk of secondary infection.

CD30+ LYMPHOPROLIFERATIVE DISEASES

Cutaneous CD30+ lymphoproliferative diseases (CD30+ LPDs) account for approximately 30% of all primary cutaneous T-cell lymphomas. CD30+ LPDs are a spectrum of disease linked by the expression of CD30 by tumor cells. The spectrum of CD30+ LPD includes lymphomatoid papulosis (LyP), primary cutaneous anaplastic large-cell lymphoma (pcALCL) and other types of

CTCL that may express CD30 antigen, and reactive infiltrates that contain CD30-positive cells.

CD30+ LPDs have a benign clinical course that belies their malignant histologic features. These diseases are difficult to differentiate histologically, and familiarity and understanding of their clinical course are required to distinguish them from more malignant systemic diseases. Recent advances in immunotherapy have identified CD30 as a therapeutic target with promising implications in the treatment of these diseases.

LYMPHOMATOID PAPULOSIS
Epidemiology

Lymphomatoid papulosis (LyP) is a rare disease first described by Macaulay in 1968 (**Fig. 2**).[35] Worldwide incidence is estimated at 1.2 to 1.9 cases per 1,000,000 population.[36] Men are more frequently affected, but there is no ethnic predisposition. The peak incidence is in the fifth decade, and its 5-year survival rate is nearly 100%.[36–38]

Although LyP has a positive prognosis,[38,39] there is a 5% to 30% risk of secondary malignancies. One study observed 52% incidence of secondary malignancy.[36] Mycosis fungoides and anaplastic large cell lymphoma are the most commonly associated secondary malignancies.[39] Male sex,[36,38] older age, and presence of a T-cell clone in LyP lesions[40] are risk factors associated with risk of secondary malignancy. Subtypes of LyP were thought to have no association with prognosis; however, Wieser and colleagues have observed a higher incidence of secondary malignancy with type B and C LyP, and lesser incidence with type A and D[36] (**Table 1**).

Pathophysiology

The pathogenesis of LyP is not fully understood, athough it is hypothesized that CD30 overexpression is implicated. CD30 and CD30 ligand (CD30L) interaction are thought to cause CD30+ neoplastic cells to undergo apoptosis.[41] Resistance to CD30L-mediated growth inhibition may be the cause of tumor progression. It has also been suggested that LyP may be triggered by herpes outbreak, with improvement upon concurrent treatment with acyclovir.[36]

Clinicopathological Presentation and Differential Diagnoses

LyP is characterized by recurrent red-to-violaceous crops of papulonodular skin lesions that spontaneously regress after weeks to months.[38,42,43] These lesions usually present at various stages of healing because of the recurrent nature of the disease. They can measure up to 20 mm, although they typically are 3 to 10 mm in diameter and often appear on the trunk or extremities.[38] Oral involvement and mucosal involvement are uncommon. About half of all patients are asymptomatic, while the other half experience pruritis and/or pain from ulcerating lesions.[38] LyP is not associated with systemic symptoms. Ulcerated lesions often leave hypo- or hyperpigmented varioliform scars. Type E (angioinvasive) LyP is more likely to develop large ulcers. The patient may present with a highly variable number of lesions at a time, from just a few to hundreds. The duration of disease is also variable, lasting from weeks to many years. The hallmark feature of LyP is self-healing lesions, which are required to make the diagnosis. Currently, the World Health Organization (WHO) classification[44] recognizes 5 histologic types of LyP, and 1 type with a specific chromosome 6p25.3 rearrangement (**Table 1**).[43] None of the subtypes has prognostic or therapeutic significance, and multiple types may coexist in a single patient.

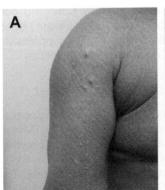
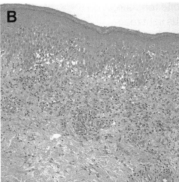
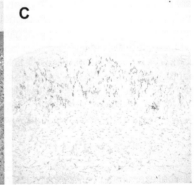

Fig. 2. Lymphomatoid papulosis. (*A*) Numerous violaceous cropped papules on arm. (*B*) Epidermotropic infiltrate of small-to-medium atypical cells with cerebriform nuclei (*C*) positive for CD30 positive (magnification 200X).

Table 1
Lymphomatoid papulosis subtypes

Subtype	Histologic Features	Phenotype	Major Histopathological Differential Diagnoses
Type A	Wedge-shaped infiltrate Large atypical CD30+ lymphocytes scattered or arranged in small clusters Mixed background of numerous inflammatory cells (histiocytes, eosinophils, neutrophils)	Primarily CD4+	• Hodgkin lymphoma • Transformed mycosis fungoides
Type B	Epidermotropic infiltrate of small- to medium-sized lymphocytes CD30 variably expressed	CD4+ (CD30 variable)	• Mycosis fungoides
Type C	Cohesive sheets of large atypical CD30+ lymphocytes Few inflammatory cells	CD4+ > CD8+	• Anaplastic large-cell lymphoma • HTLV1-associated lymphoma
Type D	Epidermotropic infiltrate of small-to-medium atypical CD8+ and CD30+ lymphocytes.	CD8+ (100%)	• Aggressive epidermotropic CD8+ cytotoxic T-cell lymphoma
Type E	Angioinvasive infiltrates of atypical CD30+ lymphocytes Hemorrhage, extensive necrosis, and ulceration	CD8+ (70%)	• NK/T-cell lymphoma • Gamma/delta lymphoma
6p25.3 rearrangement	Prominent epidermotropism overlying dense dermal infiltrates of small-to-medium CD30+ lymphocytes		• Pagetoid reticulosis

Type A is the most common histologic type, accounting for 75% of all LyP biopsies.[43] It is characterized by a wedge-shaped dermal infiltrate of mixed inflammatory cells, with scattered mostly single cells of medium-to-large size and pleomorphic and anaplastic CD30+ T cells. Type B has epidermotropic infiltrate of small-to-medium atypical cells with cerebriform nuclei that may be CD30 positive or negative, and resemble early mycosis fungoides. Type C demonstrates a nodular infiltrate of large atypical CD30+ cells with few background inflammatory cells, akin to cutaneous anaplastic large-cell lymphoma (ALCL).[45] Types D and E were recently described and are more likely to be mistaken for aggressive lymphomas.[43] Type D is also epidermotropic, with upward pagetoid spread of atypical CD8+ and CD30+ small- to medium-sized lymphocytes. These features lend to its similarity to primary cutaneous aggressive epidermotropic CD8+ cytotoxic T-cell lymphoma. Finally, LyP type E is unique with angioinvasive features.[46] Histologically, there are angiodestructive infiltrates of

medium-sized atypical lymphocytes. Hemorrhagic necrosis and prominent ulceration are often found because of vascular damage and occlusion.

Karai and colleagues[47] recently discovered a rare form of LyP with a specific chromosome rearrangement on 6p25.3 involving the *DUSP22-IRF4* locus. This variant presents with localized lesions and epidermotropism, which resembles pagetoid reticulosis over a background of dense dermal infiltrate of small- to medium-sized CD30+ lymphocytes.

Rare variants of LyP include acral and regional forms, where lesions are limited to a region of the body.[48] Persistent agminated LyP (PALP) presents with papular, spontaneously regressing lesions with concurrent mycosis fungoides-like patches. Other rare variants of LyP have been described, such as follicular, syringotropic, granulomatous, and spindle cell.[49] Follicular LyP presents with pustular lesions that resemble folliculitis[50] and are characterized by perifollicular infiltrates with CD30+ cells and folliculotropism of CD30+ atypical lymphocytes. Follicular LyP has recently been proposed as type F to highlight the importance of recognizing follicular involvement.[36,50]

Lymphoid cells of LyP display the phenotype of an activated T helper cell, expressing CD3, CD4, CD30, CD45RO, HLA-DR, and CD25.[48,51] The most common observed phenotype is CD45RO+ and CD4+. All types of LyP lymphocytes express CD30 except type B, where expression is variable.[48] Variable loss of pan-T cell antigens (CD2, CD3, CD5, and CD7) has been observed, with CD7 being most commonly absent. CD8+ phenotypes are more common in the pediatric population. Most lymphocytes express cytotoxic molecules including TIA-1 and granzyme B. CD15, a marker for Hodgkin lymphoma, is usually absent. The markers anaplastic lymphoma kinase protein (ALK-1), epithelial membrane antigen (EMA), and CD56 are suggestive of systemic lymphoma, and are usually absent. It is important to note that the phenotype of atypical lymphocytes does not affect prognosis.[48,51]

Data regarding T cell clonality is controversial. Most lymphocytes express α/β T cell receptor (TCR), but γ/δ TCR has been found, particularly in LyP type D. Steinhoff and colleagues[52] have demonstrated monoclonality in CD30+ cells, while CD30-lymphocytes were polyclonal, supporting the observation that LyP represents a monoclonal T-cell disorder. However, Gellrich and colleagues[53] have identified large, atypical, polyclonal CD30+ cells supporting a heterogenous tumor cell line. Further investigation is required to elucidate the role of T-cell clonality in LyP.

Diagnosis cannot be made by pathology alone. Histologic appearance can vary broadly and suggests malignant disease. It is important to distinguish CD30+ PCTLD from other cutaneous CD30+ disorders involving skin, which include systemic ALCL, ATLL, PTCL, MF (transformed MF), and benign disorders, including lymphomatoid drug reactions, arthropod bites, viral infections, folliculitis, PLEVA, and PLC. Lymphomatoid drug reactions have been documented with amlodipine, carbamazepine, cefuroxime, and valsartan, associated with CD30+ atypical large cells on histology. Coexpression of CD30 and CD15 in T cell lymphomas may be mistaken for classical Hodgkin lymphoma.[48]

Work-Up

The diagnosis of LyP is primarily based on the characteristic clinical presentation of self-limited papulonodular lesions, absence of lymphadenopathy, in the setting of appropriate histologic findings. A complete work-up, including CBC, CMP, and LDH, is essential to rule out other malignancies that present similarly to LyP.[42] Biopsy of suspicious lesions should be performed with immunohistochemistry to confirm diagnosis. It is important to differentiate LyP from secondary skin involvement of systemic ALCL (Table 2). It is also important to identify immunodeficiencies in the setting of CD30+ LPD, which carry a worse prognosis[38,42].

Treatment

LyP is not a malignant disorder and has an excellent prognosis. There is no cure for the disease, nor has treatment been proven to alter its course or prevent secondary malignancy. Thus, in patients with mild disease with few lesions that are small without extensive scarring or ulceration, observation is appropriate.[37,48] When treatment is offered, it is typically for symptomatic relief and to accelerate the regression of lesions. A study by the Dutch Cutaneous Lymphoma Group found that topical steroids and phototherapy are the most common first-line treatments (56% and 35%, respectively, of 118 patients).[37] CR and PR were common; however, neither treatment led to a sustained CR. Another study, a retrospective, multicenter study of 252 patients also confirmed the same first-line treatments (35% and 14% of 252 patients).[54] They reported a CR rate of 48%. Overall, estimated median disease-free survival (DFS) was 11 months, and phototherapy resulted in longer DFS (23 months, $P<.03$). Type A LyP treated with other treatment than phototherapy was associated with increased risk of early relapse. Some institutions also offer acyclovir and valacyclovir in patients with virus exposure. In patients with oral herpes, concomitant antiviral therapy was found to reduce the severity and number of lesions.[36]

Systemic therapy is only used for patients with severely symptomatic disease, stigmatizing lesions, severe pruritus, and numerous active lesions. Low-dose methotrexate is the most commonly used agent.[55] Although methotrexate is effective in suppressing lesions, retrospective studies have found a 63% relapse rate. Vonderheid and colleagues[56] examined 45 patients with LyP; 87% of patients responded to methotrexate treatment at a low dose (10 to 25 mg weekly). The median duration of treatment was greater than 39 months. After discontinuation of treatment, 25% of patients remained relapse free during a follow-up period of 24 to 227 months. Another study by the Dutch Cutaneous Lymphoma Group found that doses as low as 7.5 to 10 mg weekly were sufficient to control disease.[57] In both studies, a small number of patients progressed to systemic lymphoma, a known secondary malignancy associated with LyP, but also a known adverse effect of methotrexate therapy. Otherwise, methotrexate has been found to be safe and effective, although the disease often recurs after discontinuation of treatment. Multiagent chemotherapy was also evaluated by the Dutch Cutaneous Lymphoma Group.[37] Multiagent chemotherapy leads to resolution of lesions; however, they quickly recur, during or after treatment.

Anti-CD30 therapy is the latest development in LyP therapy, reserved for severe disease. SGN-30 (Seattle Genetics, Bothell, Washington) is a murine monoclonal antibody to CD30. Phase 2 data published by Duvic and colleagues[58] demonstrated CR or PR in 70% of 23 patients with CD30+ LPD, including LyP. Only 3 patients were diagnosed with primary LyP; each patient developed long-lasting remission. One patient was in remission for over 3 years. Brentuximab vedotin (SGN-35, Seattle Genetics) is an anti-CD30 antibody-drug conjugate composed of monomethyl auristatin E, a cytotoxic antitubulin agent, covalently bonded to chimeric monoclonal anti-CD30 antibody.[43] It is currently approved for treatment of Hodgkin lymphoma, systemic ALCL, and CD30+ cutaneous ALCL and MF with prior systemic therapy.[43] The ALCANZA trial[59] compared brentuximab vedotin to standard treatments of methotrexate or bexarotene. Treatment with brentuximab had 43.8% (95% CI 29.1–58.4) absolute improvement in ORR4 in 56.3% (36 of 64 patients) versus 12.5% (8 of 64 patients) compared with methotrexate or bexarotene treatments. Secondary endpoints also showed improvement, including patients who achieved CR and improved symptom burden. Although this study did not specifically examine brentuximab therapy for LyP, it demonstrated improved benefit for all CD30+ LPDs.

A phase 2 clinical trial[60] demonstrated 100% ORR of pcALCL and LyP patients after treatment with brentuximab. The most common dose-limiting adverse effects were peripheral neuropathy and fatigue. These findings were also corroborated in a small series[61] of 12 patients with LyP treated at MD Anderson with brentuximab vedotin. They also demonstrated 100% ORR. All patients responded after a single infusion, with several patients experiencing sustained responses.

PRIMARY CUTANEOUS ANAPLASTIC LARGE-CELL LYMPHOMA
Epidemiology

Primary cutaneous anaplastic large-cell lymphoma (pcALCL) is the second of the defined CD30+ LPD, and accounts for about 9% of all CTCLs (**Fig. 3**). Patients are older at time of diagnosis, median age of 60 years, compared with LyP patients. It is also male dominant, at a ratio of 3:1.[37,38,48] Children are rarely affected. PcALCL has a favorable prognosis, with 5-year survival between 76% and 96%.[48] PcALCL of the legs has poorer prognosis; 5-year survival is 76%.[54] Immunosuppressed patients have more aggressive disease course with worse prognosis.

Pathophysiology

The etiology of pcALCL is unknown. There may be an association with immunomodulating medications such as adalimumab and fingolimod.

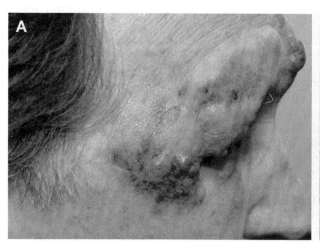
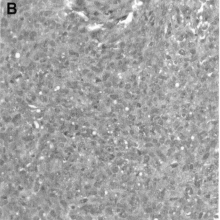

Fig. 3. Anaplastic large cell lymphoma. (*A*) Erythematous tumor and nodules on the left temporal zone. (*B*) Diffuse dermal infiltrate of large anaplastic cells with frequent mitotic figures and apoptotic bodies (magnification 400X).

Clinicopathological Presentation and Differential Diagnoses

PcALCL is defined by expression of CD30 in more than 75% of large atypical T cells. It is distinct from systemic ALCL, because the diseases behave differently. It typically presents as a solitary tumor or group of localized nodules that are often ulcerated. These lesions grow rapidly and may reach several centimeters.[48] Approximately 20% of patients present with multifocal lesions, with 2 or more lesions at different sites. Lesions are usually found in the head and neck region, or on the extremities, but may occur anywhere.[38] Tumors may spontaneously regress.[62] However, recurrence is common. Regional lymph node involvement is rare and has not been associated with worse prognosis. Extensive skin lesions on the leg and multifocal disease are associated with worse prognosis.[62]

Histologically, pcALCL is characterized by nodular and diffuse infiltrates of neoplastic T cells that extend into the deep dermis or subcutaneous tissue. Tumor cells are large in size with round to irregularly shaped nuclei and 1 or more prominent nucleoli and abundant pale cytoplasm.[48,51,62] Although the cells tend to have this anaplastic morphology, immunoblastic and pleomorphic morphology have also been reported. Eosinophil- and neutrophil-rich forms of pcALCL have been described and pose a diagnostic challenge, masquerading as other diseases. Other rare presentations include angiocentric and angiodestructive growth patterns. Keratoacanthoma-like variants exhibit pseudoepitheliomatous epidermal hyperplasia overlying CD30+ infiltrate of tumor cells, easily mistaken for squamous cell carcinoma. The sarcomatoid variant is rare, with prominent spindle-cell morphology.

The atypical cells of pcALCL show an activated T-cell phenotype and express CD2, CD4, and CD45RO, with variable loss of CD2 and CD5. CD8+, CD4+/CD8+, or CD4-/CD8- (null) phenotypes of these atypical cells have also been described. Other activation markers, such as cytotoxic proteins (TIA-1, granzyme B and perforin), CD25, and HLA-DR are expressed in half of pcALCL cases. In contrast to systemic ALCL, pcALCL is EMA and ALK-1 negative and rarely carries the t(2;5) translocation.[48,51] Tumor cells additionally express KIR3DL2, which is also found in transformed MF and Sézary syndrome. IPH4102 (Innate Pharma, Marseille, France), a new anti-KIR3DL2 humanized monoclonal antibody with antitumor activity, is currently undergoing investigation (NCT02593045).[63]

Clonal rearrangement of TCR genes is found in 90% of pcALCL cases. As mentioned previously, the t(2;5) translocation is rarely seen in pcALCL, and cells are normally ALK-negative, while ALK positivity is usually seen in systemic ALCL (Table 2). ALK-positive pcALCL has been described,[48] ultimately with complete remission and unchanged prognosis. Further investigation will be required to understand the implications of a potentially worrisome finding in a normally benign disease.

The differential diagnosis of pcALCL is broad and includes primary cutaneous and systemic large-cell lymphomas with CD30+ infiltrates, LyP, transformed mycosis fungoides, and nodular reactive lymphoid hyperplasia caused by arthropod bites, medications, or infections. It is important to differentiate systemic ALCL, which has a worse prognosis and different treatment. PcALCL expresses cutaneous lymphocyte-associated antigen (CLA), which is not expressed in systemic disease. Conversely, systemic ALCL expresses ALK, which is rarely expressed in primary cutaneous disease. ATLL histologically presents similarly; however, can be differentiated by detection of HTLV-1 in the tumor cell genome.

Work-Up

The work-up for pcALCL is more extensive than LyP because of the importance of ruling out systemic lymphomas. A complete skin examination including regional lymph nodes is the first step. Suspicious lesions and lymph nodes greater than 1.5 cm should be biopsied with immunohistochemistry, and T-cell clonality should be assessed. Laboratory tests including CBC, CMP, and lactate dehydrogenase (LDH) are performed. HTLV-1 serology should also be assessed to rule out CD30+ ATLL. Whole-body imaging should be performed, either contrast computed tomography (CT) of the chest, abdomen, and pelvis or whole-body positron emission tomography, which is preferred. Bone marrow biopsy is considered in the setting of diffuse or multifocal tumors, abnormal blood tests, or with extracutaneous involvement on imaging.[38,43]

Treatment

Surgical excision and radiotherapy[43,64] are first-line therapies for single or grouped lesions. Radiation therapy may be preferred, as there is no current recommendation for margin of resection.[38] In the study from the Dutch Cutaneous Lymphoma Group,[37] radiation therapy and surgical excision were used as initial therapy in 48% and 19% of 79 pcALCL patients, respectively. They observed CR in 100% of patients. After median follow-up

Table 2
Comparison of immunohistological profiles of lymphomatoid papulosis, primary cutaneous anaplastic large cell lymphoma, and systemic anaplastic large cell lymphoma

	LyP	pcALCL	Systemic ALCL
CD2	Variable	Variable	50%
CD3	Variable	−/lesser expression	− (<25%)
CD4	+	+	50%
CD5	Variable	Variable	− (<25%)
CD7	Variable (most commonly absent)		− (<25%)
CD8	− (type D: +, type E: 70%)	+	− (<25%)
CD25	+	50%	
CD30	+ (type B: variable)	>75% cells + (diagnostic)	+
CD45RO	+	+	+
HLA-DR	+	50%	
CD56	10%	12%–75%	+
Bcl-2	−	30%	+
Cytotoxic proteins	+	50%	+
ALK	−	Rare	50%
CLA	+	50%	−
EMA	−	−	+
t(2;5) translocation	−	<10%	60%

61 months, skin-only relapse and extracutaneous disease were reported in 41% and 10% of patients, respectively. A multicenter retrospective analysis in 56 pcALCL patients studied radiation therapy as primary therapy or after surgical resection. Ninety-five percent of patients had complete clinical response with 98% local control after median follow-up of 3.5 years.[65] CR was seen with a radiation dose as low as 6 Gy (range 6–45 Gy). Two other studies confirmed efficacy of low-dose RT (≤20 Gy) for treatment of solitary or localized PC-ALCL.[65,66]

Multiagent chemotherapy is indicated for extracutaneous tumor spread beyond locoregional lymph nodes. In their study, Bekkenk and colleagues[37] also evaluated multiagent chemotherapy in pcALCL patients. Nine of 11 patients with regional node involvement were treated with a regimen similar to CHOP as initial therapy. Eight patients (88%) had CR; however, 5 of these 8 patients had skin recurrence. Because of the high rate of relapse, multiagent chemotherapy is not first-line treatment. Low-dose methotrexate remains first-line treatment for multifocal disease if radiation therapy is not possible.

Brentuximab vedotin is safe and effective for multifocal, refractory, extracutaneous, or recurrent pcALCL.[38,59,61] In the ALCANZA trial, brentuximab vedotin was found to be superior to treatment with methotrexate and bexarotene for pcALCL[59] and is currently the preferred systemic treatment for multifocal lesions and regional node involvement.

REFERENCES

1. Boos MD, Samimi SS, Rook AH, et al. Pityriasis lichenoides and cutaneous T cell lymphoma: an update on the diagnosis and management of the most common benign and malignant cutaneous lymphoproliferative diseases in children. Curr Dermatol Rep 2013;2(4):203–11.
2. Khachemoune A, Blyumin ML. Pityriasis lichenoides: pathophysiology, classification, and treatment. Am J Clin Dermatol 2007;8(1):29–36. Available at: http://www.ncbi.nlm.nih.gov/pubmed/17298104. Accessed July 29, 2018.
3. Bowers S, Warshaw EM. Pityriasis lichenoides and its subtypes. J Am Acad Dermatol 2006;55(4): 557–72 [quiz: 573–6].
4. Koh W-L, Koh MJ-A, Tay Y-K. Pityriasis lichenoides in an Asian population. Int J Dermatol 2013;52(12): 1495–9.
5. Lane TN, Parker SS. Pityriasis lichenoides chronica in black patients. Cutis 2010;85(3):125–9. Available

at: http://www.ncbi.nlm.nih.gov/pubmed/20408509. Accessed July 29, 2018.

6. Nair PS. A clinical and histopathological study of pityriasis lichenoides. Indian J Dermatol Venereol Leprol 2007;73(2):100–2. Available at: http://www.ncbi.nlm.nih.gov/pubmed/17456915. Accessed July 29, 2018.

7. Maranda EL, Smith M, Nguyen AH, et al. Phototherapy for pityriasis lichenoides in the pediatric population: a review of the published literature. Am J Clin Dermatol 2016;17(6):583–91.

8. Zang JB, Coates SJ, Huang J, et al. Pityriasis lichenoides: long-term follow-up study. Pediatr Dermatol 2018;35(2):213–9.

9. Geller L, Antonov NK, Lauren CT, et al. Pityriasis lichenoides in childhood: review of clinical presentation and treatment options. Pediatr Dermatol 2015; 32(5):579–92.

10. Longley J, Demar L, Feinstein RP, et al. Clinical and histologic features of pityriasis lichenoides et varioliformis acuta in children. Arch Dermatol 1987;123(10):1335–9. Available at: http://www.ncbi.nlm.nih.gov/pubmed/3662566. Accessed July 29, 2018.

11. Nofal A, Alakad R, Assaf M, et al. A fatal case of febrile ulceronecrotic Mucha-Habermann disease in a child. JAAD Case Rep 2016;2(2):181–5.

12. Xing C, Shen H, Xu J, et al. A fatal case of febrile ulceronecrotic mucha-habermann disease which presenting as toxic epidermal necrolysis. Indian J Dermatol 2017;62(6):567.

13. Horie C, Mizukawa Y, Yamazaki Y, et al. Varicella zoster virus as a possible trigger for the development of pityriasis lichenoides et varioliformis acuta: retrospective analysis of our institutional cases. Clin Exp Dermatol 2018;43(6):703–7.

14. Cho E, Jun HJ, Cho SH, et al. Varicella-zoster virus as a possible cause of pityriasis lichenoides et varioliformis acuta. Pediatr Dermatol 2014;31(2):259–60.

15. Gunatheesan S, Ferguson J, Moosa Y. Pityriasis lichenoides et varioliformis acuta: a rare association with the measles, mumps and rubella vaccine. Australas J Dermatol 2012;53(4):e76–8.

16. de Castro BAC, Pereira JMM, Meyer RLB, et al. Pityriasis lichenoides et varioliformis acuta after influenza vaccine. An Bras Dermatol 2015;90(3 Suppl 1):181–4.

17. González Rodríguez AJ, Montesinos Villaescusa E, Jordá Cuevas E. Pityriasis lichenoides chronica associated with herpes simplex virus type 2. Case Rep Dermatol Med 2012;2012:737428.

18. Mutgi KAJ, Milhem M, Swick BL, et al. Pityriasis lichenoides chronica-like drug eruption developing during pembrolizumab treatment for metastatic melanoma. JAAD Case Rep 2016;2(4):343–5.

19. Wood GS, Edinger A, Hoppe RT, et al. Mycosis fungoides skin lesions contain CD8+ tumor-infiltrating lymphocytes expressing an activated, MHC-restricted cytotoxic T-lymphocyte phenotype. J Cutan Pathol 1994;21(2):151–6. Available at: http://www.ncbi.nlm.nih.gov/pubmed/8040463. Accessed July 29, 2018.

20. Wood GS, Strickler JG, Abel EA, et al. Immunohistology of pityriasis lichenoides et varioliformis acuta and pityriasis lichenoides chronica. Evidence for their interrelationship with lymphomatoid papulosis. J Am Acad Dermatol 1987;16(3 Pt 1): 559–70. Available at: http://www.ncbi.nlm.nih.gov/pubmed/2434538. Accessed July 29, 2018.

21. Magro C, Crowson AN, Kovatich A, et al. Pityriasis lichenoides: a clonal T-cell lymphoproliferative disorder. Hum Pathol 2002;33(8):788–95. Available at: http://www.ncbi.nlm.nih.gov/pubmed/12203210. Accessed July 29, 2018.

22. Magro C, Crowsen AN, Morrison C, et al. Pityriasis lichenoides chronica: stratification by molecular and phenotypic profile. Hum Pathol 2007;38(3): 479–90.

23. Tomasini D, Zampatti C, Palmedo G, et al. Cytotoxic mycosis fungoides evolving from pityriasis lichenoides chronica in a seventeen-year-old girl. Report of a case. Dermatology 2002;205(2): 176–9.

24. Pileri A, Neri I, Raone B, et al. Mycosis fungoides following pityriasis lichenoides: an exceptional event or a potential evolution. Pediatr Blood Cancer 2012; 58(2):306.

25. Clayton R, Haffenden G. An immunofluorescence study of pityriasis lichenoides. Br J Dermatol 1978;99(5):491–3. Available at: http://www.ncbi.nlm.nih.gov/pubmed/361062. Accessed July 29, 2018.

26. Karouni M, Rahal JA, Kurban M, et al. Possible role of plasmacytoid dendritic cells in pityriasis lichenoides. Clin Exp Dermatol 2018;43(4):404–9.

27. Ankad BS, Beergouder SL. Pityriasis lichenoides et varioliformis acuta in skin of color: new observations by dermoscopy. Dermatol Pract Concept 2017;7(1): 27–34.

28. Fernandes NF, Rozdeba PJ, Schwartz RA, et al. Pityriasis lichenoides et varioliformis acuta: a disease spectrum. Int J Dermatol 2010;49(3): 257–61.

29. Someshwar S, Udare S. Pityriasis lichenoides. Indian Pediatr 2012;49(11):936–7. Available at: http://www.ncbi.nlm.nih.gov/pubmed/23255714. Accessed July 29, 2018.

30. Pereira N, Brinca A, Brites MM, et al. Pityriasis lichenoides et varioliformis acuta: case report and review of the literature. Case Rep Dermatol 2012;4(1): 61–5.

31. Simon D, Boudny C, Nievergelt H, et al. Successful treatment of pityriasis lichenoides with topical tacrolimus. Br J Dermatol 2004;150(5):1033–5.

32. Fernández-Guarino M, Aboin-Gonzalez S, Ciudad Blanco C, et al. Treatment of adult diffuse pityriasis lichenoides chronica with narrowband ultraviolet B: experience and literature review. Clin Exp Dermatol 2017;42(3):303–5.

33. Fernández-Guarino M, Harto A, Reguero-Callejas ME, et al. Pityriasis lichenoides chronica: good response to photodynamic therapy. Br J Dermatol 2008;158(1):198–200.

34. Wilson LD, Hinds GA, Yu JB. Age, race, sex, stage, and incidence of cutaneous lymphoma. Clin Lymphoma Myeloma Leuk 2012;12(5):291–6.

35. Macaulay WL. Lymphomatoid papulosis. A continuing self-healing eruption, clinically benign–histologically malignant. Arch Dermatol 1968;97(1): 23–30. Available at: http://www.ncbi.nlm.nih.gov/pubmed/5634442. Accessed June 24, 2018.

36. Wieser I, Oh CW, Talpur R, et al. Lymphomatoid papulosis: treatment response and associated lymphomas in a study of 180 patients. J Am Acad Dermatol 2016;74(1):59–67.

37. Bekkenk MW, Geelen FA, van Voorst Vader PC, et al. Primary and secondary cutaneous CD30(+) lymphoproliferative disorders: a report from the Dutch Cutaneous Lymphoma Group on the long-term follow-up data of 219 patients and guidelines for diagnosis and treatment. Blood 2000;95(12): 3653–61. Available at: http://www.ncbi.nlm.nih.gov/pubmed/10845893. Accessed June 17, 2018.

38. Sauder MB, O'Malley JT, LeBoeuf NR. CD30+ lymphoproliferative disorders of the skin. Hematol Oncol Clin North Am 2017;31(2):317–34.

39. Wang HH, Myers T, Lach LJ, et al. Increased risk of lymphoid and nonlymphoid malignancies in patients with lymphomatoid papulosis. Cancer 1999;86(7): 1240–5. Available at: http://www.ncbi.nlm.nih.gov/pubmed/10506709. Accessed June 17, 2018.

40. Cordel N, Tressieres B, DIncan M, et al. Frequency and risk factors for associated lymphomas in patients with lymphomatoid papulosis. Oncologist 2016;21(1):76–83.

41. Mori M, Manuelli C, Pimpinelli N, et al. CD30-CD30 ligand interaction in primary cutaneous CD30(+) T-cell lymphomas: a clue to the pathophysiology of clinical regression. Blood 1999;94(9):3077–83. Available at: http://www.ncbi.nlm.nih.gov/pubmed/10556192. Accessed June 24, 2018.

42. Kempf W, Pfaltz K, Vermeer MH, et al. EORTC, ISCL, and USCLC consensus recommendations for the treatment of primary cutaneous CD30-positive lymphoproliferative disorders: lymphomatoid papulosis and primary cutaneous anaplastic large-cell lymphoma. Blood 2011;118(15):4024–35.

43. Kempf W, Kerl K, Mitteldorf C. Cutaneous CD30-positive T-cell lymphoproliferative disorders— clinical and histopathologic features, differential diagnosis, and treatment. Semin Cutan Med Surg 2018;37(1):24–9.

44. Swerdlow SH, Campo E, Pileri SA, et al. The 2016 revision of the World Health Organization classification of lymphoid neoplasms. Blood 2016;127(20): 2375–90.

45. El Shabrawi-Caelen L, Kerl H, Cerroni L. Lymphomatoid papulosis: reappraisal of clinicopathologic presentation and classification into subtypes A, B, and C. Arch Dermatol 2004;140(4):441–7.

46. Kempf W, Kazakov DV, Schärer L, et al. Angioinvasive lymphomatoid papulosis. Am J Surg Pathol 2013;37(1):1–13.

47. Karai LJ, Kadin ME, Hsi ED, et al. Chromosomal rearrangements of 6p25.3 define a new subtype of lymphomatoid papulosis. Am J Surg Pathol 2013; 37(8):1173–81.

48. Kempf W. A new era for cutaneous CD30-positive T-cell lymphoproliferative disorders. Semin Diagn Pathol 2017;34(1):22–35.

49. Kempf W, Mitteldorf C, Karai LJ, et al. Lymphomatoid papulosis - making sense of the alphabet soup: a proposal to simplify terminology. J Dtsch Dermatol Ges 2017;15(4):390–4.

50. Kempf W, Kazakov DV, Baumgartner H-P, et al. Follicular lymphomatoid papulosis revisited: A study of 11 cases, with new histopathological findings. J Am Acad Dermatol 2013;68(5):809–16.

51. Guitart J, Querfeld C. Cutaneous CD30 lymphoproliferative disorders and similar conditions: a clinical and pathologic prospective on a complex issue. Semin Diagn Pathol 2009;26(3):131–40.

52. Steinhoff M, Hummel M, Anagnostopoulos I, et al. Single-cell analysis of CD30+ cells in lymphomatoid papulosis demonstrates a common clonal T-cell origin. Blood 2002;100(2):578–84. https://doi.org/10.1182/blood-2001-12-0199.

53. Gellrich S, Wernicke M, Wilks A, et al. The cell infiltrate in lymphomatoid papulosis comprises a mixture of polyclonal large atypical cells (CD30-positive) and smaller monoclonal T cells (CD30-negative). J Invest Dermatol 2004;122(3):859–61.

54. Fernández-de-Misa R, Hernández-Machín B, Servitje O, et al. First-line treatment in lymphomatoid papulosis: a retrospective multicentre study. Clin Exp Dermatol 2018;43(2):137–43.

55. Newland KM, McCormack CJ, Twigger R, et al. The efficacy of methotrexate for lymphomatoid papulosis. J Am Acad Dermatol 2015;72(6):1088–90.

56. Vonderheid EC, Sajjadian A, Kadin ME. Methotrexate is effective therapy for lymphomatoid papulosis and other primary cutaneous CD30-positive lymphoproliferative disorders. J Am Acad Dermatol 1996;34(3):470–81. Available at: http://www.ncbi.nlm.nih.gov/pubmed/8609262. Accessed July 9, 2018.

57. Bruijn MS, Horváth B, van Voorst Vader PC, et al. Recommendations for treatment of lymphomatoid papulosis with methotrexate: a report from the Dutch

Cutaneous Lymphoma Group. Br J Dermatol 2015; 173(5):1319–22.

58. Duvic M, Reddy SA, Pinter-Brown L, et al. A phase II study of SGN-30 in cutaneous anaplastic large cell lymphoma and related lymphoproliferative disorders. Clin Cancer Res 2009;15(19):6217–24.

59. Prince HM, Kim YH, Horwitz SM, et al. Brentuximab vedotin or physician's choice in CD30-positive cutaneous T-cell lymphoma (ALCANZA): an international, open-label, randomised, phase 3, multicentre trial. Lancet 2017;390(10094):555–66.

60. Duvic M, Tetzlaff MT, Gangar P, et al. Results of a phase II trial of brentuximab vedotin for CD30 + cutaneous T-cell lymphoma and lymphomatoid papulosis. J Clin Oncol 2015;33(32):3759–65.

61. Lewis DJ, Talpur R, Huen AO, et al. Brentuximab vedotin for patients with refractory lymphomatoid papulosis. JAMA Dermatol 2017;153(12):1302.

62. Hughey LC. Practical management of CD30+ lymphoproliferative disorders. Dermatol Clin 2015; 33(4):819–33.

63. Bagot M, Porcu P, Ram-Wolff C, et al. First-in-human, multicenter phase I study of IPH4102, first-in-class humanized anti-KIR3DL2 monoclonal antibody, in relapsed/refractory cutaneous T-cell lymphomas: preliminary safety, exploratory and clinical activity results. Blood 2016;128(22). Available at: http://www.bloodjournal.org/content/128/22/1826?sso-checked=true. Accessed July 9, 2018.

64. Yu JB, McNiff JM, Lund MW, et al. Treatment of primary cutaneous CD30+ anaplastic large-cell lymphoma with radiation therapy. Int J Radiat Oncol 2008;70(5):1542–5.

65. Million L, Yi EJ, Wu F, et al. Radiation therapy for primary cutaneous anaplastic large cell lymphoma: an international lymphoma radiation oncology group multi-institutional experience. Int J Radiat Oncol Biol Phys 2016;95(5):1454–9.

66. Melchers RC, Willemze R, Daniëls LA, et al. Recommendations for the optimal radiation dose in patients with primary cutaneous anaplastic large cell lymphoma: a report of the Dutch cutaneous lymphoma group. Int J Radiat Oncol Biol Phys 2017;99(5): 1279–85.

Dermatofibrosarcoma Protuberans

Aubrey Allen, BA[a],*, Christine Ahn, MD[b], Omar P. Sangüeza, MD[b]

KEYWORDS

- Dermatofibrosarcoma protuberans • Fibrosarcomatous transformation
- Cutaneous soft tissue sarcoma • t(17;22) translocation • Imatinib mesylate

KEY POINTS

- Dermatofibrosarcoma protuberans (DFSP) is rare, slow-growing dermal neoplasm with a high rate of local recurrence and infiltration, but low metastatic potential.
- DFSP is associated with the COL1A1-PDGFB fusion protein that is a result of a t(17;22) chromosomal translocation; tyrosine kinase inhibitors such as imatinib mesylate target this mechanism.
- CD34, factor XIIIa, nestin, D2-40, and PDGFB protein are histologic markers that are useful in diagnosing DFSP and distinguishing it from dermatofibroma.
- Wide excision with negative margins is the mainstay of treatment; there is great utility for Mohs micrographic surgery for lesions in cosmetically sensitive areas or tumors where wide margins are unachievable.

INTRODUCTION

Dermatofibrosarcoma protuberans (DFSP) is an uncommon, cutaneous fibrohistiocytic neoplasm that was first described by Darier and Ferrand in 1924. The term DFSP was coined by Hoffman in 1925.[1] It accounts for 1% of all soft tissue sarcomas, with an incidence of 0.8 to 5 cases per million population each year. DFSP rates are highest among blacks, with a male-to-female ratio of 1:1 and a 5-year relative survival rate of 99%.[2–4] The median age at diagnosis is typically between 20 to 59 years, but congenital and pediatric cases have been described.[5] There are no specific risk factors associated with DFSP; it can arise on healthy skin or on chronically damaged areas. DFSP typically follows an indolent clinical course with a high rate of local recurrence because of its infiltrative behavior, but low metastatic potential.[1]

DFSP tumorigenesis is associated with a translocation involving chromosomes 17 and 22, leading to the fusion of collagen type 1alpha 1 (COL1A1) and platelet-derived growth factor subunit β (PDGFB) genes. This fusion protein causes a continuous activation of the receptor PDGF receptor β (PDGFRB) tyrosine kinase, which promotes DFSP cell growth. This mechanism justifies the use of tyrosine kinase inhibitors in treatment.[3] Nakamura and colleagues[6] recently described a novel fusion gene, COL1A2-PDGFB, which resulted in constitutively expressed PDGFB, indicating that DFSP tumorigenesis involves the promoter activity of the COL1A1 or COL1A2 genes that contribute to the overexpression of PDGFB.

CLINICAL FEATURES

DFSP classically presents as a slowly progressive, painless cutaneous lesion that may begin as a violet or pink plaque (Fig. 1). Patients will often report a history of the lesion being present for years,

Disclosure statement: These authors have no commercial or financial conflicts and no funding sources.
[a] Brody School of Medicine, East Carolina University, 517 Moye Boulevard, Greenville, NC 27834, USA;
[b] Departments of Dermatology and Pathology, Wake Forest School of Medicine, 4618 Country Club Road, Winston Salem, NC 27104, USA
* Corresponding author.
E-mail addresses: aubreylynnallen@gmail.com; cahn@wakehealth.edu

Fig. 1. DFSP. Ill-defined erythematous patch on the trunk of an individual.

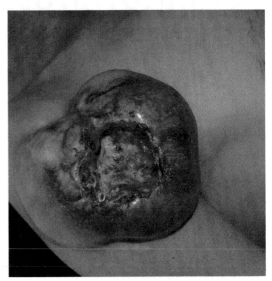

Fig. 3. Ulcerated DFSP. Pink-violaceous tumor on the proximal extremity with central ulceration and necrosis.

slow-growing, or with apparent stability in size. DFSP most commonly arises in the dermis or subcutis of the trunk (50% to 60% of cases) and upper limbs (25%), but involvement of the head and neck accounts for 10% to 15% of cases.[7] Lesions usually occur on the proximal extremities, although cases have been described on the distal extremities and acral sites.[4,8] Untreated, lesions usually progress to nodules or tumors (**Fig. 2**) and may ulcerate and/or bleed (**Fig. 3**).

DFSP rarely metastasizes. Less than 5% of patients with DFSP develop metastatic disease; when distant recurrences do occur, they are found in regional lymph nodes and the lung.[4,7] The development of metastasis from DFSP is a poor prognostic sign, and the highest rate of mortality is within 2 years of visceral involvement. In nearly all cases, metastases are preceded by local recurrences.[7] Recurrent lesions are more prone to

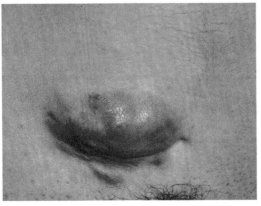

Fig. 2. DFSP. Pink nodule on the trunk with areas of hyperpigmentation.

sarcomatous transformation, a factor that may increase the risk for metastasis.

DFSP is a deep dermal neoplasm. The growth of DFSP is usually asymmetric, with finger-like projections; lateral or deep extension is unpredictable and can vary from 0.3 to 12 cm over the macroscopic borders.[9] If not completely resected, these projections lead to local recurrence. For this reason, it is crucial for the pathologist to evaluate the peripheral and deep margins of resection specimens.

HISTOLOGY

Microscopic examination will reveal a monomorphous spindle cell proliferation in a storiform pattern, often surrounding and trapping subcutaneous fat to form a honeycomb appearance (**Fig. 4**).[1] A punch biopsy containing subcutaneous fat is needed for an accurate diagnosis; however, excisional biopsy is preferable. Ninety percent of all DFSPs are low-grade lesions, while sarcomatous transformation is seen in 10% to 15% of all cases, usually to a low-grade fibrosarcoma. This histologic difference has been associated with increased aggressiveness of the tumor. The fibrosarcomatous DFSP subtype is an adverse predictor of recurrence-free survival. Therefore, this subtype is considered to have a more aggressive growth pattern and a higher rate of local recurrence and metastasis.[4] Single-institution retrospective reviews report 5-year recurrence-free survival rates of between 42% and 52% for fibrosarcomatous DFSP, and a 10% to 15% risk of

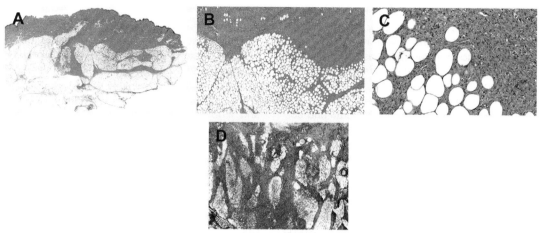

Fig. 4. DFSP. (*A*) Low-magnification view demonstrating infiltrative growth of spindle cells into the subcutaneous fat in a honeycomb pattern (H&E, 2x). (*B*) Dense proliferation of spindle cells in a storiform pattern dissecting through and entrapping adipocytes (H&E, 8x). (*C*) Spindle cells with bland cytomorphology surrounding adipocytes (H&E, 40x). (*D*) Spindle cells stain strongly positive for CD34 (CD34, 40x).

metastasis.[10–13] The transformed lesion has histologic differences, including a fascicular or herringbone pattern of growth, increased mitotic rate, and greater nuclear pleomorphism and hyperchromasia.[1]

The histopathologic features of DFSP are usually characteristic, but immunohistochemical staining can aid in ruling out benign entities, such as a cellular dermatofibroma (CDF). Additionally, biopsy specimens that do not extend to the subcutaneous fat can lead to misdiagnosis as dermatofibroma or CDF. CD34 is usually positive in DFSP (positive in 92% to 100% of cases), while factor XIII-a is negative, with the converse staining pattern found in CDF.[1] Some cases of CDF stain positive for CD34; however, the areas of staining are less diffuse and usually seen at the periphery of the neoplasm. Expression of CD34 is often decreased or lost in DFSP with fibrosarcomatous transformation.[14] Bandarchi and colleagues[15] used D2-40 to distinguish dermatofibroma from DFSP, with the protein being universally expressed in 56 cases of dermatofibroma, and negative staining in 29 cases of DFSP.

Nestin is a class 4 intermediate filament protein that is expressed in mesenchymal stem cells of the bone marrow, lungs, muscle, and pancreas. DFSP has been shown to be a nestin-positive tumor. Mori and colleagues[16] found in 2008 that nestin was expressed in 94% of DFSP cases, but just 13% of dermatofibromas. More results have been reported that show strong nestin staining in all cases of DFSP.[17,18] High levels of nestin expression have been associated with poorer prognosis in certain tumors, and Serra-Guillen and colleagues[14] examined the correlation

between nestin expression and depth of invasion in a large series of DFSP. In this study, high nestin expression was associated with invasion of the tumor into the fascia and the presence of larger and longer-standing tumors, suggesting its use as possible indicator of tumor invasion. Although CD34 staining in fibrosarcomatous areas of DFSP is expected to be absent or decreased, nestin levels remained unaltered. Thus, staining with nestin can be used in conjunction with CD34 in cases of DFSP with fibrosarcomatous transformation.[14]

The expression of PDGFB protein is also a possible histologic marker for DFSP, with 1 study detecting expression in 28 (93%) of 30 cases. Whereas CD34 and nestin are typically expressed throughout the tumor mass, PDGFB was not homogeneously expressed. PDGFB protein is a highly specific marker for DFSP. In 1 study, PDGFB expression was absent in 47 (98%) of 48 patients with non-DFSP mesenchymal tumors.[6] Fluorescence in situ hybridization or polymerase chain reaction can be performed to detect the t17:22 (COL1A1-PDGFB) translocation, which is present in 72% to 96% of cases of DFSP.[1]

TREATMENT

The mainstay of treatment for DFSP is complete surgical excision with histologically negative margins. Because of its storiform growth pattern and pseudopod-like extensions, incomplete excisions are common. Recurrence rates as high as 50% have been described in literature. Recurrence is most common for tumors of the head and neck, likely because it is difficult to achieve wide margins in these areas.[1] Adequate primary resection is important, as the recurring tumor is usually more locally destructive at the time of re-excision, with a higher likelihood of sarcomatous transformation and invasion into the underlying fascia.[1]

Wide local excision (WLE) is the most common method of excision, with studies suggesting 2 to 3 cm margins.[1,19–21] In a study by Harati and colleagues,[4] 16 patients with DFSP underwent excision with negative histologic margins greater than 1 cm. One-hundred percent of patients in this series had recurrence-free survival during follow-up (5 years). However, this study reported on histologic assessed margin width, and thus it did not establish what surgical margins from the tumor were obtained for these results. Based on these results, the authors conclude that the lateral safety margins of 2 to 3 cm are justified whenever achievable. Although preoperative margins of 2 to 3 cm are commonly suggested, various studies have suggested that lower recurrence rates are possible without excessively wide margins, and in many cases, margins less than 2 to 3 cm are adequate and provide better aesthetic outcomes.[1,22–24] Parker and Zitelli[20] attempted to determine necessary margins for DFSP excision using Mohs micrographic surgery (MMS) and determined that tumors less than 2 cm in size were completely cleared with a 1.5 cm margin. The available data suggest that emphasis should be placed on the need for meticulous examination of the margins, including CD34 immunohistochemistry when necessary.[1,25]

Mohs micrographic surgery is an alternative to wide local excision, as it allows the clinician to analyze 100% of the tumor margins, identify microscopic extensions, and remove them while conserving healthy tissue. Although recurrence rates for standard surgical resection and WLE have been reported at 26% to 60% and 0% to 41% respectively, the rate of recurrence after MMS has been reported at 0% to 8.3%.[3,7,26] Reported recurrence rates for DFSP treated with MMS are significantly lower than those treated with WLE, especially in head and neck sites (1.9% with MMS, 51.8% with WLE), but there is controversy over the 2 methods. There is a lack of randomized controlled trials, and few comparative studies. Lowe and colleagues[27] found that in patients with primary DFSP as opposed to recurrent disease, the recurrence-free survival in patients who received wide excision compared with MMS was the same at 5, 10, and 15 years. Disadvantages of MMS are that tumor cells can be confused with normal spindle cells of the dermis in frozen sections, and CD34 staining of frozen sections has high variability. Some authors do not consider the technique entirely reliable.[19,28,29] Another limitation is the ability to clear the deep margin, especially if the tumor has invaded the underlying fascia or muscle.[1] MMS is also complex, time consuming, and possibly costly. It can require a long procedure for patients and reconstruction. WLE may be the preferred treatment for trunk and limb lesions. Head and neck tumors may have greater benefit from MMS, allowing for tissue conservation and a better aesthetic outcome.

Veronese and colleagues[3] completed a retrospective study of 135 patients treated between 1997 and 2014 comparing WLE with Mohs Tubingen technique (MTT). This surgical variant was adopted for the treatment of DFSP at Tubingen's University in Germany in 1988 and utilizes a 3-dimensional visualization of the excision margins, the Tubingen cake, and it is particularly useful for large and deep excision of skin cancers. In contrast to MMS, which requires sectioning the tumor several times horizontally and mapping the specimen on paper, the MTT technique analyzes all margins and deep side of the specimen at the first cut. This technique was determined to have a recurrence rate between 0% to 5.5% and may be an acceptable alternative to MMS with comparable efficacy and less time needed.[3]

Radiation therapy can be used in combination with resection when wide surgical margins are not possible, or as adjuvant therapy after resection in recurrent DFSP.[1,19] Adverse effects of radiation therapy increase the risk of wound complications and include fibrosis, necrosis, edema, and skin graft failures. Because of these adverse effects, radiotherapy is not indicated in cases of resection with negative margins.[19]

Systemic therapy has not been studied extensively for the treatment of DFSP because of the low rate of metastasis. However, for large tumors in cosmetically sensitive locations or metastatic disease, systemic therapy can be utilized. The fusion protein responsible for DFSP cell growth can be targeted by tyrosine kinase inhibitors such as imatinib mesylate. Imatinib has shown to be effective in patients with the t(17;22) translocation, but lacks activity against t(17;22)-negative DFSP. Detection of the COL1A1-PDGFB translocation fusion is recommended using FISH or reverse transcriptase polymerase chain reaction prior to the start of imatinib therapy.[19] The overall responses of imatinib is reported around 43%, with 73% reporting partial response and 90% reporting stable disease.[30–32] Imatinib has also been used as neoadjuvant therapy before MMS, with the rate of tumor shrinkage reported at 20% and 31.5% over 2 and 3 months, respectively.[33,34] Sunitinib malate, a multityrosine kinase inhibitor, can be used as a second-line agent for the treatment of imatinib-resistant tumors. A study by Fu and colleagues[35] examined the use of sunitinib malate as a second-line agent after imatinib resistance. Of 95 patients initially treated with imatinib, 30 patients developed resistance and were switched to sunitinib. The median follow-up rate was 2.5 years, and the overall rate of disease control was 80% (which included patients demonstrating complete response, partial response, and stable disease). Sorafenib, another tyrosine kinase inhibitor, has also been suggested as a potential therapy, with 1 case report describing patient who responded to sorafenib after failing imatinib.

SUMMARY

In the treatment of DFSP, the focus should be on complete surgical resection of the tumor with histologically confirmed negative margins. Based on available data, there is no universally accepted minimum margin of excision. WLE remains the mainstay of treatment. MMS should be considered in cases involving cosmetically sensitive areas or in locations where tissue conservation is critical, such as the face or ears. MTT can be considered as an alternative to MMS, as it has demonstrated low rates of tumor recurrence and is less time-consuming. Information about the tumor size, location, and histology should guide clinical decision making regarding excision method and width of initial surgical margins. In cases where complete resection is not possible or in metastatic disease, radiation or systemic imatinib therapy should be considered. The clinician should be aware that fibrosarcomatous transformation of DFSP is a higher-risk tumor, and the goal of treatment is complete resection with negative surgical margins.

REFERENCES

1. Luu C, Messina JL, Brohl AS, et al. Dermatofibrosarcoma protuberans. In: Raghavan D, Ahluwalia MS, Blanke CD, editors. Textbook of uncommon cancer. 5th edition. Oxford: Wiley-Blackwell; 2017. p. 994–1001.
2. Rouhani P, Fletcher CD, Devesa SS, et al. Cutaneous soft tissue sarcoma incidence patterns in the US. Cancer 2008;113(3):616–27.
3. Veronese F, Boggio P, Tiberio R, et al. Wide local excision vs. Mohs Tübingen technique in the treatment of dermatofibrosarcoma protuberans: a two-centre retrospective study and literature review. J Eur Acad Dermatol Venereol 2017;31(12): 2069–76.
4. Harati K, Lange K, Goertz O, et al. A single-institutional review of 68 patients with dermatofibrosarcoma protuberans: wide re-excision after inadequate previous surgery results in a high rate of local control. World J Surg Oncol 2017;15(1):5.
5. Saiag P, Grob JJ, Lebbe C, et al. Diagnosis and treatment of dermatofibrosarcoma protuberans. European consensus-based interdisciplinary guideline. Eur J Cancer 2015;51(17):2604–8.
6. Nakamura I, Kariya Y, Okada E, et al. A novel chromosomal translocation associated with COL1A2-PDGFB gene fusion in dermatofibrosarcoma protuberans: PDGF expression as a new diagnostic tool. JAMA Dermatol 2015;151(12):1330–7.
7. Paradisi A, Abeni D, Rusciani A, et al. Dermatofibrosarcoma protuberans: wide local excision vs. Mohs micrographic surgery. Cancer Treat Rev 2008;34: 728–36.
8. Shah KK, McHugh JB, Folpe AL, et al. Dermatofibrosarcoma protuberans of distal extremities and acral sites. Am J Surg Pathol 2018;42(3):413–9.
9. Ratner D, Thomas CO, Johnson TM, et al. Mohs micrographic surgery for the treatment of dermatofibrosarcoma protuberans: results of a multiinstitutional series with an analysis of the extent of microscopic spread. J Am Acad Dermatol 1997; 37(4):600–13.
10. Palmerini E, Gambarotti M, Staals EL, et al. Fibrosarcomatous changes and expression of CD34+ and apolipoprotein–D in dermatofibrosarcoma protuberans. Clin Sarcoma Res 2012;2:4.
11. Hoesly PM, Lowe GC, Lohse CM, et al. Prognostic impact of fibrosarcomatous transformation in dermatofibrosarcoma protuberans: a cohort study. J Am Acad Dermatol 2015;72:419–25.
12. Abbott JJ, Oliveira AM, Nascimento AG. The prognostic significance of fibrosarcomatous transformation in dermatofibrosarcoma protuberans. Am J Surg Pathol 2006;30:436–43.
13. Stacchiotti S, Pedeutour F, Negri T, et al. Dermatofibrosarcoma protuberans-derived fibrosarcoma: clinical history, biological profile and sensitivity to imatinib. Int J Cancer 2011;129:1761–72.
14. Serra-Guillén C, Llombart B, Nagore E, et al. High immunohistochemical nestin expression is associated with greater depth of infiltration in dermatofibrosarcoma protuberans: a study of 71 cases. J Cutan Pathol 2013;40(10):871–8.
15. Bandarchi B, Ma L, Marginean C, et al. D2-40, a novel immunohistochemical marker in differentiating dermatofibroma from dermatofibrosarcoma protuberans. Mod Pathol 2010;23:434–8.
16. Mori T, Misago N, Yamamoto O, et al. Expression of nestin in dermatofibrosarcoma protuberans in comparison to dermatofibroma. J Dermatol 2008;35(7): 419–25.

17. Sellheyer K, Nelson P, Patel RM. Expression of embryonic stem cell markers SOX2 and nestin in dermatofibrosarcoma protuberans and dermatofibroma. J Cutan Pathol 2011;38:415.

18. Sellheyer K, Nelson P, Krahl D. Dermatofibrosarcoma protuberans: a tumour of nestin-positive cutaneous mesenchymal stem cells? Br J Dermatol 2009;161(6):1317–22.

19. Acosta AE, Santa Vélez C. Dermatofibrosarcoma protuberans. Curr Treat Options Oncol 2017; 18(9):56.

20. Parker TL, Zitelli JA. Surgical margins for excision of dermatofibrosarcoma protuberans. J Am Acad Dermatol 1995;32:233–6.

21. Farma JM, Ammori JB, Zager JS, et al. Dermatofibrosarcoma protuberans: how wide should we resect? Ann Surg Oncol 2010;17:2112–8.

22. Fields RC, Hameed M, Qin LX, et al. Dermatofibrosarcoma protuberans (DFSP): predictors of recurrence and the use of systemic therapy. Ann Surg Oncol 2011;18:328–36.

23. Hersant B, May P, Battistella M, et al. Reducing surgical margins in dermatofibrosarcoma protuberans using the pathological analysis technique 'vertical modified technique': a 5-year experience. J Plast Reconstr Aesthet Surg 2013;66:617–22.

24. Woo KJ, Bang SI, Mun GH, et al. Long-term outcomes of surgical treatment for dermatofibrosarcoma protuberans according to width of gross resection margin. J Plast Reconstr Aesthet Surg 2016;69:395–401.

25. Criscito MC, Martires KJ, Stein JA. Prognostic factors, treatment, and survival in dermatofibrosarcoma protuberans. JAMA Dermatol 2016;152:1398–9.

26. Snow SN, Gordon EM, Larson PO, et al. Dermatofibrosarcoma protuberans: a report on 29 patients treated by Mohs micrographic surgery with long-term follow-up and review of the literature. Cancer 2004;101:28–38.

27. Lowe GC, Onajin O, Baum CL, et al. A comparison of Mohs micrographic surgery and wide local excision for treatment of dermatofibrosarcoma protuberans with long-term follow-up: the Mayo Clinic experience. Dermatol Surg 2017;43:98–106.

28. Massey RA, Tok J, Strippoli BA, et al. A comparison of frozen and paraffin sections in dermatofibrosarcoma protuberans. Dermatol Surg 1998;24(9): 995–8.

29. Garcia C, Viehman G, Hitchcock M, et al. Dermatofibrosarcoma protuberans treated with Mohs surgery. A case with CD34 immunostaining variability. Dermatol Surg 1996;22(2):177–9.

30. McArthur GA, Demetri GD, van Oosterom A, et al. Molecular and clinical analysis of locally advanced dermatofibrosarcoma protuberans treated with imatinib: Imatinib Target Exploration Consortium Study B2225. J Clin Oncol 2005;23(4):866–73.

31. Rutkowski P, Van Glabbeke M, Rankin CJ, et al. Imatinib mesylate in advanced dermatofibrosarcoma protuberans: pooled analysis of two phase II clinical trials. J Clin Oncol 2010;28(10):1772–9.

32. Rutkowski P, Debiec-Rychter M, Nowecki Z, et al. Treatment of advanced dermatofibrosarcoma protuberans with imatinib mesylate with or without surgical resection. J Eur Acad Dermatol Venereol 2011; 25(3):264–70.

33. Misset J, Kerob D, Porcher R, et al. Imatinib mesylate as a preoperative therapy in dermatofibrosarcoma: results of a multicentric phase II study on 25 patients. J Clin Oncol 2007;25(18_suppl):10032.

34. Ugurel S, Mentzel T, Utikal J, et al. Neoadjuvant imatinib in advanced primary or locally recurrent dermatofibrosarcoma protuberans: a multicenter phase II DeCOG trial with long-term follow-up. Clin Cancer Res 2014;20:499–510.

35. Fu Y, Kang H, Zhao H, et al. Sunitinib for patients with locally advanced or distantly metastatic dermatofibrosarcoma protuberans but resistant to imatinib. Int J Clin Exp Med 2015;8:8288–94.

Updates on Merkel Cell Carcinoma

Drew A. Emge, MD, MSc[a], Adela R. Cardones, MD, MHSc[b],*

KEYWORDS

• Merkel cell carcinoma • Cancer • Skin • Polyomavirus

KEY POINTS

• Merkel cell carcinoma is a rare cancer, but its incidence and mortality are increasing.
• Most Merkel cell carcinoma tumors are linked to the common Merkel cell Polyomavirus.
• Novel disease detection and monitoring could take advantage of Merkel cell Polyomavirus T-antigen oncoproteins, which have been found to correlate with disease activity.
• Ultraviolet radiation exposure and immunosuppressed state are important risk factors for Merkel cell carcinoma.
• Immunotherapy with programmed cell death ligand-1/programmed cell death protein-1 and cytotoxic T lymphocyte–associated protein 4 inhibitors is promising in late-stage Merkel cell carcinoma. Avelumab and pembrolizumab have recently been approved by the United States Food and Drug Administration for Merkel cell carcinoma. Clinical trials of immunotherapies are ongoing.

INTRODUCTION

Merkel cell carcinoma (MCC) is a rare, rapidly progressing, and difficult-to-treat neuroendocrine tumor of the skin that is associated with high mortality. In the last few decades, the medical community has made advances in the understanding of the epidemiology and pathophysiology of MCC. The Merkel cell polyomavirus (MCPyV) causes up to 80% of MCC tumors in North America and Europe, but advanced age, exposure to ultraviolet (UV) radiation, and immunosuppressed state are important risk factors.[1–15] Surgery, with or without adjuvant radiation therapy, remains the mainstay of treatment, but immunotherapies such as programmed cell death ligand-1 (PD-L1) and programmed cell death protein-1 (PD-1) inhibitors have recently shown promise in advanced disease and are now approved for advanced-stage MCC.[16–18] The focus of this article is the new and potential diagnostic and treatment modalities for MCC.

EPIDEMIOLOGY

MCC incidence is highest in the eighth decade of life.[2,12,13,19–22] Countries with growing percentages of the population more than 65 years old are likely to see an increase in the incidence of MCC in the coming years. This increase has been linked to prolonged exposure to risk factors that are associated with MCC,[20,23] as well as an altered immune system.[3,18,24–26]

UV radiation is a risk factor for MCC.[2,8,27] Tumors commonly appear on areas of skin with significant UV radiation exposure; the incidence of MCC correlates with UVB radiation index and other skin cancers resulting from sun exposure.[2,8,10,28,29] White patients are more commonly affected than other races.[2,8,12,20] Immunosuppressed patients, such as those with hematologic malignancies, acquired immunodeficiency syndrome (AIDS), autoimmune disease, and history of solid organ transplant, are at higher risk for developing MCC.[2,3,30–37]

Disclosure: The authors have nothing to disclose.
[a] Department of Dermatology, Duke University, Durham, NC, USA; [b] Department of Dermatology, Duke University, Duke Cancer Institute, Durham VA Medical Center, Durham, NC, USA
* Corresponding author. DUMC Box 3135, Room 3307, Purple Zone, Duke South, 200 Trent Drive, Durham, NC 27710.
E-mail address: adela.cardones@duke.edu

Dermatol Clin 37 (2019) 489–503
https://doi.org/10.1016/j.det.2019.06.002

Recent analyses of the Surveillance, Epidemiology, and End Results (SEER) registry in the United States revealed an incidence of 0.7 cases per 100,000 person years in 2013, a 95% annual increase since 2000.[20,38] The mortality per 100,000 people increased from 0.03 to 0.43 from 1986 to 2011.[20] Several European countries, Australia, and China have also seen increasing incidence of MCC in the past several decades.[9,39–42]

PATHOPHYSIOLOGY
Merkel Cell Polyomavirus

Nearly 80% of MCC in the United States and other northern hemisphere countries is associated with the ubiquitous MCPyV.[1,43] In contrast, only about 25% of MCC in Australia has been attributed to MCPyV.[4,44] The MCPyV integrates its DNA into the host cells' DNA, which results in aberrant oncogenic gene expression.[45] The retinoblastoma tumor suppressor protein (RB1) is inhibited by MCPyV integration, thereby causing MCC cell proliferation.[46] This pathway is specific to MCPyV but is not the only MCC-causing mutation.[46] An accumulation of inactivation mutations in the tumor suppressor gene, p53, have also been implicated in MCC pathogenesis.[47]

Ultraviolet Radiation

The remaining MCC is thought to be a result of UV exposure, because MCPyV-negative MCC cells show UV-associated DNA damage.[2,7,25,45] An array of loss-of-function mutations in the tumor suppressor, DNA repair, and activating genes have been implicated in MCPyV-negative MCC.[5,45] Many of these pathways, such as mammalian target of rapamycin (mTOR), are under investigation as potential targets for therapeutic agents.[48] The MCPyV-negative tumors have a higher mutational burden, neoantigen expression, and inactivation of tumor suppressor genes RB1 and p53.[49] However, no clinically significant difference in outcomes between MCPyV-positive and MCPyV-negative tumors has been identified at this time.

DIAGNOSIS
Clinical Appearance

MCC tumors are usually firm, painless, and rapidly growing, on the sun-exposed areas of the head, neck, or extremities[2] (**Fig. 1**). These tumors can be various shades of red, pink, or flesh colored.[2] The AEIOU (asymptomatic, expanding rapidly, immune suppression, older than 50 years, and UV-exposed location on a person with lighter skin

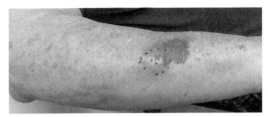

Fig. 1. MCC presenting as a smooth, bland nodule on the extensor, sun-exposed, forearm.

color) mnemonic is often used as a clinical tool to aid in diagnosis, because 89% of patients with MCC have at least 3 of the 5 characteristics.[2]

Histology, Pathology, and Immunohistochemistry

The diagnosis of MCC often requires incisional or excisional biopsy and confirmation by histology and immunohistochemistry.[50] The progenitor cell in MCC remains unidentified and controversial, but it is likely derived from a cell population such as dermal fibroblasts that enter the Merkel cell differentiation pathway before or during neoplastic transformation. The MCPyV can infect dermal fibroblasts, whereas UV radiation induces the signaling pathway that stimulates the expression of genes in fibroblasts that are responsible for encoding matrix metalloproteinases driving MCC development.[51]

The MCC's nodular growth involves the dermis and subcutaneous tissue.[52] High-grade neuroendocrine morphologic features such as undifferentiated small round blue cells with large lobulated nuclei and scant cytoplasm, high mitotic figures and apoptotic bodies, and necrosis are seen on hematoxylin-eosin (H&E) staining (**Figs. 2** and **3**).[53–55] Expression of cytokeratin-20 (CK20) in a

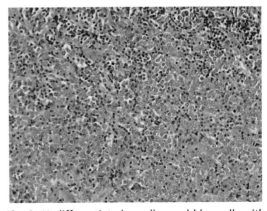

Fig. 2. Undifferentiated, small round blue cells with large lobulated nuclei and scant cytoplasm, high mitotic figures, and apoptotic bodies (H&E, original magnification ×200).

punctate pattern (**Fig. 4**) and neuroendocrine markers such as neuron-specific enolase, synaptophysin (**Fig. 5**), and chromogranin A are characteristic of MCC on immunohistochemistry.[55–60] Electron microscopy shows characteristic neurosecretory granules within cytoplasmic extensions.[61]

The American Joint Committee on Cancer (AJCC), the College of American Pathologists (CAP), and the National Comprehensive Cancer Network (NCCN), recommend that pathology reports contain the minimum needed for oncologists to determine the T of the tumor, node, metastasis (TNM) staging system: maximum tumor dimension less than or equal to or greater than 2 cm and invasion into bone, muscle, fascia, or cartilage.[62] The CAP and NCCN make further recommendations on reporting other details of the biopsy specimen, including but not limited to peripheral and deep margins, Breslow depth, and mitotic rate.[16,63] At this time, the value of factors such as Breslow depth and mitotic rate have yet to be fully determined.

Detection of Merkel Cell Polyomavirus

The MCPyV can be detected through standard techniques such as polymerase chain reaction (PCR) or immunohistochemistry.[49,64] Antibodies to the MCPyV viral capsid reflect prior exposure to the virus but do not necessarily indicate tumor formation or burden.[65–67]

The MCPyV-associated MCC cells persistently express T-antigen (T-Ag) oncoproteins that are thought to be required for cell proliferation and viral replication.[68–70] The T-Ag is specific to MCC and may be a useful indicator of disease status.[65,71] The small T-Ag promotes transcription and gene expression to transform fibroblasts.[72]

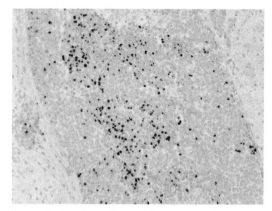

Fig. 4. Expression of CK20 in a punctate pattern, which appears brown (CK20, original magnification ×200).

The large T-Ag is thought to promote cell division in MCC through inhibition of the tumor suppressor, RB1, thereby leading to tumor progression and proliferation.[73–75] Testing for T-Ag may be considered in the initial management of MCC based on updated NCCN guidelines.[16]

Potential Diagnostic Tools for Merkel Cell Carcinoma

There are several assays that could be more specific than immunohistochemistry or PCR techniques in detecting MCPyV. The RNA in situ hybridization (RNA-ISH) technique, targeting MCPyV T-Ag transcripts on tissue microarrays and whole-tissue sections, was 100% sensitive and specific in detecting MCPyV in 57 confirmed MCC samples.[76] Next-generation sequencing (NSG) can confirm the presence of tumor-specific MCPyV.[77] Neither RNA-ISH nor NSG have been integrated into current recommendations on MCC diagnosis but both have the

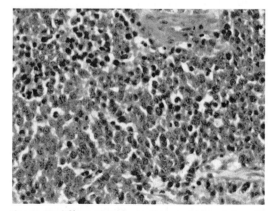

Fig. 3. Undifferentiated, small round blue cells with large lobulated nuclei and scant cytoplasm, high mitotic figures, and apoptotic bodies (H&E, original magnification ×400).

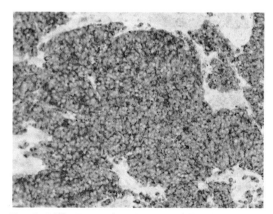

Fig. 5. Diffuse cytoplasmic synaptophysin (immunoperoxidase, original magnification ×200).

potential to improve MCC diagnosis on old and new tissue samples.

A recent study described MCPyV-derived peptide–major histocompatibility complex (MHC) multimers on cytotoxic CD8+ lymphocytes that are specific to patients with MCC compared with healthy controls.[78] High-throughput screening techniques that identify these multimers allow the mapping of cancer-specific T cells and could be used to recognize and treat MCC.[79]

In addition, microRNAs (small, noncoding RNA molecules involved in silencing and posttranscriptional regulation of gene expression) can be overexpressed by cancers such as MCC.[80] Circulating cell-free miR-375 can distinguish patients with and without MCC tumors and is a potential surrogate marker of disease activity regardless of MCPyV status.[81] Repeated miR-375 quantification throughout the patients' therapeutic interventions reflected the dynamic change in tumor burden when correlated to PET/computed tomography (CT) imaging.[81]

PROGNOSTIC FACTORS
Patient-Related Characteristics

MCC is a highly aggressive tumor. Older age, male gender, black race, advanced stage or increasing number of metastatic sites, primary tumor on the head/neck or trunk, and immunosuppression are associated with lower survival rates.[12,14,82–85] Pathologic, rather than clinical, node involvement is associated with poorer prognosis.[10,83,86–88]

Patients living in areas with an increased density of dermatologists were more likely to survive than those in areas without dermatologists.[89] These areas also have a higher median household income, are more metropolitan, and have increased density of hospitals, primary care physicians, and oncologists.[89]

Pathophysiologic Factors

Increasing size, infiltrative versus nodular tumor growth pattern, and lymph node involvement have also been associated with lower survival rates.[52,83] Evidence is conflicting on how MCPyV infection and tumor depth of invasion at initial biopsy relate to prognosis.[49,73,83,90–92]

Merkel Cell Polyomavirus Oncoprotein (T Antigen) Antibodies

An immunologic response to the MCPyV (T-Ag) oncoproteins may be important in primary tumor regression. High titers of antibodies to T-Ag at diagnosis have been associated with decreased recurrence and increased survival.[66,71,93,94] Serial

evaluation showed that T-Ag antibody titers decreased in patients who were treated for MCC and did not have cancer recurrence.[65,66,71,93] In addition, T-Ag antibody titers increased rapidly in those with progressive, metastatic disease before clinical detection and had a positive predictive value of 66% for clinically evident disease recurrence.[65,71]

Other Immune Response to Merkel Cell Carcinoma

Cytotoxic CD8+ T lymphocytes have been found in the MCC tumor microenvironment.[11,78,95–97] The presence of these tumor-infiltrating lymphocytes (TILs) indicates high tumor immunogenicity and confers a survival benefit.[3,24,98–100] Augmenting the natural role of TILs in MCC disease progression provides the potential for future therapeutics in MCC.

Immunohistochemistry

There are currently no standard prognostic immunohistologic markers for MCC, but there are potential candidates. Tumor protein p63, cell survival protein Bcl-2, and calcium-dependent intercellular adhesion protein E-cadherin have been investigated. The results of such studies have been mixed. Although p63 expression has overall been shown to portend lower survival than when it is absent, studies have shown variable clinical and statistical strength between p63 positivity and lower rates of survival.[90,91,101–103] There is less evidence supporting the roles of Bcl-2 and E-cadherin in disease progression, recurrence, or survival.[104–106] The oncogene survivin, which inhibits apoptosis, and chemokine receptor, CXCR4, are potential markers of tumor progression in MCC but need further investigation.[106–108]

A recent study has shown that enhancer of zeste homolog 2 (EZH2), a histone methyltransferase that influences tumorigenesis by epigenetic silencing, is aberrantly expressed in MCC tumors.[109–111] Nodal metastases had higher expression of EZH2 compared with the primary tumors.[112] Higher expression of EZH2 was associated with disease progression and worse outcome.[112] Inhibition of this oncogene is a potential target for therapy.

Staging

Recently, the AJCC released the eighth edition of its Manual for Cancer Staging. The manual includes updates on MCC. Patients with MCC are now characterized by the extent of the disease at diagnosis and whether or not there is clinical or pathologic involvement for more accurate determination of recurrence rates and survival probability. There is also now a distinction in staging based on whether the primary tumor is known or unknown.[113]

Imaging

The role of imaging in MCC has yet to be fully defined. Work-up and monitoring of MCC may include imaging when clinically indicated for suspected metastatic or unresectable disease.[16] MRI, CT, and PET-CT are the most common imaging modalities used in MCC. Although MCC can be detected in many anatomic locations by these imaging modalities, not all MCC tumors are detected. Studies have shown that imaging with MRI, CT, or PET-CT affects MCC staging and can influence management decisions in some cases, including radiation field placement and dose selection.[114-117] However, generalizable data are lacking on the sensitivity and specificity of imaging, as well as the utility of imaging in clinical management decisions and disease outcomes. Imaging remains secondary to sentinel lymph node biopsy (SLNB) for staging at this time because of its inability to identify subclinical nodal disease.

Sentinel Lymph Node Biopsy

SLNB is recommended for all patients who are able to tolerate the procedure[16] because of the large proportion of patients with metastasis at presentation and SLNB's ability to detect pathologic nodal involvement.[10,16,50,87,88,118] However, the current NCCN[16] recommendations on management and treatment are still based on clinically detectable nodal involvement because of conflicting evidence on the survival benefit of SLNB in patients without clinical nodal involvement.[14,119]

MANAGEMENT
Surgery

MCC requires a multidisciplinary approach to care, which involves dermatologists, medical and radiation oncologists, pathologists, and surgeons.[120] The goal of surgical treatment is negative histologic margin.[16] Surgical excision with 1-cm to 2-cm margins remains the preferred first step in the management and treatment of the primary tumor.[16,50] Mohs micrographic surgery (MMS) can be considered when tissue sparing and/or a more comprehensive histologic evaluation of margins is required.[121,122] Retrospective analyses of data from the National Comprehensive Database (NCDB) suggest no difference in the overall and relative survival of patients with stage I to II MCC who were treated with wide local excision versus MMS.[123,124] Larger cohorts and prospective studies are needed to determine the optimal surgical treatment choice for early-stage MCC.

Radiotherapy

Radiotherapy (RT) has a significant role in MCC treatment, but the full benefit of radiation therapy has yet to be defined. Radiation monotherapy is inferior to surgical resection because of the risk of distant MCC recurrence,[125-128] but it can be used when surgery is contraindicated[125-127,129-135] and for palliation in metastatic disease.[132,133,136-138]

Conflicting data exist on the survival benefit from adjuvant radiation in early-stage MCC with or without local lymphatic invasion or a positive SLNB.[14,50,128,133,139-148] A large, single-center retrospective study showed low rates of regional recurrence and no survival benefit of adjuvant RT among SLNB-negative patients.[149] However, a more recent, retrospective study using the NCDB showed improved survival among patients with stage I to II disease who were treated with wide local excision (WLE) and chemotherapy plus radiation (CRT) compared with those who had WLE, with or without chemotherapy, but no RT.[123] Survival of patients with head and neck MCC who were treated with WLE and CRT or RT was superior to that of patients who underwent excision alone.[84] Current NCCN guidelines recommend patients with MCC have either postoperative adjuvant radiation therapy for the primary tumor site or observation alone if the SLNB is negative.[16]

Adjuvant radiation therapy can be applied to the primary site plus draining nodal basin if the SLNB is positive and lymph node dissection is positive.[16] Adjuvant radiation has been applied in immunosuppressed patients or if the patient has extensive lymphovascular invasion.[150] The NCCN recommends considering adjuvant radiation therapy if the SLNB is not done, the SLNB is not successful, or lymphovascular invasion is confirmed by fine-needle aspiration or core biopsy.[16]

Adjuvant chemoradiation is not currently recommended for localized disease, although some investigators suggest it may be beneficial.[84] In advanced-stage disease, adjuvant radiation therapy is recommended on a case-by-case basis because it has failed to provide a universal benefit.[143] However, for widely metastatic disease, adjuvant chemoradiation is not widely accepted as beneficial and toxicities are common.[114,151-153] Adjuvant radiation with immunotherapy might be beneficial as a short course in widely metastatic disease.[154-156]

Chemotherapy

Chemotherapy with a platinum-based agent combined with etoposide or taxanes and anthracyclines alone or in combination have been shown to be initially effective in a wide range (20%–75%) of patients but does not produce a lasting response and lacks a survival benefit; the median progression-free survival is a mere 3 to 8 months, and duration of partial response is only 3 months for first-line therapy.[50,139,143,157–162] However, late-stage disease traditionally involved cytotoxic chemotherapy and referral for clinical trial because other evidence-based treatment options were limited.[50,161] Chemotherapy is now only suggested to be considered in patients who are not candidates for immunotherapy.[16]

Immunotherapy

Immunotherapies that target the immune checkpoint pathway have emerged as effective, evidence-based treatments for MCC. MCC cells upregulate the PD-1/PD-L1 axis through the oncogenic mutations that are linked to both MCPyV integration and UV radiation damage.[5,44,96,163–165] Avelumab is now approved as first-line therapy for advanced MCC in the United States, Canada, Australia, the European Union, Norway, Iceland, and Japan.[166]

AVELUMAB
JAVELIN Merkel 200 Trial

Avelumab, a human monoclonal antibody that inhibits PD-L1, has been approved by the US Food and Drug Administration (FDA), European Union, Canada, and Japan for the treatment of advanced MCC based on the JAVELIN Merkel 200 trial,[18] a phase II, open-label, multicenter trial investigating the clinical activity and safety of avelumab in patients with MCC. Twenty-eight of 88 patients with stage IV MCC who had previously received chemotherapy, or 31.8% (95% confidence interval [CI], 21.9–43.1), had objective responses, defined as either partial or complete response, over approximately 10.4 months of follow-up.[18] The 6-month estimate of avelumab durability was 92% compared with 6% to 7% of patients who were treated with chemotherapy in observational studies.[160]

The same trial is evaluating the clinical activity and safety of avelumab as first-line therapy for patients with stage IV MCC.[17] In a preplanned interim analysis of 29 patients, the confirmed objective response rate (ORR) was 62.1% (95% CI, 42.3%–79.3%); 14 of 18 (77.8%) responses were ongoing at the time of analysis.[17] Nearly all of the patients had a good duration of response: 93% (95% CI, 61%–99%) of patients had at least 3 months and 83% (95% CI, 46%–96%) had at least 6 months of response.[17] Overall, avelumab was found to have earlier responses, higher response rates, and a more manageable safety profile compared with the traditional cytotoxic chemotherapies.[17,18]

An update of the JAVELIN Merkel 200 trial was presented at the American Society of Clinical Oncology's annual meeting in June 2018. With more than 2 years of follow-up, avelumab showed continued durable responses and meaningful survival outcomes.[167] In 88 patients, the confirmed ORR was 33% (95% CI, 23.3–43.8) and progression-free survival was 26% to 29% through 2 years.[167]

Other Avelumab Trials

The Adjuvant Avelumab in Merkel Cell Cancer (ADAM) trial is evaluating the clinical activity of avelumab after definitive therapy with surgery with or without adjuvant radiation (NCT03271372). Other studies are investigating the use of avelumab and radiation or interferon beta, with or without adoptive transfer of MCPyV T-Ag–specific polyclonal autologous CD8+ T cells, for metastatic MCC (NCT02584829). In addition, recruiting is ongoing in a phase Ib/II study investigating avelumab, bevacizumab, and other agents, such as 5-fluorouracil, as a combination therapy in patients with MCC who have progressed on or after anti–PD-L1 therapy (NCT03167164).

Pembrolizumab

The PD-1 inhibitor, pembrolizumab, has recently been granted approval by the FDA for adult and pediatric patients with recurrent locally advanced or metastatic MCC.[168] Pembrolizumab has been shown to be highly effective in a phase II, noncontrolled study of adults with advanced MCC who had received no previous systemic therapy.[25] There was an ORR of 56% (95% CI, 35–76), with responses observed in patients with MCPyV-positive and MCPyV-negative tumors.[25] The response duration ranged from 2.2 to 9.7 months.[25] The rate of progression-free survival at 6 months was 67% (95% CI, 49–86).[25]

Preliminary data from a phase II multicenter study investigating pembrolizumab as a first-line systemic therapy for patients with unresectable or metastatic MCC (NCT02267603) showed an ORR of 50% (95% CI, 34.2–65.8) among 42 patients with at least a 21-week follow-up. A complete response was seen in 19% of patients and a partial response was seen in 31%.[169] The overall survival (OS) rate at 18 months was 68%, which was higher than in control patients receiving chemotherapy.[169]

Nivolumab

Nivolumab, another PD-1 inhibitor, is also under investigation as a potential therapy for metastatic MCC. Preliminary results suggest that nivolumab alone and in combination with ipilimumab, relatlimab, and daratumumab in virus-associated MCC tumors can induce a durable and rapid regression (NCT02488759).[170] Nivolumab is also being investigated in combination with ipilimumab, a cytotoxic T lymphocyte–associated protein 4 (CTLA-4) inhibitor, both with and without stereotactic body radiation therapy (NCT03071406). Nivolumab is also being investigated and compared with ipilimumab and observation as an adjuvant therapy for completely resected MCC (NCT02196961). These trials are either recruiting or underway.

Ipilimumab, Tremelimumab/Durvalumab, and Utomilumab

Ipilimumab disrupts the CTLA-4 receptors on cytotoxic T lymphocytes, thereby potentiating an antitumor response.[171] Ipilimumab could be a promising treatment of MCC in boosting the immune response, particularly in cases in which PD-1 blockade has been ineffective. Ipilimumab is currently undergoing investigation in multiple clinical trials, as previously mentioned.[165,172]

There is also a new phase I/II trial of which the focus is metastatic solid tumors such as MCC using the CTLA-4 inhibitor, tremelimumab, and PD-L1 inhibitor, durvalumab (NCT02643303). These immunotherapies are combined with poly-lysine and carboxymethylcellulose (poly-ICLC), a toll-like receptor-3 ligand. In addition, utomilumab, an agonist of cluster of differentiation (CD) 137 (4-1BB) that stimulates antitumor immunity, has been shown to be well tolerated in a phase I trial that is currently ongoing (NCT01307267).[173]

Drawbacks to Immunotherapy

A significant proportion of patients with advanced MCC fail to respond to PD-L1/PD-1 inhibition.[17,18,25] Failure to respond with immunotherapies could be caused by immune reactivity within the tumor, which is based on the frequency of TIL and PD-L1 expression. A high number of TILs and high expression of PD-L1 by the MCC cells could be more immune resistant because their mutation burden is higher.[5–7,45,48,174,175]

A potential work-around to boost the effectiveness of immunotherapies could be targeting the immune escape mechanisms of MCC. For instance, there are epigenetic changes in histone acetylation after MCPyV viral integration into the human cells; this malignant transformation inhibits or halts the expression of MHC class I chain-related protein (MIC), which signals distress to immune cells.[176] Impairing histone changes by inhibiting histone deacetylases (HDACs) reinduces MIC expression, which could boost the natural immune response against MCC by HDAC inhibitors.[176]

Potential and Pipeline Therapies

Other treatment modalities under investigation as either single or adjuvant therapy for MCC include Toll-like receptor antagonists,[177] interleukin (IL)-12,[172,178] and inhibitors of the mTOR pathway.[179,180] Tyrosine kinase inhibitors (TKIs) such as cabozantinib, pazopanib, and imatinib have had mixed and disappointing results.[181–186]

Cytotoxic cluster of differentiation 8+ T lymphocytes

Harnessing the cytotoxic CD8+ T lymphocytes in the fight against MCC has great potential. A phase I/II trial of localized radiation therapy or recombinant interferon beta and avelumab with or without cellular adoptive immunotherapy in metastatic MCC has recently concluded (NCT02584829).[187] The investigators used ex vivo expanded MCPyV-specific T cells plus human leukocyte antigen (HLA) upregulation (radiation or interferon) with (triple therapy) and without (double therapy) avelumab in 4 patients.[187] All participants had objective responses.[187]

An additional phase I/II trial is also currently underway using autologous, tumor-infiltrating, polyclonal lymphocytes that are MCPyV T-Ag specific (NCT01758458). The lymphocytes, in conjunction with recombinant interferon beta and RT, are used to stimulate the host's immune system. A case report has described 1 patient's favorable response to this therapy.[188]

Natural killer cells

Natural killer (NK) cells are a subset of cytotoxic T lymphocytes that attack cells with aberrant expression of their antigen-presenting HLA class I molecules.[189] A subset of activated NK (aNK) cells derived from a human IL-2–dependent NK cell line have been shown to have antitumor effects ex vivo.[190] A recent phase II trial using aNK cells and modified IL-15 has reported that the initial 3 patients had no major toxicities, with at least 1 patient having a partial response and clinical resolution of macroscopic MCC tumors (NCT02465957).[191] Participants in this study had few toxicities. One participant who had previously failed PD-1 inhibitor therapy had a response to the aNK.[191] This therapy may be a solution for patients who have contraindications to or fail immunotherapies such as PD-L1/PD-1 inhibitors.

Somatostatin Analogues

Many MCC tumors have been found to have somatostatin receptors regardless of MCPyV status.[192,193] Cases of MCC successfully treated with radiolabeled and nonradiolabeled somatostatin analogues lanreotide, pasireotide, and octreotide have been reported,[194,195] and it has been suggested that somatostatin analogues could be beneficial in combination with TKIs.[186] In a phase I study, octreotide in combination with cixutumumab, an insulinlike growth factor 1 receptor, and everolimus was not tolerated well in participants despite most having stable disease.[196] Results from clinical trials on somatostatin analogues are either underway or have recently been completed (NCT02351128, NCT01652547, NCT01237457, NCT02936323). Results of these trials have yet to be published.

Oncolytic Viruses

Several phase II studies are currently recruiting patients to investigate intralesional talimogene laherparepvec (T-VEC) with or without hypofractionated RT and nivolumab, respectively (NCT02819843 and NCT02978625). The T-VEC is a modified herpes simplex virus type 1 that has been designed to select, replicate in, lyse, and promote tumor cell immunity.[197] It has shown promise in melanoma but has yet to be tested in MCC.[198]

SUMMARY

In summary, MCC is a rare and aggressive cancer with increasing incidence. There have been many advances in the last several decades in the etiology and management of MCC, but much about its natural history and most effective treatment remains unknown. Surgical excision with margins of 1 to 2 cm remains the recommended first-line therapy for early-stage disease, but larger, prospective studies are needed to confirm the potential benefits and role of MMS. Robust evidence supporting immunotherapy for patients with advanced disease has led to recent approval of immune checkpoint inhibitors in the treatment of advanced MCC. However, immunotherapies are not effective or not tolerated in a minor subset of patients. The need remains for additional adjuvant therapies.

REFERENCES

1. Feng H, Shuda M, Chang Y, et al. Clonal integration of a polyomavirus in human Merkel cell carcinoma. Science 2008;319(5866):1096–100.
2. Heath M, Jaimes N, Lemos B, et al. Clinical characteristics of Merkel cell carcinoma at diagnosis in 195 patients: the AEIOU features. J Am Acad Dermatol 2008;58(3):375–81.
3. Paulson KG, Iyer JG, Blom A, et al. Systemic immune suppression predicts diminished merkel cell carcinoma–specific survival independent of stage. J Invest Dermatol 2013;133(3):642–6.
4. Garneski KM, Warcola AH, Feng Q, et al. Merkel cell polyomavirus is more frequently present in North American than Australian Merkel cell carcinoma tumors. J Invest Dermatol 2009;129(1):246.
5. Goh G, Walradt T, Markarov V, et al. Mutational landscape of MCPyV-positive and MCPyV-negative Merkel cell carcinomas with implications for immunotherapy. Oncotarget 2016;7(3):3403.
6. Harms PW, Vats P, Verhaegen ME, et al. The distinctive mutational spectra of polyomavirus-negative merkel cell carcinoma. Cancer Res 2015;75(18):3720–7.
7. Wong SQ, Waldeck K, Vergara IA, et al. UV-associated mutations underlie the etiology of MCV-negative merkel cell carcinomas. Cancer Res 2015;75(24):5228–34.
8. Agelli M, Clegg LX. Epidemiology of primary Merkel cell carcinoma in the United States. J Am Acad Dermatol 2003;49(5):832–41.
9. Youlden DR, Soyer HP, Youl PH, et al. Incidence and survival for Merkel cell carcinoma in Queensland, Australia, 1993-2010. JAMA Dermatol 2014; 150(8):864–72.
10. Lemos BD, Storer BE, Iyer JG, et al. Pathologic nodal evaluation improves prognostic accuracy in Merkel cell carcinoma: analysis of 5823 cases as the basis of the first consensus staging system. J Am Acad Dermatol 2010;63(5):751–61.
11. Miller NJ, Church CD, Dong L, et al. Tumor-infiltrating merkel cell polyomavirus-specific T cells are diverse and associated with improved patient survival. Cancer Immunol Res 2017;5(2):137–47.
12. Tarantola TI, Vallow LA, Halyard MY, et al. Prognostic factors in Merkel cell carcinoma: analysis of 240 cases. J Am Acad Dermatol 2013;68(3): 425–32.
13. Albores-Saavedra J, Batich K, Chable-Montero F, et al. Merkel cell carcinoma demographics, morphology, and survival based on 3870 cases: a population based study. J Cutan Pathol 2010; 37(1):20–7.
14. Sridharan V, Muralidhar V, Margalit DN, et al. Merkel cell carcinoma: a population analysis on survival. J Natl Compr Canc Netw 2016;14(10): 1247–57.
15. Ezaldein HH, Ventura A, DeRuyter NP, et al. Understanding the influence of patient demographics on disease severity, treatment strategy, and survival outcomes in merkel cell carcinoma: a surveillance,

epidemiology, and end-results study. Oncoscience 2017;4(7–8):106–14.

16. Bichakjian CK, Olencki T, Aasi SZ, et al. Merkel cell carcinoma, Version 1.2018, NCCN clinical practice guidelines in oncology. J Natl Compr Canc Netw 2018;16(6):742–74.

17. D'Angelo SP, Russell J, Lebbe C, et al. Efficacy and safety of first-line avelumab treatment in patients with stage iv metastatic merkel cell carcinoma: a preplanned interim analysis of a clinical trial. JAMA Oncol 2018;4(9):e180077.

18. Kaufman HL, Russell J, Hamid O, et al. Avelumab in patients with chemotherapy-refractory metastatic Merkel cell carcinoma: a multicentre, single-group, open-label, phase 2 trial. Lancet Oncol 2016;17(10):1374–85.

19. Hodgson NC. Merkel cell carcinoma: changing incidence trends. J Surg Oncol 2005;89(1):1–4.

20. Fitzgerald TL, Dennis S, Kachare SD, et al. Dramatic Increase in the Incidence and Mortality from Merkel Cell Carcinoma in the United States. Am Surg 2015;81(8):802–6.

21. Reichgelt BA, Visser O. Epidemiology and survival of Merkel cell carcinoma in the Netherlands. A population-based study of 808 cases in 1993–2007. Eur J Cancer 2011;47(4):579–85.

22. Girschik J, Thorn K, Beer TW, et al. Merkel cell carcinoma in Western Australia: a population-based study of incidence and survival. Br J Dermatol 2011;165(5):1051–7.

23. Colby SL, Ortman JM. Projections of the size and composition of the US population: 2014 to 2060: population estimates and projections. Washington, DC: United States Department of Commerce; 2017.

24. Paulson KG, Iyer JG, Simonson WT, et al. CD8+ lymphocyte intratumoral infiltration as a stage-independent predictor of Merkel cell carcinoma survival: a population-based study. Am J Clin Pathol 2014;142(4):452–8.

25. Nghiem PT, Bhatia S, Lipson EJ, et al. PD-1 blockade with pembrolizumab in advanced merkel-cell carcinoma. N Engl J Med 2016; 374(26):2542–52.

26. Goronzy JJ, Weyand CM. Understanding immunosenescence to improve responses to vaccines. Nat Immunol 2013;14:428.

27. Lunder EJ, Stern RS. Merkel-cell carcinomas in patients treated with methoxsalen and ultraviolet A radiation. N Engl J Med 1998;339(17):1247–8.

28. Howard RA, Dores GM, Curtis RE, et al. Merkel cell carcinoma and multiple primary cancers. Cancer Epidemiol Biomarkers Prev 2006;15(8):1545–9.

29. Popp S, Waltering S, Herbst C, et al. UV-B-type mutations and chromosomal imbalances indicate common pathways for the development of Merkel and skin squamous cell carcinomas. Int J Cancer 2002;99(3):352–60.

30. Engels EA, Frisch M, Goedert JJ, et al. Merkel cell carcinoma and HIV infection. Lancet 2002; 359(9305):497–8.

31. Vlad R, Woodlock TJ. Merkel cell carcinoma after chronic lymphocytic leukemia: case report and literature review. Am J Clin Oncol 2003;26(6):531–4.

32. Buell J, Trofe J, Hanaway M, et al. Immunosuppression and Merkel cell cancer. Paper presented at: Transplant Proc 2002;34(5):1780–1. Available at: http://www.sciencedirect.com/science/article/pii/S0041134502030658. Accessed August 1.

33. Penn I, First MR. Merkel's cell carcinoma in organ recipients: report of 41 cases. Transplantation 1999;68(11):1717–21.

34. Kassem A, Technau K, Kurz AK, et al. Merkel cell polyomavirus sequences are frequently detected in nonmelanoma skin cancer of immunosuppressed patients. Int J Cancer 2009;125(2):356–61.

35. Lanoy E, Dores GM, Madeleine MM, et al. Epidemiology of non-keratinocytic skin cancers among persons with acquired immunodeficiency syndrome in the US. AIDS 2009;23(3):385.

36. Sahi H, Sihto H, Artama M, et al. History of chronic inflammatory disorders increases the risk of Merkel cell carcinoma, but does not correlate with Merkel cell polyomavirus infection. Br J Cancer 2017; 116(2):260–4.

37. Koljonen V, Sahi H, Bohling T, et al. Post-transplant Merkel Cell Carcinoma. Acta Derm Venereol 2016; 96(4):442–7.

38. Paulson KG, Park SY, Vandeven NA, et al. Merkel cell carcinoma: Current US incidence and projected increases based on changing demographics. J Am Acad Dermatol 2018;78(3): 457–63.e2.

39. Fondain M, Du Thanh A, Bessaoud F, et al. Epidemiological trends in Merkel cell carcinoma in southern France: a registry-based study. Br J Dermatol 2017;176(5):1379–81.

40. Zaar O, Gillstedt M, Lindelöf B, et al. Merkel cell carcinoma incidence is increasing in Sweden. J Eur Acad Dermatol Venereol 2016;30(10): 1708–13.

41. Eisemann N, Jansen L, Castro FA, et al. Survival with nonmelanoma skin cancer in Germany. Br J Dermatol 2016;174(4):778–85.

42. Song PI, Liang H, Wei W-Q, et al. The clinical profile of Merkel cell carcinoma in mainland China. Int J Dermatol 2012;51(9):1054–9.

43. Becker JC, Houben R, Ugurel S, et al. MC polyomavirus is frequently present in Merkel cell carcinoma of European patients. J Invest Dermatol 2009;129(1):248–50.

44. Schadendorf D, Nghiem P, Bhatia S, et al. Immune evasion mechanisms and immune checkpoint inhibition in advanced merkel cell carcinoma. Oncoimmunology 2017;6(10):e1338237.

45. Erstad DJ, Cusack JC Jr. Mutational analysis of merkel cell carcinoma. Cancers (Basel) 2014;6(4): 2116–36.

46. Hesbacher S, Pfitzer L, Wiedorfer K, et al. RB1 is the crucial target of the Merkel cell polyomavirus Large T antigen in Merkel cell carcinoma cells. Oncotarget 2016;7(22):32956–68.

47. Starrett GJ, Marcelus C, Cantalupo PG, et al. Merkel cell polyomavirus exhibits dominant control of the tumor genome and transcriptome in virus-associated merkel cell carcinoma. MBio 2017;8(1) [pii:e02079-16].

48. Cohen PR, Tomson BN, Elkin SK, et al. Genomic portfolio of Merkel cell carcinoma as determined by comprehensive genomic profiling: implications for targeted therapeutics. Oncotarget 2016;7(17): 23454–67.

49. Moshiri AS, Doumani R, Yelistratova L, et al. Polyomavirus-negative merkel cell carcinoma: a more aggressive subtype based on analysis of 282 cases using multimodal tumor virus detection. J Invest Dermatol 2017;137(4):819–27.

50. Lebbe C, Becker JC, Grob J-J, et al. Diagnosis and treatment of Merkel Cell Carcinoma. European consensus-based interdisciplinary guideline. Eur J Cancer 2015;51(16):2396–403.

51. Liu W, Yang R, Payne AS, et al. Identifying the target cells and mechanisms of merkel cell polyomavirus infection. Cell Host Microbe 2016;19(6): 775–87.

52. Andea AA, Coit DG, Amin B, et al. Merkel cell carcinoma. Cancer 2008;113(9):2549–58.

53. Fried I, Cerroni L. Merkel cell carcinoma. Pathologe 2014;35(5):467–75 [in German].

54. Skelton HG, Smith KJ, Hitchcock CL, et al. Merkel cell carcinoma: analysis of clinical, histologic, and immunohistologic features of 132 cases with relation to survival. J Am Acad Dermatol 1997;37(5 Pt 1):734–9.

55. Llombart B, Monteagudo C, Lopez-Guerrero J, et al. Clinicopathological and immunohistochemical analysis of 20 cases of Merkel cell carcinoma in search of prognostic markers. Histopathology 2005;46(6):622–34.

56. Tilling T, Wladykowski E, Failla AV, et al. Immunohistochemical analyses point to epidermal origin of human Merkel cells. Histochem Cell Biol 2014; 141(4):407–21.

57. Chan JK, Suster S, Wenig BM, et al. Cytokeratin 20 immunoreactivity distinguishes Merkel cell (primary cutaneous neuroendocrine) carcinomas and salivary gland small cell carcinomas from small cell carcinomas of various sites. Am J Surg Pathol 1997;21(2):226–34.

58. Fantini F, Johansson O. Neurochemical markers in human cutaneous Merkel cells. An immunohistochemical investigation. Exp Dermatol 1995;4(6):365–71.

59. Heenan PJ, Cole JM, Spagnolo DV. Primary cutaneous neuroendocrine carcinoma (Merkel cell tumor). An adnexal epithelial neoplasm. Am J Dermatopathol 1990;12(1):7–16.

60. Gu J, Polak JM, Van Noorden S, et al. Immunostaining of neuron-specific enolase as a diagnostic tool for Merkel cell tumors. Cancer 1983;52(6):1039–43.

61. Goepfert H, Remmler D, Silva E, et al. Merkel cell carcinoma (endocrine carcinoma of the skin) of the head and neck. Arch Otolaryngol 1984; 110(11):707–12.

62. Amin MB, Greene FL, Edge SB, et al. The Eighth Edition AJCC Cancer Staging Manual: Continuing to build a bridge from a population-based to a more "personalized" approach to cancer staging. CA Cancer J Clin 2017;67(2):93–9.

63. Smoller B, Bichakjian C, Brown J, et al. Protocol for the examination of specimens from patients with Merkel cell carcinoma of the skin, version 4.0.0.1. College of American Pathologists Cancer Protocol Templates; 2017. Available at: https://www. cap.org/protocols-and-guidelines/cancer-reporting-tools/cancer-protocol-templates.

64. Tolstov YL, Pastrana DV, Feng H, et al. Human Merkel cell polyomavirus infection II. MCV is a common human infection that can be detected by conformational capsid epitope immunoassays. Int J Cancer 2009;125(6):1250–6.

65. Paulson KG, Carter JJ, Johnson LG, et al. Antibodies to merkel cell polyomavirus T antigen oncoproteins reflect tumor burden in merkel cell carcinoma patients. Cancer Res 2010;70(21): 8388–97.

66. Samimi M, Molet L, Fleury M, et al. Prognostic value of antibodies to Merkel cell polyomavirus T antigens and VP1 protein in patients with Merkel cell carcinoma. Br J Dermatol 2016;174(4):813–22.

67. Pastrana DV, Tolstov YL, Becker JC, et al. Quantitation of human seroresponsiveness to Merkel cell polyomavirus. PLoS Pathog 2009;5(9):e1000578.

68. Vandeven N, Nghiem P. Rationale for immune-based therapies in Merkel polyomavirus-positive and -negative Merkel cell carcinomas. Immunotherapy 2016;8(8):907–21.

69. Houben R, Shuda M, Weinkam R, et al. Merkel cell polyomavirus-infected Merkel cell carcinoma cells require expression of viral T antigens. J Virol 2010;84(14):7064–72.

70. Shuda M, Arora R, Kwun HJ, et al. Human Merkel cell polyomavirus infection I. MCV T antigen expression in Merkel cell carcinoma, lymphoid tissues and lymphoid tumors. Int J Cancer 2009; 125(6):1243–9.

71. Paulson KG, Lewis CW, Redman MW, et al. Viral oncoprotein antibodies as a marker for recurrence of Merkel cell carcinoma: A prospective validation study. Cancer 2017;123(8):1464–74.

72. Berrios C, Padi M, Keibler MA, et al. Merkel cell polyomavirus small T antigen promotes pro-glycolytic metabolic perturbations required for transformation. PLoS Pathog 2016;12(11):e1006020.

73. Bhatia K, Goedert JJ, Modali R, et al. Immunological detection of viral large T antigen identifies a subset of Merkel cell carcinoma tumors with higher viral abundance and better clinical outcome. Int J Cancer 2010;127(6):1493–6.

74. Houben R, Adam C, Baeurle A, et al. An intact retinoblastoma protein-binding site in Merkel cell polyomavirus large T antigen is required for promoting growth of Merkel cell carcinoma cells. Int J Cancer 2012;130(4):847–56.

75. Borchert S, Czech-Sioli M, Neumann F, et al. High-affinity Rb binding, p53 inhibition, subcellular localization, and transformation by wild-type or tumor-derived shortened Merkel cell polyomavirus large T antigens. J Virol 2014;88(6):3144–60.

76. Wang L, Harms PW, Palanisamy N, et al. Age and gender associations of virus positivity in merkel cell carcinoma characterized using a novel rna in situ hybridization assay. Clin Cancer Res 2017; 23(18):5622–30.

77. Duncavage EJ, Magrini V, Becker N, et al. Hybrid capture and next-generation sequencing identify viral integration sites from formalin-fixed, paraffin-embedded tissue. J Mol Diagn 2011;13(3):325–33.

78. Lyngaa R, Pedersen NW, Schrama D, et al. T-cell responses to oncogenic merkel cell polyomavirus proteins distinguish patients with merkel cell carcinoma from healthy donors. Clin Cancer Res 2014; 20(7):1768–78.

79. Bentzen AK, Marquard AM, Lyngaa R, et al. Large-scale detection of antigen-specific T cells using peptide-MHC-I multimers labeled with DNA barcodes. Nat Biotechnol 2016;34(10):1037–45.

80. Daily K, Coxon A, Williams JS, et al. Assessment of cancer cell line representativeness using microarrays for Merkel cell carcinoma. J Invest Dermatol 2015;135(4):1138–46.

81. Fan K, Ritter C, Nghiem P, et al. Circulating cell-free miR-375 as surrogate marker of tumor burden in Merkel cell carcinoma. Clin Cancer Res 2018; 24(23):5873–82.

82. Madankumar R, Criscito MC, Martires KJ, et al. A population-based cohort study of the influence of socioeconomic factors and race on survival in Merkel cell carcinoma. J Am Acad Dermatol 2017;76(1):166–7.

83. Harms KL, Healy MA, Nghiem P, et al. Analysis of Prognostic Factors from 9387 Merkel Cell Carcinoma Cases Forms the Basis for the New 8th Edition AJCC Staging System. Ann Surg Oncol 2016;23(11):3564–71.

84. Chen MM, Roman SA, Sosa JA, et al. The role of adjuvant therapy in the management of head and neck merkel cell carcinoma: an analysis of 4815 patients. JAMA Otolaryngol Head Neck Surg 2015;141(2):137–41.

85. van Veenendaal LM, van Akkooi ACJ, Verhoef C, et al. Merkel cell carcinoma: clinical outcome and prognostic factors in 351 patients. J Surg Oncol 2018;117(8):1768–75.

86. Mehrany K, Otley CC, Weenig RH, et al. A meta-analysis of the prognostic significance of sentinel lymph node status in Merkel Cell Carcinoma. Dermatol Surg 2002;28(2):113–7.

87. Allen PJ, Bowne WB, Jaques DP, et al. Merkel Cell carcinoma: prognosis and treatment of patients from a single institution. J Clin Oncol 2005;23(10): 2300–9.

88. Iyer JG, Storer BE, Paulson KG, et al. Relationships among primary tumor size, number of involved nodes, and survival for 8044 cases of Merkel cell carcinoma. J Am Acad Dermatol 2014;70(4):637–43.

89. Criscito MC, Martires KJ, Stein JA. A population-based cohort study on the association of dermatologist density and Merkel cell carcinoma survival. J Am Acad Dermatol 2017;76(3):570–2.

90. Dabner M, McClure RJ, Harvey NT, et al. Merkel cell Polyomavirus and p63 status in Merkel cell carcinoma by immunohistochemistry: Merkel cell Polyomavirus positivity is inversely correlated with sun damage, but neither is correlated with outcome. Pathology 2014;46(3):205–10.

91. Asioli S, Righi A, de Biase D, et al. Expression of p63 is the sole independent marker of aggressiveness in localised (stage I–II) Merkel cell carcinomas. Mod Pathol 2011;24:1451.

92. Brummer GC, Bowen AR, Bowen GM. Merkel Cell Carcinoma: current issues regarding diagnosis, management, and emerging treatment strategies. Am J Clin Dermatol 2016;17(1):49–62.

93. Touzé A, Le Bidre E, Laude H, et al. High levels of antibodies against merkel cell polyomavirus identify a subset of patients with merkel cell carcinoma with better clinical outcome. J Clin Oncol 2011; 29(12):1612–9.

94. Vandeven N, Lewis CW, Makarov V, et al. Merkel Cell carcinoma patients presenting without a primary lesion have elevated markers of immunity, higher tumor mutation burden, and improved survival. Clin Cancer Res 2018;24(4):963–71.

95. Sihto H, Bohling T, Kavola H, et al. Tumor infiltrating immune cells and outcome of Merkel cell carcinoma: a population-based study. Clin Cancer Res 2012;18(10):2872–81.

96. Afanasiev OK, Yelistratova L, Miller N, et al. Merkel polyomavirus-specific T cells fluctuate with merkel cell carcinoma burden and express therapeutically targetable PD-1 and Tim-3 exhaustion markers. Clin Cancer Res 2013;19(19):5351–60.

97. Iyer JG, Afanasiev OK, McClurkan C, et al. Merkel cell polyomavirus-specific CD8+ and CD4+ T-cell

responses identified in Merkel cell carcinomas and blood. Clin Cancer Res 2011;1513:2011.

98. Feldmeyer L, Hudgens CW, Ray-Lyons G, et al. Density, distribution, and composition of immune infiltrates correlate with survival in Merkel cell carcinoma. Clin Cancer Res 2016;22(22):5553–63.

99. Inoue T, Yoneda K, Manabe M, et al. Spontaneous regression of merkel cell carcinoma: a comparative study of TUNEL index and tumor-infiltrating lymphocytes between spontaneous regression and non-regression group. J Dermatol Sci 2000;24(3):203–11.

100. Paulson KG, Iyer JG, Tegeder AR, et al. Transcriptome-wide studies of merkel cell carcinoma and validation of intratumoral CD8+ lymphocyte invasion as an independent predictor of survival. J Clin Oncol 2011;29(12):1539–46.

101. Stetsenko GY, Malekirad J, Paulson KG, et al. p63 expression in Merkel cell carcinoma predicts poorer survival yet may have limited clinical utility. Am J Clin Pathol 2013;140(6):838–44.

102. Hall BJ, Pincus LB, Yu SS, et al. Immunohistochemical prognostication of Merkel cell carcinoma: p63 expression but not polyomavirus status correlates with outcome. J Cutan Pathol 2012;39(10):911–7.

103. Fleming KE, Ly TY, Pasternak S, et al. Support for p63 expression as an adverse prognostic marker in Merkel cell carcinoma: report on a Canadian cohort. Hum Pathol 2014;45(5):952–60.

104. Sahi H, Koljonen V, Kavola H, et al. Bcl-2 expression indicates better prognosis of Merkel cell carcinoma regardless of the presence of Merkel cell polyomavirus. Virchows Arch 2012;461(5):553–9.

105. Vujic I, Marker M, Posch C, et al. Merkel cell carcinoma: mitoses, expression of Ki-67 and bcl-2 correlate with disease progression. J Eur Acad Dermatol Venereol 2015;29(3):542–8.

106. Knapp CF, Sayegh Z, Schell MJ, et al. Expression of CXCR4, E-cadherin, Bcl-2, and survivin in Merkel cell carcinoma: an immunohistochemical study using a tissue microarray. Am J Dermatopathol 2012;34(6):592–6.

107. Kim J, McNiff JM. Nuclear expression of survivin portends a poor prognosis in Merkel cell carcinoma. Mod Pathol 2008;21:764.

108. Arora R, Shuda M, Guastafierro A, et al. Survivin is a therapeutic target in Merkel cell carcinoma. Sci Transl Med 2012;4(133):133ra156.

109. Kim KH, Roberts CWM. Targeting EZH2 in cancer. Nat Med 2016;22:128.

110. Harms PW, Patel RM, Verhaegen ME, et al. Distinct gene expression profiles of viral- and nonviral-associated merkel cell carcinoma revealed by transcriptome analysis. J Invest Dermatol 2013;133(4):936–45.

111. Veija T, Koljonen V, Bohling T, et al. Aberrant expression of ALK and EZH2 in Merkel cell carcinoma. BMC Cancer 2017;17(1):236.

112. Harms KL, Chubb H, Zhao L, et al. Increased expression of EZH2 in Merkel cell carcinoma is associated with disease progression and poorer prognosis. Hum Pathol 2017;67:78–84.

113. Amin M, Greene F, Edge S, et al. The Eighth Edition AJCC Cancer Staging Manual: Continuing to build a bridge from a population-based to a more "personalized" approach to cancer staging. CA Cancer J Clin 2017;67:93–9.

114. Sundaresan P, Hruby G, Hamilton A, et al. Definitive radiotherapy or chemoradiotherapy in the treatment of Merkel cell carcinoma. Clin Oncol 2012;24(9):e131–6.

115. Bedi C, Seel M, Ramdave S, et al. The use of FDG-PET Scanning (PET) in the management of merkel cell carcinoma. Int J Radiat Oncol Biol Phys 2008;72(1):S107.

116. Belhocine T, Pierard GE, Frühling J, et al. Clinical added-value of 18FDG PET in neuroendocrine-Merkel cell carcinoma. Oncol Rep 2006;16(2):347–52.

117. Poulsen M, Macfarlane D, Veness M, et al. Prospective analysis of the utility of 18-FDG PET in Merkel cell carcinoma of the skin: A Trans Tasman Radiation Oncology Group Study, TROG 09:03. J Med Imaging Radiat Oncol 2018;62(3):412–9.

118. Kachare SD, Wong JH, Vohra NA, et al. Sentinel lymph node biopsy is associated with improved survival in Merkel cell carcinoma. Ann Surg Oncol 2014;21(5):1624–30.

119. Fields RC, Busam KJ, Chou JF, et al. Recurrence and survival in patients undergoing sentinel lymph node biopsy for merkel cell carcinoma: analysis of 153 patients from a single institution. Ann Surg Oncol 2011;18(9):2529.

120. Prieto I, de la Fuente TP, Medina S, et al. Merkel cell carcinoma: An algorithm for multidisciplinary management and decision-making. Crit Rev Oncol Hematol 2016;98:170–9.

121. Kline L, Coldiron B. Mohs micrographic surgery for the treatment of Merkel Cell carcinoma. Dermatol Surg 2016;42(8):945–51.

122. O'Connor WJ, Roenigk RK, Brodland DG. Merkel cell carcinoma: comparison of Mohs micrographic surgery and wide excision in eighty-six patients. Dermatol Surg 1997;23(10):929–33.

123. Singh B, Qureshi MM, Truong MT, et al. Demographics and outcomes of stage I and II Merkel cell carcinoma treated with Mohs micrographic surgery compared with wide local excision in the National Cancer Database. J Am Acad Dermatol 2018;79(1):126–34.e123.

124. Su C, Bai HX, Christensen S. Relative survival analysis in patients with stage I-II Merkel cell carcinoma

treated with Mohs micrographic surgery or wide local excision. J Am Acad Dermatol 2018. Epub ahead of print.

125. Pape E, Rezvoy N, Penel N, et al. Radiotherapy alone for Merkel cell carcinoma: a comparative and retrospective study of 25 patients. J Am Acad Dermatol 2011;65(5):983–90.

126. Veness M, Foote M, Gebski V, et al. The role of radiotherapy alone in patients with merkel cell carcinoma: reporting the Australian Experience of 43 patients. Int J Radiat Oncol Biol Phys 2010;78(3): 703–9.

127. Fang LC, Lemos B, Douglas J, et al. Radiation monotherapy as regional treatment for lymph node-positive Merkel cell carcinoma. Cancer 2010;116(7):1783–90.

128. Gupta SG, Wang LC, Penas PF, et al. Sentinel lymph node biopsy for evaluation and treatment of patients with Merkel cell carcinoma: the Dana-Farber experience and meta-analysis of the literature. Arch Dermatol 2006;142(6):685–90.

129. Gunaratne DA, Howle JR, Veness MJ. Definitive radiotherapy for Merkel cell carcinoma confers clinically meaningful in-field locoregional control: a review and analysis of the literature. J Am Acad Dermatol 2017;77(1):142–8.e1.

130. Veness MJ, Morgan GJ, Gebski V. Adjuvant locoregional radiotherapy as best practice in patients with Merkel cell carcinoma of the head and neck. Head Neck 2005;27(3):208–16.

131. Strom T, Naghavi AO, Messina JL, et al. Improved local and regional control with radiotherapy for Merkel cell carcinoma of the head and neck. Head Neck 2017;39(1):48–55.

132. Veness M, Howle J. Radiotherapy alone in patients with Merkel cell carcinoma: The Westmead Hospital experience of 41 patients. Australas J Dermatol 2015;56(1):19–24.

133. Koh CS, Veness MJ. Role of definitive radiotherapy in treating patients with inoperable Merkel cell carcinoma: The Westmead Hospital experience and a review of the literature. Australas J Dermatol 2009; 50(4):249–56.

134. Harrington C, Kwan W. Outcomes of merkel cell carcinoma treated with radiotherapy without radical surgical excision. Ann Surg Oncol 2014; 21(11):3401–5.

135. Leonard JH, Ramsay JR, Kearsley JH, et al. Radiation sensitivity of merkel cell carcinoma cell lines. Int J Radiat Oncol Biol Phys 1995;32(5):1401–7.

136. Hao S, Zhao S, Bu X. Radioactive seed implantation in treatment of an eyelid primary Merkel cell carcinoma. Can J Ophthalmol 2016;51(1): e31–3.

137. Cotter SE, Devlin PM, Sahni D, et al. Treatment of cutaneous metastases of merkel cell carcinoma with surface-mold computer-optimized high-dose-rate brachytherapy. J Clin Oncol 2010;28(27): e464–6.

138. Garibyan L, Cotter SE, Hansen JL, et al. Palliative treatment for in-transit cutaneous metastases of Merkel cell carcinoma using surface-mold computer-optimized high-dose-rate brachytherapy. Cancer 2013;19(4):283.

139. Garneski KM, Nghiem P. Merkel cell carcinoma adjuvant therapy: Current data support radiation but not chemotherapy. J Am Acad Dermatol 2007;57(1):166–9.

140. Takagishi SR, Marx TE, Lewis C, et al. Postoperative radiation therapy is associated with a reduced risk of local recurrence among low risk Merkel cell carcinomas of the head and neck. Adv Radiat Oncol 2016;1(4):244–51.

141. Lewis KG, Weinstock MA, Weaver AL, et al. Adjuvant local irradiation for Merkel cell carcinoma. Arch Dermatol 2006;142(6):693–700.

142. Cassler NM, Merrill D, Bichakjian CK, et al. Merkel cell carcinoma therapeutic update. Curr Treat Options Oncol 2016;17(7):36.

143. Bhatia S, Storer BE, Iyer JG, et al. Adjuvant radiation therapy and chemotherapy in Merkel cell carcinoma: survival analyses of 6908 cases from the National Cancer Data Base. J Natl Cancer Inst 2016;108(9) [pii:djw042].

144. Mojica P, Smith D, Ellenhorn JDI. Adjuvant radiation therapy is associated with improved survival in Merkel cell carcinoma of the skin. J Clin Oncol 2007;25(9):1043–7.

145. Jouary T, Leyral C, Dreno B, et al. Adjuvant prophylactic regional radiotherapy versus observation in stage I Merkel cell carcinoma: a multicentric prospective randomized study. Ann Oncol 2011; 23(4):1074–80.

146. Hasan S, Liu L, Triplet J, et al. The role of postoperative radiation and chemoradiation in merkel cell carcinoma: a systematic review of the literature. Front Oncol 2013;3:276.

147. Kim JA, Choi AH. Effect of radiation therapy on survival in patients with resected Merkel cell carcinoma: a propensity score surveillance, epidemiology, and end results database analysis. JAMA Dermatol 2013;149(7):831–8.

148. Bishop AJ, Garden AS, Gunn GB, et al. Merkel cell carcinoma of the head and neck: Favorable outcomes with radiotherapy. Head Neck 2016; 38(S1):E452–8.

149. Grotz TE, Joseph RW, Pockaj BA, et al. Negative sentinel lymph node biopsy in merkel cell carcinoma is associated with a low risk of same-nodal-basin recurrences. Ann Surg Oncol 2015;22(12):4060–6.

150. Bichakjian CK, Harms KL, Schwartz JL. Selective use of adjuvant therapy in the management of Merkel cell carcinoma. JAMA Oncol 2015;1(8): 1162–3.

151. Poulsen M, Rischin D, Walpole E, et al. High-risk merkel cell carcinoma of the skin treated with synchronous carboplatin/etoposide and radiation: a trans-tasman radiation oncology group study—TROG 96:07. J Clin Oncol 2003;21(23):4371–6.

152. Poulsen M, Rischin D, Walpole E, et al. Analysis of toxicity of Merkel cell carcinoma of the skin treated with synchronous carboplatin/etoposide and radiation: a Trans-Tasman Radiation Oncology Group study. Int J Radiat Oncol Biol Phys 2001;51(1):156–63.

153. Bajetta E, Celio L, Platania M, et al. Single-institution series of early-stage Merkel cell carcinoma: long-term outcomes in 95 patients managed with surgery alone. Ann Surg Oncol 2009;16(11):2985–93.

154. Twyman-Saint Victor C, Rech AJ, Maity A, et al. Radiation and dual checkpoint blockade activate nonredundant immune mechanisms in cancer. Nature 2015;520:373.

155. Iyer JG, Parvathaneni U, Gooley T, et al. Single-fraction radiation therapy in patients with metastatic Merkel cell carcinoma. Cancer Med 2015;4(8):1161–70.

156. Cimbak N, Barker CA. Short-course radiation therapy for merkel cell carcinoma: relative effectiveness in a "Radiosensitive" tumor. Int J Rad Oncol Biol Phys 2016;96(2, Supplement):S160.

157. Satpute SR, Ammakkanavar NR, Einhorn LH. Role of platinum-based chemotherapy for Merkel cell tumor in adjuvant and metastatic settings. J Clin Oncol 2014;32(15):9049.

158. Desch L, Kunstfeld R. Merkel cell carcinoma: chemotherapy and emerging new therapeutic options. J Skin Cancer 2013;2013:327150.

159. Tai PT, Yu E, Winquist E, et al. Chemotherapy in neuroendocrine/Merkel cell carcinoma of the skin: case series and review of 204 cases. J Clin Oncol 2000;18(12):2493–9.

160. Iyer JG, Blom A, Doumani R, et al. Response rates and durability of chemotherapy among 62 patients with metastatic Merkel cell carcinoma. Cancer Med 2016;5(9):2294–301.

161. Asgari MM, Sokil MM, Warton EM, et al. Effect of host, tumor, diagnostic, and treatment variables on outcomes in a large cohort with Merkel cell carcinoma. JAMA Dermatol 2014;150(7):716–23.

162. Cowey CL, Mahnke L, Espirito J, et al. Real-world treatment outcomes in patients with metastatic Merkel cell carcinoma treated with chemotherapy in the USA. Future Oncol 2017;13(19):1699–710.

163. Lipson EJ, Vincent JG, Loyo M, et al. PD-L1 expression in the Merkel cell carcinoma microenvironment: association with inflammation, Merkel cell polyomavirus, and overall survival. Cancer Immunol Res 2013;1(1):54–63.

164. Terheyden P, Becker JC. New developments in the biology and the treatment of metastatic Merkel cell carcinoma. Curr Opin Oncol 2017;29(3):221–6.

165. Winkler JK, Dimitrakopoulou-Strauss A, Sachpekidis C, et al. Ipilimumab has efficacy in metastatic Merkel cell carcinoma: a case series of five patients. J Eur Acad Dermatol Venereol 2017;31(9):e389–91.

166. Baker M, Cordes L, Brownell I. Avelumab: a new standard for treating metastatic Merkel cell carcinoma. Expert Rev Anticancer Ther 2018;18(4):319–26.

167. Nghiem P, Bhatia S, Brohl AS, et al. Two-year efficacy and safety update from JAVELIN Merkel 200 part A: A registrational study of avelumab in metastatic Merkel cell carcinoma progressed on chemotherapy. J Clin Oncol 2018;36(15):9507.

168. US FDA. FDA approves pembrolizumab for Merkel cell carcinoma 2019. Available at: https://www.fda.gov/Drugs/InformationOnDrugs/ApprovedDrugs/ucm628867.htm. Accessed August 21, 2019.

169. Nghiem P, Bhatia S, Lipson EJ, et al. Durable tumor regression and overall survival (OS) in patients with advanced Merkel cell carcinoma (aMCC) receiving pembrolizumab as first-line therapy. J Clin Oncol 2018;36(15):9506.

170. Topalian SL, Bhatia S, Hollebecque A, et al. Abstract CT074: non-comparative, open-label, multiple cohort, phase 1/2 study to evaluate nivolumab (NIVO) in patients with virus-associated tumors (CheckMate 358): Efficacy and safety in Merkel cell carcinoma (MCC). Cancer Res 2017;77(13 Supplement):CT074.

171. Schwartz RH. Costimulation of T lymphocytes: the role of CD28, CTLA-4, and B7/BB1 in interleukin-2 production and immunotherapy. Cell 1992;71(7):1065–8.

172. Colunga A, Pulliam T, Nghiem P. Merkel cell carcinoma in the age of immunotherapy: facts and hopes. Clin Cancer Res 2018;24(9):2035–43.

173. Segal NH, He AR, Doi T, et al. Phase I study of single-agent utomilumab (PF-05082566), a 4-1BB/CD137 agonist, in patients with advanced cancer. Clin Cancer Res 2018;24(8):1816–23.

174. Veija T, Sarhadi VK, Koljonen V, et al. Hotspot mutations in polyomavirus positive and negative Merkel cell carcinomas. Cancer Genet 2016;209(1–2):30–5.

175. Harms KL, Lazo de la Vega L, Hovelson DH, et al. Molecular profiling of multiple primary merkel cell carcinoma to distinguish genetically distinct tumors from clonally related metastases. JAMA Dermatol 2017;153(6):505–12.

176. Ritter C, Fan K, Paulson KG, et al. Reversal of epigenetic silencing of MHC class I chain-related protein A and B improves immune recognition of Merkel cell carcinoma. Sci Rep 2016;6:21678.

177. Bhatia S, Miller NJ, Lu H, et al. Intratumoral G100, a TLR4 agonist, induces anti-tumor immune responses and tumor regression in patients with Merkel cell carcinoma. Clin Cancer Res 2019;25(4):1185–95.

178. Bhatia S, Iyer J, Ibrani D, et al. 504 Intratumoral delivery of Interleukin-12 DNA via in vivo electroporation leads to regression of injected and non-injected tumors in Merkel cell carcinoma: Final Results of a phase 2 study. Eur J Cancer 2015;51:S104.

179. Iwasaki T, Matsushita M, Nonaka D, et al. Comparison of Akt/mTOR/4E-BP1 pathway signal activation and mutations of PIK3CA in Merkel cell polyomavirus–positive and Merkel cell polyomavirus–negative carcinomas. Hum Pathol 2015;46(2):210–6.

180. Kannan A, Lin Z, Shao Q, et al. Dual mTOR inhibitor MLN0128 suppresses Merkel cell carcinoma (MCC) xenograft tumor growth. Oncotarget 2016;7(6):6576–92.

181. Rabinowits G, Lezcano C, Catalano PJ, et al. Cabozantinib in patients with advanced merkel cell carcinoma. Oncologist 2018;23(7):814–21.

182. Frenard C, Peuvrel L, Brocard A, et al. Dramatic response of an inoperable Merkel cell carcinoma with imatinib. JAAD Case Rep 2016;2(1):16–8.

183. Samlowski WE, Moon J, Tuthill RJ, et al. A phase II trial of imatinib mesylate in merkel cell carcinoma (neuroendocrine carcinoma of the skin): A Southwest Oncology Group study (S0331). Am J Clin Oncol 2010;33(5):495–9.

184. Davids M, Charlton A, Ng S-S, et al. Response to a novel multitargeted tyrosine kinase inhibitor pazopanib in metastatic Merkel cell carcinoma. J Clin Oncol 2009;27(26):e97–100.

185. Nathan PD, Gaunt P, Wheatley K, et al. UKMCC-01: a phase II study of pazopanib (PAZ) in metastatic Merkel cell carcinoma. J Clin Oncol 2016;34(15_suppl):9542.

186. Tarabadkar ES, Thomas H, Blom A, et al. Clinical benefit from tyrosine kinase inhibitors in metastatic merkel cell carcinoma: a case series of 5 patients. Am J Case Rep 2018;19:505.

187. Paulson KG, Perdicchio M, Kulikauskas R, et al. Augmentation of adoptive T-cell therapy for Merkel cell carcinoma with avelumab. J Clin Oncol 2017;35(15_suppl):3044.

188. Chapuis AG, Afanasiev OK, Iyer JG, et al. Regression of metastatic Merkel cell carcinoma following transfer of polyomavirus-specific T cells and therapies capable of re-inducing HLA class-I. Cancer Immunol Res 2014;2(1):27–36.

189. Ritter C, Fan K, Paschen A, et al. Epigenetic priming restores the HLA class-I antigen processing machinery expression in Merkel cell carcinoma. Sci Rep 2017;7(1):2290.

190. Klingemann HG, Wong E, Maki G. A cytotoxic NK-cell line (NK-92) for ex vivo purging of leukemia from blood. Biol Blood Marrow Transplant 1996;2(2):68–75.

191. Bhatia S, Burgess M, Zhang H, et al. Adoptive cellular therapy (ACT) with allogeneic activated natural killer (aNK) cells in patients with advanced Merkel cell carcinoma (MCC): preliminary results of a phase II trial. Paper presented at: Society for Immunotherapy of Cancer, 31st Annual Meeting. National Harbor, MD, November 9–13, 2016.

192. Gardair C, Samimi M, Touzé A, et al. Somatostatin receptors 2A and 5 are expressed in merkel cell carcinoma with no association with disease severity. Neuroendocrinology 2015;101(3):223–35.

193. Buder K, Lapa C, Kreissl MC, et al. Somatostatin receptor expression in Merkel cell carcinoma as target for molecular imaging. BMC Cancer 2014;14:268.

194. Basu S, Ranade R. Favorable response of metastatic merkel cell carcinoma to targeted 177Lu-DOTA-TATE therapy: will PRRT evolve to become an important approach in receptor-positive cases? J Nucl Med Technol 2016;44(2):85–7.

195. Fakiha M, Letertre P, Vuillez J, et al. Remission of Merkel cell tumor after somatostatin analog treatment. J Cancer Res Ther 2010;6(3):382–4.

196. Dasari A, Phan A, Gupta S, et al. Phase I study of the anti-IGF1R antibody cixutumumab with everolimus and octreotide in advanced well-differentiated neuroendocrine tumors. Endocr Relat Cancer 2015;22(3):431–41.

197. Hu JC, Coffin RS, Davis CJ, et al. A phase I study of OncoVEXGM-CSF, a second-generation oncolytic herpes simplex virus expressing granulocyte macrophage colony-stimulating factor. Clin Cancer Res 2006;12(22):6737–47.

198. Andtbacka R, Kaufman HL, Collichio F, et al. Talimogene laherparepvec improves durable response rate in patients with advanced melanoma. J Clin Oncol 2015;33(25):2780–8.

Kaposi Sarcoma Updates

Shervin A. Etemad, BS, Anna K. Dewan, MD, MHS*

KEYWORDS

• Kaposi sarcoma • AIDS • HIV • Immunosuppression • HHV8 • Sarcoma

KEY POINTS

- Kaposi sarcoma (KS) is a multifocal mesenchymal neoplasm caused by Kaposi sarcoma-related herpesvirus (KSHV), which is also known as human herpes virus type-8 (HHV-8).
- The 4 epidemiologic variants of KS are classic, African (endemic), immunosuppression-related (iatrogenic), and AIDS-related.
- KS typically presents on the skin as pink to purple macules, patches, and plaques. The most common extracutaneous locations are the oral mucosa, gastrointestinal tract, and lymph nodes.
- The cornerstone of treatment of AIDS KS is combined antiretroviral therapy, and immunosuppression-related KS may be managed with modifications to the immunosuppressive regimen.
- Checkpoint inhibitors represent an exciting new treatment modality for all variants of KS.

INTRODUCTION

Kaposi sarcoma (KS) is an angioproliferative neoplasm that is caused by infection with Kaposi sarcoma-related herpesvirus (KSHV) (also known as human herpesvirus 8 (HHV8)). The 4 epidemiologic subtypes of KS include classic, African endemic, immunosuppression-related, and AIDS-related KS. Treatment principles rest on consideration of the subtype and the extent of tumor involvement.

EPIDEMIOLOGY

Since its original description in 1872, 4 clinical variants of KS have been characterized.

Classic KS (CKS) is an indolent disease and most frequently occurs on the lower extremities of men of Mediterranean, eastern European, or Middle Eastern descent in the sixth decade.[1] Never smoking, diabetes, and oral corticosteroid use have been associated with increased risk of CKS.[2]

African endemic KS is an aggressive subtype occurring among HIV-negative individuals in sub-Saharan Africa. There was a dramatic increase in KS following the HIV epidemic in Africa, and it is now the most common cancer among males and second most common among females.[3]

Patients who are immunosuppressed, such as after organ transplant, are at increased risk for immunosuppression-related KS (IKS). Risk factors for the development of IKS include male sex, nonwhite race, non-US citizenship, lung transplant, HLA-B mismatch, and older age at transplant.[4] The incidence is highest within the first year after transplant.[4] KS arising in the context of stem cell transplantation has been described.[5] Infection with KSHV may rarely occur by way of donor organ.[6] The choice of immunosuppressive therapy may influence the risk of KS; switching from a calcineurin inhibitor to an mTOR inhibitor may prevent progression and result in regression of IKS.[7,8] Beyond transplantation, there are reports of KS developing in the context of

Disclosure Statement: S.A. Etemad and A.K. Dewan: No relevant financial relationships with any commercial interest that pertains to the content of this publication.
Department of Dermatology, Vanderbilt University Medical Center, 719 Thompson Lane, One Hundred Oaks, Suite 26300, Nashville, TN 37204, USA
* Corresponding author.
E-mail address: anna.dewan@vumc.org

0733-8635/19/© 2019 Elsevier Inc. All rights reserved.

derm.theclinics.com

immunosuppression with corticosteroids and bio-logic therapies such as infliximab.[9]

AIDS-related KS occurs most commonly in HIV-infected men who have sex with men (MSM). After the introduction of 3-drug antiretroviral therapy (ART) in the mid-1990s, the incidence of AIDS-related KS has decreased among populations with access to ART. However, there has been a recent increase in KS incidence among HIV-infected African American men in the southern United States.[10] There is an inverse relationship of CD4 count and risk of AIDS KS,[11] but up to one-third of cases may present in the context of nondetectable HIV viral load and CD4 counts of greater than 300 cells/mm[3].[12] A nonepidemic, indolent variant of KS has recently been proposed that occurs primarily in younger MSM without immunodeficiency.[13]

Patients with KS are at increased risk for solid-organ malignancies as well as Hodgkin lymphoma and acute lymphocytic lymphoma.[14] In addition, KSHV-associated multicentric Castleman disease, plasmablastic lymphoma, and primary effusion lymphoma occur with greater incidence in patients with KS.

PATHOGENESIS

In 1994, KSHV, also known as HHV-8, was identi-fied.[15] KSHV is necessary, but not sufficient, for the development of all forms of KS. Seroconversion often occurs after salivary transmission, but may occur through blood and sexual intercourse.[16] KSHV primarily affects endothelial cells, and controversy exists regarding whether the endothelial phenotype is vascular, lymphatic, or both.[17] Like other herpesviruses, KSHV has a life cycle that consists of latent and lytic phases.[18] Acute infection is followed by a latent program, characterized by persistent infection, restricted oncogene expression, and avoidance of host immune surveillance.[19] The switch to a lytic program is critical for progression from an asymptomatic seropositive state to clinically evident KS. Factors that influence tumorigenesis include hypoxia, oxidative stress, viral coinfection, epigenetic modification, immune suppression, and hyperglycemia.[20,21]

CLINICAL FEATURES

Cutaneous lesions in KS range from scattered pink to purple patches and papules (**Figs. 1** and **2**) to rapidly progressive, multicentric, ulcerated plaques and nodules (**Figs. 3–5**) with dissemination to visceral organs. Extracutaneous involvement may be seen (**Table 1**). There are 4 subgroups of

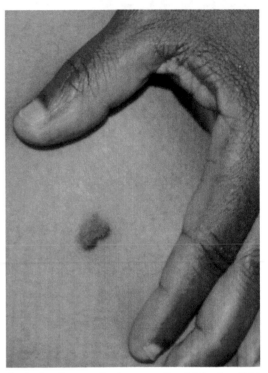

Fig. 1. Purple smooth plaque on the thigh of an African man with AIDS KS.

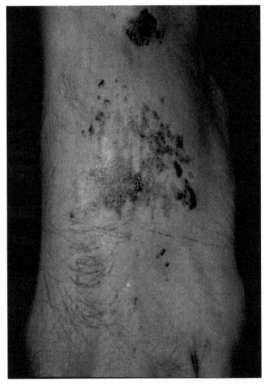

Fig. 2. Nonblanching red to purple vascular macules coalescing into a patch on the dorsal foot of a patient with classic KS.

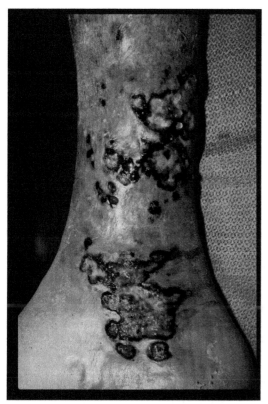

Fig. 3. Clustered purple nodules and "punched out" ulcerations with violaceous borders on the lower extremity of a patient with classic KS.

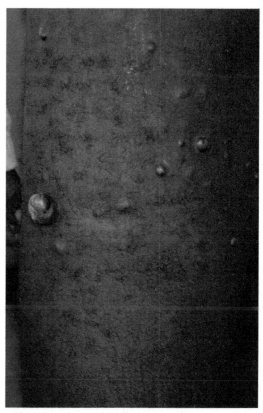

Fig. 5. Diffuse induration and edema with associated exophytic red nodules in a patient with AIDS KS.

African endemic KS: nodular, florid, infiltrative, and lymphadenopathic. Nodular KS is an indolent disease limited to skin involvement. Florid KS is typically exophytic and locally aggressive, and infiltrative lesions are deep with extensive cutaneous disease and involvement of bone. Lymphadenopathic KS (Fig. 6) is a particularly aggressive and rapidly fatal variant that occurs in children. In AIDS-related KS, visceral disease is more frequent. Oral mucosal KS (Fig. 7) is an important prognostic factor in patients who do not receive HAART (highly active antiretroviral therapy), because it is associated with a poor prognosis.[22] Unique features of all subtypes of pediatric KS described recently include primary lymph node involvement, few cutaneous lesions, fulminant progression, cytopenias, and relatively normal CD4 count.[23]

STAGING

In the pre-ART era, the NIH AIDS Clinical Trials Group (ACTG) developed a staging system for AIDS-related KS that stratified patients based on tumor extent (T), immune status according to

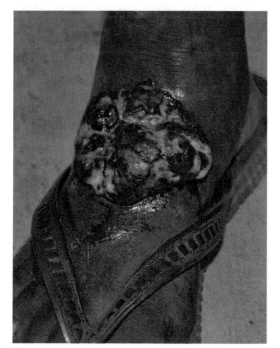

Fig. 4. Exophytic ulcerating tumor on the dorsal foot of an African patient with AIDS KS.

Table 1
Extracutaneous manifestations of KS

Organ System[a]	Symptoms	Clinical Evaluation
Gastrointestinal Tract	Asymptomatic, abdominal pain, weight loss, vomiting, bloody diarrhea, obstructive symptoms	Endoscopy + biopsy
Pulmonary	Nonproductive cough, hemoptysis, dyspnea, weight loss, fever, hypoxemia	Chest radiograph or CT Bronchoscopy + biopsy or bronchoalveolar lavage
Lymphatic	Lymphadenopathy	Fine-needle aspiration Biopsy
Liver	Hepatomegaly	Ultrasonography CT

[a] KS has been described less frequently in the adrenal glands, pancreas, heart, testes, bone marrow, bone, and skeletal muscle.

Data from Bhutani M, Polizzotto MN, Uldrick TS, et al. Kaposi sarcoma-associated herpesvirus-associated malignancies: epidemiology, pathogenesis, and advances in treatment. Semin Oncol. 2015;42(2):223–46.

CD4 count (I), and extent of systemic illness (S).[24] A separate pediatric-specific staging system has been proposed to guide therapy given the distinct clinical features of pediatric KS in sub-Saharan Africa.[23]

PATHOLOGY

Pathology remains the gold standard for diagnosis of KS. The patch, plaque, and nodular stages share similar histologic findings (**Fig. 8 and 9**). Patch stage disease is characterized by a perivascular dermal lymphocytic infiltrate with scattered plasma cells. A promontory sign, or proliferation of oddly shaped, endothelial cell-lined vascular channels surrounding existing vasculature, is a characteristic finding. These irregular channels become more prominent and CD31/34+ spindle cells proliferate in the dermis as lesions transition to the plaque stage of development. Histopathology of nodular lesions shows a dermal mass of spindle cells; extravasated red blood cells are noted in the slitlike vascular spaces. Other,

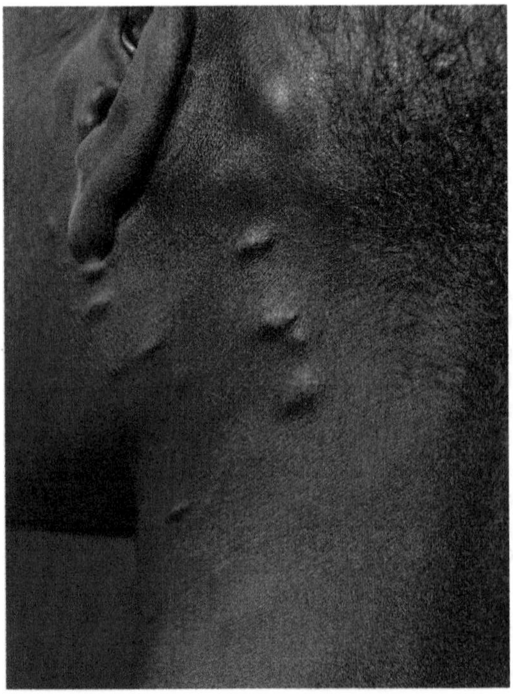

Fig. 6. Multiple hyperpigmented to purple nodules with associated prominent lymphadenopathy in an African patient with AIDS KS.

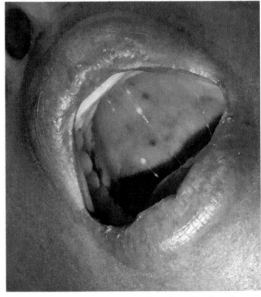

Fig. 7. Purple macules on the hard and soft palate of an African patient with AIDS KS.

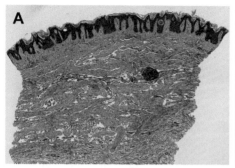
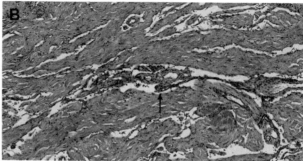

Fig. 8. (*A*) Subtle perivascular dermal lymphocytic infiltrate with irregular vascular channels (stain: hematoxylin and eosin; original magnification, ×2). (*B*) Proliferation of oddly shaped, endothelial cell-lined vascular channels surrounding existing vasculature, also known as the "promontory sign," as indicated by the black arrow (stain: hematoxylin and eosin, original magnification, ×10).

more rare, histopathologic variants have been described.[25] A commercially available immunohistochemical stain against KSHV latent nuclear antigen-1 (LNA-1) has been shown to be both sensitive and specific for the diagnosis of KS[26] (**Fig. 10**).

TREATMENTS

Overall management considerations for KS include clinical variant, extent and rate of tumor growth, immune system status, comorbidities, and symptomatology. Localized therapies should be considered for limited disease, and systemic therapies are indicated in cases of extensive or painful cutaneous disease, visceral disease, or rapid progression.[27] Treatment options for the classic and African endemic variants of KS range from observation to localized and systemic chemotherapy. KS arising in the context of immunosuppression typically regresses with a decrease or discontinuation of immunosuppressive medications.[28] Patients on calcineurin inhibitors may benefit from a switch to a sirolimus-based regimen if possible.[7] Combination ART is the mainstay of treatment of patients with AIDS KS, with response rates ranging from 20%[29] to 76%[30] with ART alone. A subset of patients clinically worsen after initiation of ART therapy as part of immune reconstitution syndrome (IRIS). KS IRIS occurs in approximately 16% of patients in the United States within the first year of initiating ART.[31] Preexisting lung involvement is a risk factor. Recommended treatment includes continuing ART with the addition of adjunctive chemotherapeutic agents.[32]

Intravenous pegylated liposomal doxorubicin is approved by the United States Food and Drug Administration (FDA) for use in AIDS KS, may be administered as first-line systemic chemotherapy, and is more effective than ART alone.[29] Paclitaxel is also FDA approved for AIDS KS and may be considered as a second-line agent.[33] Doxorubicin, bleomycin, vincristine, and etoposide are commonly used in resource-poor settings.[34]

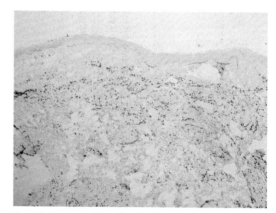

Fig. 10. Immunohistochemical staining against KSHV LNA-1, showing spindled cells infected with KSHV (stain: immunoperoxidase; original magnification, ×2).

Fig. 9. Dermal mass of spindle cells with extravasated red blood cells and cellular atypia (stain: hematoxylin and eosin, original magnification, ×10).

Table 2
Skin-directed and systemic treatments for KS

Treatment	Dose/Regimen	KS Subtype[a]	Side Effects[b]	Evidence Level[c]	Best Response
Skin-Directed Therapy					
Cryotherapy	11–60 s freeze cycles 2–3 freeze-thaw cycles Up to 3 sessions	**AIDS**[40]	Pain, blistering	B	Complete
Laser therapy	Nd: YAG laser every 4 wk for 2–4 sessions	Classic[41]	Mild atrophic scarring	D	Complete
Radiation therapy	6–40 Gy	AIDS[42] **Classic**[43]	Pain Infection Desquamation Hyperpigmentation Swelling Edema	B	Complete
Brachytherapy	24–35 Gy in 4–6 fractions over 12 d	AIDS[44] Classic[45] Endemic[46]	Erythema Hypopigmentation Telangiectasia Bleeding	C	Complete
Intralesional Therapy					
Bleomycin	0.75 mg/mL 1.5 mg per lesion Median period between injections 1 mo Median dose per patient 8 mg	AIDS[47]	Pain Hypopigmentation Hyperpigmentation	C	Complete
Doxorubicin	2 mg/mL diluted 1:1 with saline 4 treatments every 6 wk	Classic[48]	Pain Skin necrosis	D	Complete
Interferon-alpha	1 million units 3 times weekly for 6 wk	AIDS[49] **Classic**[50]	Pain Flulike symptoms	B	Complete
Sodium tetradecyl sulfate (STS)	0.2 mg/mL per 1 cm² of 0.3% STS	**AIDS (oral)**[51]	Pain Ulceration	B	Complete
Vinblastine	0.5 mg/mL One treatment	**AIDS**[52] Classic[53]	Hyperpigmentation Pain	B	Complete

Vincristine	0.03–0.08 mL of 1 μg/mL	Classic[54]	Pain Erythema Pruritus Ulceration	B	Complete
Topical Therapy					
Diphencyprone (DPCP)	Sensitization with 2% DPCP solution followed by once weekly at-home application of 0.2% solution with 24 h of occlusion	Classic[55]	Eczematous reaction	D	Complete
Imiquimod	5% imiquimod 3 times per week for 24 wk	AIDS[56] **Classic**[57] Iatrogenic[58] **Endemic**[57]	Erythema Pruritus	B	Complete
Rapamycin	0.5% ointment compounded by crushing tablets and adding mineral oil and petrolatum to make 20 g of ointment at 0.5% concentration Twice a day for 16 wk	Classic[59]		D	Complete
Silver nitrate	Weekly cauterization	Classic[60]		C	Complete
Timolol	0.1%–0.5% solution or gel Twice a day for 16 wk	AIDS[61] Classic[62] Iatrogenic[63]		D	Complete
Antiviral Therapy					
Antiretroviral therapy (ART)	Combination ART	AIDS[64]	Initial exacerbation of KS due to IRIS	C	Complete
Valganciclovir	900 mg oral twice daily	Classic[65]		D	Complete
Other					
9-*cis*-Retinoic acid	40–140 mg/m² oral	AIDS[66]	Headache Xerosis Rash Alopecia Hyperlipidemia	B	Complete

(continued on next page)

Table 2
(continued)

Treatment	Dose/Regimen	KS Subtype[a]	Side Effects[b]	Evidence Level[c]	Best Response
Bevacizumab	15 mg/kg intravenous (IV) on days 1 + 8 and then every 3 wk	AIDS[67]	Hypertension Neutropenia Cellulitis Headache	B	Complete
COL-3 (MMP Inhibitor)	50 mg/d	AIDS[68]	Photosensitivity Rash	B	Complete
IL-12	100–500 ng/kg Subcutaneous Twice weekly up to 6 mo	AIDS[69]	Flulike symptoms	B	Complete
Imatinib	400 mg/d	AIDS[70,71]	Hypersensitivity Dehydration Nausea Hypophosphatemia Creatine kinase increased Mood alterations	B	Complete
IM immunoglobulin	7 + injections of 800 mg	Classic[41]		D	Complete
Lenalidomide	Oral 25 mg days 1–21 with 7 d washout over 24 wk	AIDS[72]	Neutropenia Thrombocytopenia Anemia Asthenia	B	Partial
Liposomal tretinoin	IV 60–12 mg/m^2 1–3 times per week	AIDS[73]	Headache Xerosis	B	Partial
Nivolumab	3 mg/kg IV every 2 wk	AIDS[36] Endemic[35]	Fatigue Pruritus Onycholysis	C	Complete
Pazopanib	400 mg daily	Classic[74]	Thrombocytopenia	D	Partial
Pembrolizumab	200 mg IV every 3 wk	AIDS[36] Classic[39]	Fatigue Pruritus Onycholysis	C	Complete

Pomalidomide	Oral 5 mg daily Aspirin 81 mg per day for thromboprophylaxis	AIDS[75] Classic[75]	Neutropenia Constipation Anemia Fatigue Rash	B	Complete
Sirolimus	0.04–0.06 mg/kg/d	Iatrogenic[7]		C	Complete
Sorafenib	200 mg daily	AIDS[76]	Increased lipase Thrombocytopenia Hand-foot syndrome	B	Partial
Thalidomide	100–1000 mg per day for up to 1 year	AIDS[77] Classic[78] Iatrogenic[78]	Hypersensitivity Dehydration Nausea Cellulitis Creatinine kinase elevation Hypophosphatemia Depression	C	Complete

Current Clinical Trials[d]

Agent	ClinicalTrials.Gov Identifier
Digoxin	NCT02212639
EphB4-HAS fusion protein	NCT02799485
Intralesional nivolumab	NCT03316274
Nelfinavir	NCT03077451
Nivolumab and ipilimumab	NCT03219671
Pembrolizumab	NCT03469804
Pomalidomide	NCT01495598, NCT03601806
Selumetinib	NCT01752569
Valganciclovir	NCT03296553

[a] KS subtypes in bold type indicate subtypes for which the highest level of evidence exists.

[b] All listed side effects correspond to side effects reported in cited studies.

[c] Evidence levels are as follows: (A) double-blind, randomized, placebo-controlled trial, (B) lesser quality randomized controlled trial or prospective study, (C) case-control study or retrospective study, (D) case series or case reports, (E) expert opinion.

[d] Clinical trials were included if they were recruiting, not yet recruiting, active not recruiting, or enrolling by invitation in November 2018.

A review of systemic and skin-directed therapies for all KS variants can be found in **Table 2**. A description of chemotherapy regimens for KS is beyond the scope of this article and has been omitted. There are several systemic treatments for KS currently in clinical trials. There are reports of patients with endemic KS[35] and patients with HIV-associated KS[36] responding to immune checkpoint inhibitors. PD-1 is upregulated on CD8+ T cells in HIV and has been shown to be associated with T cell exhaustion during chronic viral infection.[37] Blocking the PD-1/L1 interaction is therefore hypothesized to decrease viremia, decrease immunosuppression, and result in tumor regression due to increased immune surveillance of malignancy.[37,38] Although some conjecture that a high tumor mutational burden may be predictive of response,[39,40] patients with sarcomas with low mutational burden lacking PD-L1 expression have also been successfully treated.[36]

SUMMARY

KS, with its distinct clinical variants, presents a unique challenge for clinical care. The advent of ART in the mid-1990s was a major advance in the treatment of AIDS KS, and the incorporation of cytotoxic chemotherapies has been a mainstay for advanced or rapidly progressive disease. A summary of treatment options is presented in **Table 2**. Exciting new developments in immunotherapy, including the use of checkpoint inhibitors, mark the first new advances in systemic therapies for KS in many years. However, there continue to be major health care disparities with regard to access to care and survival both globally and within the United States.

ACKNOWLEDGMENTS

The authors gratefully acknowledge Jo-David Fine, MD, MPH; Jeffrey P. Zwerner, MD, PhD; Abigail Koch, MD; and Badri Modi, MD for contribution of clinical and pathologic images.

REFERENCES

1. Marcoval J, Bonfill-Orti M, Martinez-Molina L, et al. Evolution of Kaposi sarcoma in the past 30 years in a tertiary hospital of the European Mediterranean basin. Clin Exp Dermatol 2019. https://doi.org/10.1111/ced.13605.
2. Anderson LA, Lauria C, Romano N, et al. Risk factors for classical Kaposi sarcoma in a population-based case-control study in Sicily. Cancer Epidemiol Biomarkers Prev 2008;17(12):3435–43.
3. Parkin DM, Sitas F, Chirenje M, et al. Part I: Cancer in Indigenous Africans–burden, distribution, and trends. Lancet Oncol 2008;9(7):683–92.
4. Cahoon EK, Linet MS, Clarke CA, et al. Risk of Kaposi sarcoma after solid organ transplantation in the United States. Int J Cancer 2018;143(11):2741–8.
5. Ramzi M, Vojdani R, Haghighinejad H. Kaposi sarcoma after allogeneic hematopoietic stem cell transplant: a rare complication. Exp Clin Transplant 2018. https://doi.org/10.6002/ect.2017.0075.
6. Dollard SC, Douglas D, Basavaraju SV, et al. Donor-derived Kaposi's sarcoma in a liver-kidney transplant recipient. Am J Transplant 2018;18(2):510–3.
7. Stallone G, Schena A, Infante B, et al. Sirolimus for Kaposi's sarcoma in renal-transplant recipients. N Engl J Med 2005;352(13):1317–23.
8. Detroyer D, Deraedt K, Schöffski P, et al. Resolution of diffuse skin and systemic Kaposi's sarcoma in a renal transplant recipient after introduction of everolimus: a case report. Transpl Infect Dis 2015;17(2):303–7.
9. Ursini F, Naty S, Mazzei V, et al. Kaposi's sarcoma in a psoriatic arthritis patient treated with infliximab. Int Immunopharmacol 2010;10(7):827–8.
10. Royse KE, El chaer F, Amirian ES, et al. Disparities in Kaposi sarcoma incidence and survival in the United States: 2000-2013. PLoS One 2017;12(8):e0182750.
11. Lodi S, Guiguet M, Costagliola D, et al. Kaposi sarcoma incidence and survival among HIV-infected homosexual men after HIV seroconversion. J Natl Cancer Inst 2010;102(11):784–92.
12. Maurer T, Ponte M, Leslie K. HIV-associated Kaposi's sarcoma with a high CD4 count and a low viral load. N Engl J Med 2007;357(13):1352–3.
13. Hinojosa T, Lewis DJ, Liu M, et al. Nonepidemic Kaposi sarcoma: a recently proposed category. JAAD Case Rep 2017;3(5):441–3.
14. Mukhtar F, Ilozumba M, Utuama O, et al. Change in pattern of secondary cancers after Kaposi sarcoma in the era of antiretroviral therapy. JAMA Oncol 2018; 4(1):48–53.
15. Chang Y, Cesarman E, Pessin MS, et al. Identification of herpesvirus-like DNA sequences in AIDS-associated Kaposi's sarcoma. Science 1994; 266(5192):1865–9.
16. Hladik W, Dollard SC, Mermin J, et al. Transmission of human herpesvirus 8 by blood transfusion. N Engl J Med 2006;355(13):1331–8.
17. Wang HW, Trotter MW, Lagos D, et al. Kaposi sarcoma herpesvirus-induced cellular reprogramming contributes to the lymphatic endothelial gene expression in Kaposi sarcoma. Nat Genet 2004; 36(7):687–93.
18. Hussein HAM, Okafor IB, Walker LR, et al. Cellular and viral oncogenes: the key to unlocking unknowns of Kaposi's sarcoma-associated herpesvirus pathogenesis. J Arch Virol 2018. https://doi.org/10.1007/s00705-018-3918-3.

19. Zhong W, Wang H, Herndier B, et al. Restricted expression of Kaposi sarcoma-associated herpesvirus (human herpesvirus 8) genes in Kaposi sarcoma. Proc Natl Acad Sci U S A 1996;93(13): 6641–6.

20. Ye F, Zeng Y, Sha J, et al. High glucose induces reactivation of latent Kaposi's sarcoma-associated herpesvirus. J Virol 2016. https://doi.org/10.1128/JVI.01049-16.

21. Aneja KK, Yuan Y. Reactivation and lytic replication of Kaposi's sarcoma-associated herpesvirus: an update. Front Microbiol 2017;8:613.

22. Rohrmus B, Thoma-greber EM, Bogner JR, et al. Outlook in oral and cutaneous Kaposi's sarcoma. Lancet 2000;356(9248):2160.

23. El-mallawany NK, Mcatee CL, Campbell LR, et al. Pediatric Kaposi sarcoma in context of the HIV epidemic in sub-Saharan Africa: current perspectives. Pediatr Health Med Ther 2018;9:35–46.

24. Krown SE, Metroka C, Wernz JC. Kaposi's sarcoma in the acquired immune deficiency syndrome: a proposal for uniform evaluation, response, and staging criteria. AIDS Clinical Trials Group Oncology Committee. J Clin Oncol 1989;7(9):1201–7.

25. Grayson W, Pantanowitz L. Histological variants of cutaneous Kaposi sarcoma. Diagn Pathol 2008;3: 31.

26. Patel RM, Goldblum JR, Hsi ED. Immunohistochemical detection of human herpes virus-8 latent nuclear antigen-1 is useful in the diagnosis of Kaposi sarcoma. Mod Pathol 2004;17(4):456–60.

27. Yarchoan R, Uldrick TS. HIV-associated cancers and related diseases. N Engl J Med 2018;378(11): 1029–41.

28. Moosa MR. Kaposi's sarcoma in kidney transplant recipients: a 23-year experience. QJM 2005;98(3): 205–14.

29. Martin-carbonero L, Barrios A, Saballs P, et al. Pegylated liposomal doxorubicin plus highly active antiretroviral therapy versus highly active antiretroviral therapy alone in HIV patients with Kaposi's sarcoma. AIDS 2004;18(12):1737–40.

30. Bower M, Weir J, Francis N, et al. The effect of HAART in 254 consecutive patients with AIDS-related Kaposi's sarcoma. AIDS 2009;23(13): 1701–6.

31. Achenbach CJ, Harrington RD, Dhanireddy S, et al. Paradoxical immune reconstitution inflammatory syndrome in HIV-infected patients treated with combination antiretroviral therapy after AIDS-defining opportunistic infection. Clin Infect Dis 2012;54(3): 424–33.

32. Speicher DJ, Sehu MM, Johnson NW, et al. Successful treatment of an HIV-positive patient with unmasking Kaposi's sarcoma immune reconstitution inflammatory syndrome. J Clin Virol 2013;57(3): 282–5.

33. Cianfrocca M, Lee S, Von Roenn J, et al. Randomized trial of paclitaxel versus pegylated liposomal doxorubicin for advanced human immunodeficiency virus-associated Kaposi sarcoma: evidence of symptom palliation from chemotherapy. Cancer 2010;116(16):3969–77.

34. Robey RC, Bower M. Facing up to the ongoing challenge of Kaposi's sarcoma. Curr Opin Infect Dis 2015;28(1):31–40.

35. Delyon J, Bizot A, Battistella M, et al. PD-1 blockade with nivolumab in endemic Kaposi sarcoma. Ann Oncol 2018;29(4):1067–9.

36. Galanina N, Goodman AM, Cohen PR, et al. Successful treatment of HIV-associated Kaposi sarcoma with immune checkpoint blockade. Cancer Immunol Res 2018;6(10):1129–35.

37. Day CL, Kaufmann DE, Kiepiela P, et al. PD-1 expression on HIV-specific T cells is associated with T-cell exhaustion and disease progression. Nature 2006;443(7109):350–4.

38. Paydas S, Bagir EK, Deveci MA, et al. Clinical and prognostic significance of PD-1 and PD-L1 expression in sarcomas. Med Oncol 2016;33(8):93.

39. Saller J, Walko CM, Millis SZ, et al. Response to checkpoint inhibitor therapy in advanced classic Kaposi sarcoma: a case report and immunogenomic study. J Natl Compr Canc Netw 2018;16(7): 797–800.

40. Tappero JW, Berger TG, Kaplan LD, et al. Cryotherapy for cutaneous Kaposi's sarcoma (KS) associated with acquired immune deficiency syndrome (AIDS): a phase II trial. J Acquir Immune Defic Syndr 1991;4(9):839–46.

41. Özdemir M, Balevi A. Successful treatment of classic Kaposi sarcoma with long-pulse neodymium-doped yttrium aluminum garnet laser: a preliminary study. Dermatol Surg 2017;43(3):366–70.

42. Caccialanza M, Marca S, Piccinno R, et al. Radiotherapy of classic and human immunodeficiency virus-related Kaposi's sarcoma: results in 1482 lesions. J Eur Acad Dermatol Venereol 2008;22(3): 297–302.

43. Yildiz F, Genc M, Akyurek S, et al. Radiotherapy in the management of Kaposi's sarcoma: comparison of 8 Gy versus 6 Gy. J Natl Med Assoc 2006;98(7): 1136–9.

44. Evans MD, Yassa M, Podgorsak EB, et al. Surface applicators for high dose rate brachytherapy in AIDS-related Kaposi's sarcoma. Int J Radiat Oncol Biol Phys 1997;39(3):769–74.

45. Ruiz MÁG, Rivero JQ, García JLM, et al. High-dose-rate brachytherapy in the treatment of skin Kaposi sarcoma. J Contemp Brachytherapy 2017;9(6): 561–5.

46. Kasper ME, Richter S, Warren N, et al. Complete response of endemic Kaposi sarcoma lesions with high-dose-rate brachytherapy: treatment method,

results, and toxicity using skin surface applicators. Brachytherapy 2013;12(5):495–9.

47. Poignonec S, Lachiver LD, Lamas G, et al. Intralesional bleomycin for acquired immunodeficiency syndrome-associated cutaneous Kaposi's sarcoma. Arch Dermatol 1995;131(2):228.

48. Mirza YA, Altamura D, Hirbod T, et al. Long-term response of classic Kaposi's sarcoma to intralesional doxorubicin: a case report. Case Rep Dermatol 2015;7(1):17–9.

49. Dupuy J, Price M, Lynch G, et al. Intralesional interferon-alpha and zidovudine in epidemic Kaposi's sarcoma. J Am Acad Dermatol 1993;28(6):966–72.

50. Trattner A, Reizis Z, David M, et al. The therapeutic effect of intralesional interferon in classical Kaposi's sarcoma. Br J Dermatol 1993;129(5):590–3.

51. Lucatorto FM, Sapp JP. Treatment of oral Kaposi's sarcoma with a sclerosing agent in AIDS patients. A preliminary study. Oral Surg Oral Med Oral Pathol 1993;75(2):192–8.

52. Boudreaux AA, Smith LL, Cosby CD, et al. Intralesional vinblastine for cutaneous Kaposi's sarcoma associated with acquired immunodeficiency syndrome. A clinical trial to evaluate efficacy and discomfort associated with infection. J Am Acad Dermatol 1993;28(1):61–5.

53. Kim BR, Park JT, Byun SY, et al. Treatment of classic Kaposi's sarcoma showing a discretely scattered distribution with intralesional vinblastine injections. Ann Dermatol 2016;28(1):113–4.

54. Brambilla L, Bellinvia M, Tourlaki A, et al. Intralesional vincristine as first-line therapy for nodular lesions in classic Kaposi sarcoma: a prospective study in 151 patients. Br J Dermatol 2010;162(4):854–9.

55. Pagliarello C, Stanganelli I, Fabrizi G, et al. Topical diphencyprone immunotherapy for painful nodular acral recurrence of Kaposi sarcoma. JAMA Dermatol 2016. https://doi.org/10.1001/jamadermatol.2016.4301.

56. Lebari D, Gohil J, Patnaik L, et al. Isolated penile Kaposi's sarcoma in a HIV-positive patient stable on treatment for three years. Int J STD AIDS 2014;25(8):607–10.

57. Célestin Schartz NE, Chevret S, Paz C, et al. Imiquimod 5% cream for treatment of HIV-negative Kaposi's sarcoma skin lesions: A phase I to II, open-label trial in 17 patients. J Am Acad Dermatol 2008;58(4):585–91.

58. Prinz Vavricka BM, Hofbauer GF, Dummer R, et al. Topical treatment of cutaneous Kaposi sarcoma with imiquimod 5% in renal-transplant recipients: a clinicopathological observation. Clin Exp Dermatol 2012;37(6):620–5.

59. Díaz-Ley B, Grillo E, Ríos-Buceta L, et al. Classic Kaposi's sarcoma treated with topical rapamycin. Dermatol Ther 2015;28(1):40–3.

60. Brambilla L, Tourlaki A. Silver nitrate for Kaposi's sarcoma nodules: A new look at an old treatment. J Dermatolog Treat 2017;28(2):152–4.

61. Abdelmaksoud A, Filoni A, Giudice G, et al. Classic and HIV-related Kaposi sarcoma treated with 0.1% topical timolol gel. J Am Acad Dermatol 2017;76(1):153–5.

62. Alcántara-Reifs CM, Salido-Vallejo R, Garnacho-Saucedo GM, et al. Classic Kaposi's sarcoma treated with topical 0.5% timolol gel. Dermatol Ther 2016;29(5):309–11.

63. Chap S, Vu M, Robinson AJ, et al. Treatment of cutaneous iatrogenic Kaposi sarcoma with topical timolol. Australas J Dermatol 2017;58(3):242–3.

64. Paparizos VA, Kyriakis KP, Papastamopoulos V, et al. Response of AIDS-associated Kaposi sarcoma to highly active antiretroviral therapy alone. J Acquir Immune Defic Syndr 2002;30(2):257–8.

65. Murphy C, Hawkes E, Chionh F, et al. Durable remission of both multicentric Castleman's disease and Kaposi's sarcoma with valganciclovir, rituximab and liposomal doxorubicin in an HHV-8-positive, HIV-negative patient. J Clin Pharm Ther 2017;42(1):111–4.

66. Aboulafia DM, Norris D, Henry D, et al. 9-cis-retinoic acid capsules in the treatment of AIDS-related Kaposi sarcoma: results of a phase 2 multicenter clinical trial. Arch Dermatol 2003;139(2):178–86.

67. Uldrick TS, Wyvill KM, Kumar P, et al. Phase II study of bevacizumab in patients with HIV-associated Kaposi's sarcoma receiving antiretroviral therapy. J Clin Oncol 2012;30(13):1476–83.

68. Dezube BJ, Krown SE, Lee JY, et al. Randomized phase II trial of matrix metalloproteinase inhibitor COL-3 in AIDS-related Kaposi's sarcoma: an AIDS Malignancy Consortium Study. J Clin Oncol 2006;24(9):1389–94.

69. Little RF, Pluda JM, Wyvill KM, et al. Activity of subcutaneous interleukin-12 in AIDS-related Kaposi sarcoma. Blood 2006;107(12):4650–7.

70. Cao W, Vyboh K, Routy B, et al. Imatinib for highly chemoresistant Kaposi sarcoma in a patient with long-term HIV control: a case report and literature review. Curr Oncol 2015;22(5):e395–9.

71. Koon HB, Krown SE, Lee JY, et al. Phase II trial of imatinib in AIDS-associated Kaposi's sarcoma: AIDS malignancy consortium protocol 042. J Clin Oncol 2014;32(5):402–8.

72. Pourcher V, Desnoyer A, Assoumou L, et al. Phase II trial of Lenalidomide in HIV-infected patients with previously treated Kaposi's sarcoma: results of the ANRS 154 Lenakap trial. AIDS Res Hum Retroviruses 2017;33(1):1–10.

73. Bernstein ZP, Chanan-khan A, Miller KC, et al. A multicenter phase II study of the intravenous administration of liposomal tretinoin in patients

with acquired immunodeficiency syndrome-associated Kaposi's sarcoma. Cancer 2002; 95(12):2555–61.

74. Harris BHL, Walsh JL, Neciunaite R, et al. Ring a ring o'roses, a patient with Kaposi's? Pazopanib, pazopanib, it might go away. Mediterranean (classic) Kaposi sarcoma responds to the tyrosine kinase inhibitor pazopanib after multiple lines of standard therapy. Clin Exp Dermatol 2018; 43(2):234–6.

75. Polizzotto MN, Uldrick TS, Wyvill KM, et al. Pomalidomide for symptomatic Kaposi's sarcoma in people with and without HIV infection: a phase I/II study. J Clin Oncol 2016;34(34):4125–31.

76. Uldrick TS, Gonçalves PH, Wyvill KM, et al. A phase Ib study of Sorafenib (BAY 43-9006) in patients with Kaposi sarcoma. Oncologist 2017;22(5):505-e49.

77. Little RF, Wyvill KM, Pluda JM, et al. Activity of thalidomide in AIDS-related Kaposi's sarcoma. J Clin Oncol 2000;18(13):2593–602.

78. Ben m'barek L, Fardet L, Mebazaa A, et al. A retrospective analysis of thalidomide therapy in non-HIV-related Kaposi's sarcoma. Dermatology (Basel) 2007;215(3):202–5.

Basal Cell Carcinoma, Squamous Cell Carcinoma, and Cutaneous Melanoma in Skin of Color Patients

Latrice Hogue, BA[a,1], Valerie M. Harvey, MD, MPH[b,c],*

KEYWORDS

- Skin of color • Skin cancer • Ethnic skin • Basal cell carcinoma • Squamous cell carcinoma
- Melanoma • Health disparities

KEY POINTS

- Basal cell carcinomas in black, Hispanic, and Asian individuals tend to be pigmented and are often misdiagnosed. Therefore, clinicians should maintain a high index of suspicion.
- Squamous cell carcinoma in skin of color has strong associations with chronic scarring and inflammatory skin conditions.
- Infection with the human papilloma virus types 16 and 18 may be an important factor for squamous cell carcinoma in black and Hispanic individuals.
- Minority patients diagnosed with melanoma are more likely to present with regional and distant metastases.
- Early detection and research are important to help reduce disparities in skin cancer–related outcomes.

INTRODUCTION

Basal cell carcinoma (BCC), squamous cell carcinoma (SCC), and melanoma combined are the most common malignancies in the United States.[1,2] Although precise numbers are difficult to determine, approximately 5.4 million cases of BCC and SCC are diagnosed every year.[1] In 2018, an estimated 91,270 cases of melanoma were diagnosed and 9320 deaths were expected as a result of this disease.[1] Although melanoma comprises only 1% of all skin cancers, it accounts for approximately 82% of skin cancer mortality.[1] Although skin cancer is far more common in fair-skinned individuals, Hispanic, Asian, and black individuals account for 4% to 5%, 2% to 4%, and 1% to 2% of skin cancer cases, respectively.[3,4]

LIMITATIONS OF CURRENT SKIN CLASSIFICATIONS

Health researchers have used several classification systems as surrogates to define groups of people. Race is a social and biological construct based largely on the phenotypic features of skin and hair color.[5] Ethnicity reflects a convergence of biological factors, cultural factors, and geographic origins.[5] Although some argue for

Disclosure Statement: Dr L. Hogue has nothing to disclose. Dr V.M. Harvey is on the speaker board for Aclaris and a consultant at Novartis and L'Oréal.
[a] Department of Dermatology, Wake Forest School of Medicine, Winston Salem, NC, USA; [b] Hampton University Skin of Color Research Institute, Hampton, VA, USA; [c] TPMG Hampton Roads Center for Dermatology, Newport News, VA, USA
[1] Present address: 1321 Campus Court, Winston Salem, NC 27127.
* Corresponding author. 31 E Tyler Street, Hampton, VA 23669.
E-mail address: valerieharvey10@gmail.com

Dermatol Clin 37 (2019) 519–526
https://doi.org/10.1016/j.det.2019.05.009

abandoning variables like race and ethnicity in medical research, others fear that omitting these categories could conceal important disparities and inequities in health care quality and delivery.[5]

The Fitzpatrick phototype system (FPS), widely used by dermatologists, was initially developed for fair skin individuals to gauge sun sensitivity based on the self-report of erythema and ability to tan following ultraviolet (UV) exposure.[6,7] Patients with skin of color are commonly assumed to fall into Fitzpatrick skin phototypes 4 through 6.[8] The FPS often can be inaccurate given the heterogeneity in complexions within broadly defined groups, particularly those with increased mixed ancestry, such as African American and Hispanic.[9] Del Bino and Bernerd[7] used a colorimetric classification system to objectively measure skin pigmentation in 423 patients from various ethnic backgrounds and categorized skin color into 6 groups from very light to dark. They found significant overlap across racial and ethnic categories, with white skin ranging from light to tan, black skin from intermediate to dark, Hispanic skin from light to brown, and Asian skin from light to dark.[6,7] The investigators concluded that a more precise measure of skin color was needed when assessing the risks of sun exposure.[7]

In this review, we use the terms "skin of color" and "people of color" to describe patients from various nonwhite racial and ethnic groups. Although we acknowledge that this terminology is less than precise, we believe it to be the most appropriate approach for summarizing the literature on this topic.

RISK FACTORS

Numerous studies, conducted mostly in fair-skinned individuals, have shown that exposure to UV radiation is the major modifiable risk factor driving skin cancer development.[8,10–13] However, the role of UV exposure as an etiologic factor has been understudied in individuals with skin of color. It is also unknown if nonmodifiable risk factors in white individuals, such as fair skin tone, hair and eye color, number of nevi, propensity toward sunburns, and family history of melanoma, also influence melanoma risks in nonwhites.[14] Thus far, the limited data show conflicting results.[14] The tendency for melanomas and SCCs to develop in sun-protected areas of those with skin of color suggests that UV radiation may play a nonsignificant role for these malignancies.[9] Eide and Weinstock[15] found that increased residential UV exposure was not significantly associated with melanoma in black, Hispanic, Asian, and Native

American individuals. In contrast, Hu and colleagues[16] found a positive correlation of melanoma incidence with UV index, in white, Hispanic, and black individuals. However, this correlation reached significance only in white men, white women, and black men.[16] In support of this epidemiologic finding, experimental studies demonstrate that UV-induced DNA damage occurs to varying degrees across all skin types.[17] However, skin from subjects with higher melanin content can more efficiently repair solar-induced DNA damage than skin from those with fair skin[17] (**Table 1**).

PERCEIVED SKIN CANCER RISK, KNOWLEDGE, AND BEHAVIORS

There is a general underestimation of the risk of skin cancer in those with skin of color.[18] Kim and colleagues[19] examined how black, Hispanic, and Asian individuals perceived their risk of skin cancer and found that 65% of participants viewed themselves as having no risk. Similarly, Pichon and colleagues[20] found that 46% of black participants believed they had no risk of developing skin cancer and 30% believed they had low risk. In this same study, only 35% of subjects who reported an ability to sunburn perceived themselves as having any risk of developing skin cancer.[19] Black and Hispanic patients are also less likely to believe that behavioral practices can affect skin cancer risk and are less likely to participate in sun-protective behaviors.[21–23]

Friedman and colleagues[24] found that Caucasian (58%) and Hispanic (47%) individuals were more likely than black individuals (4%) to report wearing sunscreen within the past year. Consistent with other studies, Summers and colleagues[25] found that black patients who reported severe sunburns were 7 times less likely to wear sunscreen than non-Hispanic white patients with a history of severe sunburns.[26,27] Lower rates of sunscreen application in minority populations may stem from the belief that sun protection is not needed to prevent skin cancers, infrequent familial and community experiences with skin cancer, and the lack of dialogue with health care providers regarding skin cancer prevention.[25,28]

A survey conducted by Korta and colleagues[29] found that 5% of black, Hispanic, and Asian respondents, compared with 49% of white participants, reported receiving a total body skin examination by a physician at any point in their life. Physicians are also less likely to recommend sunscreen to persons with skin of color.[22] One study found that physicians did not universally offer advice on photoprotection to their nonwhite

Table 1
Basal cell carcinoma, squamous cell carcinoma, and melanoma in individuals with skin of color

Skin Cancer	Incidence	Clinical Presentation	Risk Associations
BCC	• Approximately 80% of skin cancers • Most common skin cancer in Hispanic and Asian individuals • Second most common skin cancer in black individuals	• Solitary papule with rolled borders (pearly nature and telangiectasias may be less conspicuous) • Pigmented variant more prevalent	• UV radiation, albinism, scars, ulcers, exposure to ionizing radiation, arsenic ingestion, oral methoxsalen (psoralen), xeroderma pigmentosum, HIV, and iatrogenic immunosuppression
SCC	• Approximately 20% of skin cancers • Most common skin cancer in black individuals • Second most common skin cancer in Hispanic and Asian individuals	• Ill-defined, rough, pink patches to well-circumscribed hyperkeratotic papules or plaques • Scaly brown or black hyperpigmented plaques, papules or nodules • Hypopigmented, hyper-pigmented, or mottled perilesional appearance	• Chronic scarring processes, inflammatory conditions, HPV, immunosuppression, burn scars, sites of radiation therapy, albinism, epidermodysplasia verruciformis, and chemical carcinogens
Melanoma	• Least common in black, Asian, and Hispanic individuals • Incidence for every 100,000 people is 4 in Hispanic, 1 in black, and 1 in Asian individuals	• Hyperpigmented macule or patch with history of rapid changes • Acral lentiginous melanoma (of palms, soles, nailbeds) involves radial and vertical growth phases	• Role of UV exposure unclear

Abbreviations: BCC, basal cell carcinoma; HIV, human immunodeficiency virus; HPV, human papilloma virus; SCC, squamous cell carcinoma.

patients, but instead used patient inquiry as a gauge of whether to provide counseling.[30]

BASAL CELL CARCINOMA

BCCs account for 80% of skin cancers.[31] They are the most common skin cancer in Asian and Hispanic individuals and the second most common in black individuals.[8] Estimates of US incidence rates for BCCs are imprecise because cancer registries do not collect data on BCCs.[1] The most reliable approximations of their occurrence among minority patients stems from single-center and multi-institutional studies. Although the timing, intensity, and pattern of UV radiation (UVR) exposure are important for estimating the BCC risk in fair skin individuals, less is known about the role of solar exposure in skin of color. Other factors associated with BCC development include albinism, scars, ulcers, exposure to ionizing radiation, arsenic ingestion, oral methoxsalen (psoralen), xeroderma pigmentosum, human immunodeficiency virus, and iatrogenic immunosuppression, such as in organ transplant recipients.[32–34] Burns

and colleagues[35] proposed that decreased cellular immunity and altered tumor surveillance may be particularly critical in black patients diagnosed with BCC. Impaired tumor surveillance may explain why Mora and Burris[36] found that 16.5% of black patients with BCCs also had a concurrent noncutaneous malignancy.

Clinical Characteristics

The mean age at diagnosis for BCC is 60 years in black individuals, and 2 studies found a female predominance in incidence.[36,37] Similar to non-Hispanic whites, BCCs in those with skin of color characteristically develop in sun-exposed areas of the head and neck region (**Fig. 1**).[8,9] The frequency of BCC may correlate with the degree of skin pigmentation.[3] In a clinical series set in an urban academic medical center, BCCs were more likely to occur in light versus darkly pigmented black patients; 67% of 23 patients were categorized as having "fair" or "olive" skin tone.[38] McLeod and colleagues[39] found a trend toward contralateral distribution of nonmelanoma skin cancers (most of which were BCCs) for older

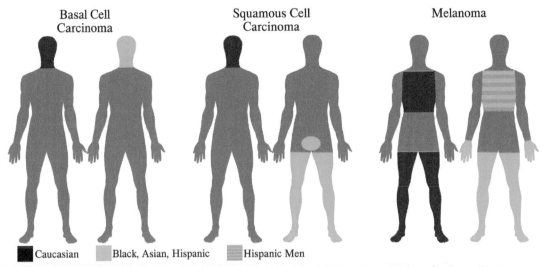

Basal Cell   Squamous Cell   Melanoma
Carcinoma   Carcinoma

■ Caucasian   ■ Black, Asian, Hispanic   ■ Hispanic Men

Fig. 1. Major anatomic distribution of BCC, SCC, and melanoma in Caucasian and skin of color patients.

non-Hispanic white patients. Hispanic patients were significantly more likely to have right-sided versus left-sided lesions.[39] The investigators speculate that differences in sun exposure patterns may account for their finding.[39]

The classic BCC presentation of a pearly papule with rolled borders and telangiectasias may be difficult to visualize in darker skin tones.[8] More than 50% of BCCs are pigmented in nonwhite versus only 5% in white individuals (**Fig. 2**).[8,37,40] In Hispanic patients, the likelihood of a pigmented BCC is twice as frequent as in white patients.[40] The pigmentation in Asian patients has been described as having a brown to glossy black appearance.[33] The presence of pigment in BCCs can make diagnosis challenging; therefore, clinicians should have a high index of suspicion.[4]

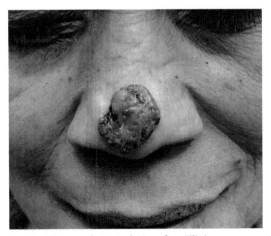

Fig. 2. BCC on the nasal tip of a Filipino woman. (*Courtesy of* C. Ahn, MD, New York NY.)

Metastatic BCC is rare, with a reported incidence of 0.0028% to 0.99%, and a poor prognosis, with mean survival of 8 months to 3.6 years.[32,33] There are no differences in BCC-associated morbidity in black when compared with white individuals.[4] Loh and colleagues[41] found no significant differences in preoperative lesion size and the number of Mohs stages required for excisions among white, Hispanic, and Asian patients with BCC.

SQUAMOUS CELL CARCINOMA

SCC accounts for approximately 20% of skin cancers.[31] It is the most common skin cancer in black individuals and the second most common in Hispanic and Asian individuals.[4,33] Mora and Perniciaro[42] found that SCCs were 20% more common than BCCs in black patients. Although epidemiologic studies have found UVR to be a major cause of SCC in white patients, UVR is not considered an important etiologic factor in black patients.[4] The strongest association for SCC development in black and Asian individuals are scarring processes and inflammatory conditions, such as burn scars, chronic ulcers (**Fig. 3**), discoid lupus erythematosus, and hidradenitis suppurativa.[4,33,42] Human papilloma virus (HPV) also may play a role in development of SCC.[43] Pritchett and colleagues[44] examined skin cancer in organ transplant recipients and found that 85.7% of black patients and 66.7% of Hispanic patients with SCC had a positive history of HPV, including subtypes 16 and 18 in the groin. This association was not identified in Asian transplant recipients.[44] Other conditions associated with the development of SCC in black patients include burn scars, sites

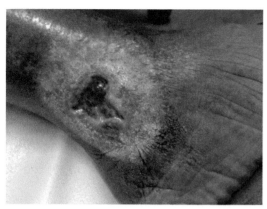

Fig. 3. SCC in a longstanding scar of the right lateral ankle in a black patient.

of radiation therapy, albinism, epidermodysplasia verruciformis, and chemical carcinogens, such as arsenic and tar.[4]

Clinical Characteristics

The mean age at diagnosis for SCC is 69 years for blacks, with a female predominance in incidence.[45,46] Although the most common distribution for SCC in white individuals is the head and neck region, sun-protected areas including the lower limbs and anogenital area are more common among black patients (see **Fig. 1**).[4] The lower limbs comprised up to 66% of SCCs in black patients in multiple case reviews, followed by head and neck.[4]

Clinically, SCC can have varied presentations from ill-defined, rough, pink patches to well-circumscribed hyperkeratotic papules or plaques.[33] In black individuals, SCC commonly presents as scaly brown or black hyperpigmented plaques, papules, or nodules.[33] The perilesional skin may have a dyspigmented or mottled appearance.[4,33] SCC in sun-protected areas and those that arise from scars may behave more aggressively than SCCs that arise in sun-exposed skin.[4] In a retrospective review of 163 black patients with SCC, Mora and Perniciaro[42] reported a mortality rate of 18.4%. SCC that developed within scarring processes had a higher mortality rate of 24% in this same cohort of black patients.[42]

MELANOMA

In 2018, the annual incidence rate of melanoma per 100,000 was 26 in non-Hispanic white individuals compared with 4, 1, and 1 in Hispanic, black, and Asian individuals, respectively.[1,47] Garnett and colleagues[48] reported a decline in the incidence of melanoma among US Hispanic

individuals between 2003 to 2012, an observation that contrasts with earlier state-level studies in California and Florida that found small but significant increases in melanoma incidence. Discrepancies in incidence trends may reflect period effects or variations in state-level reporting of melanoma. Incidence rates for black and Asian individuals remain stable over time.[49]

Despite their overall lower incidence, patients with skin of color who develop melanoma are significantly more likely to present with regional and distant metastases.[47] Cormier and colleagues[50] found that Hispanic individuals (odds ratio [OR], 3.6), African American individuals (OR, 4.2), and Asian individuals (OR, 2.4), were more likely than white individuals to have stage IV melanoma at the time of presentation. Among minority patients, differences in late-stage presentation are gender-based.[47] Hispanic men had a higher proportion of advanced disease than Hispanic women, and Asian and black women had a higher proportion of advanced melanoma than their male counterparts.[47] Cress and Holly[47] found that the rates of late-stage diagnoses in men were 21% in Hispanic, 20% in Asian, and 24% in black individuals, compared with 12% in white men. For women, late-stage melanoma was present in 13% of Hispanic, 26% of Asian, and 19% of black individuals, compared with 8% of white women.[47] Disparities also exist in the diagnosis of childhood melanoma. Hispanic children and adolescents with a diagnosis of melanoma are 3 times more likely than their non-Hispanic white counterparts to present with advanced disease.[51] Advanced disease at presentation likely contributes to the worse survival outcomes observed in minority patients.[52]

Clinical Characteristics

The mean age of diagnosis for black patients with melanoma is 60 years in men and 62 years in women.[47] For Asian patients, the mean age at presentation is 61 years for men and 55 years for women.[47] The mean age for melanoma diagnosis in Hispanic individuals is 56 years.[48] Incidence does not differ significantly between genders for Asian and black patients.[47] Incidence is higher in female individuals for younger Hispanic patients, but higher in male individuals in older Hispanic patients.[48]

Cress and Holly[47] found that the lower extremity was the most common location for melanoma in black men at 50%, Asian men at 36%, black women at 63%, Asian women at 55%, and Hispanic women at 27% (see **Fig. 1**). However, truncal melanomas predominate in Hispanic men (see **Fig. 1**).[47] The proportion of melanomas involving the head and neck increases with age for both Hispanic men and women.[47]

For melanomas in which the histologic type is known, the superficial spreading subtype is most common among Hispanic and Asian individuals.[8] Acral lentiginous melanoma is the most common subtype in black individuals (**Figs. 4 and 5**).[8]

DISCUSSION

Skin cancers are relatively uncommon in patients with skin of color; however, the large disparities in patient outcomes, particularly for melanoma, make them an important public health concern. Unfortunately, large gaps in our skin cancer knowledge exist for these rapidly growing segments of the US population. For example, the literature on BCC, SCC, and melanoma epidemiology in minority patients derives mainly from retrospective chart reviews and secondary analyses of state-level and national cancer registries. These data sources often lack critical data or have insufficient patient-level information (eg, self-identified race and ethnicity). In addition, our current paradigms for skin color classification limit the ability of researchers to collect important phenotypic information on skin cancer cases. Thus, there is a need for improved data collection methods.

The phenotypic attributes of skin cancer risk factors in non-Hispanic white individuals have been well characterized. However, the relevance

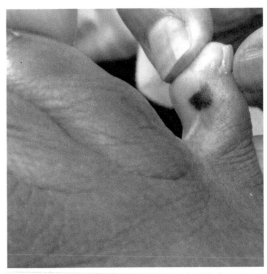

Fig. 5. Melanoma in situ on the toe of a black patient.

of such risk factors in skin of color for BCC, SCC, and melanoma has not been widely investigated. Until we have better-defined skin cancer risk profiles among nonwhite patients, public health messages targeting minority patients and the clinicians who care for them will be of utmost importance, even with their inherent limitations. Regrettably, the persistence of late-stage presentation of melanoma among black, Hispanic, and Asian individuals highlights the deficiencies of current secondary prevention efforts.[52]

The benefits of primary prevention efforts in improving skin cancer outcomes in minority patients are also unknown. There is a paucity of data supporting specific sun protection factor (SPF) recommendations in individuals with skin of color.[8] Commercial SPF testing is mainly conducted in fair-skinned individuals, rendering SPF measurements less reliable in those with skin of color.[8,53] Regardless, in 2014, the American Academy of Dermatology published guidelines for skin cancer prevention in people with skin of color. Their recommendations echoed those for fair-skinned individuals, including the daily application of broad-spectrum sunscreen with an SPF 30 or greater; the use of protective clothing, sunglasses, and wide brim hats; and regular self-skin examinations.[8]

Critical research is needed to address the most urgent questions regarding risks and reasons of disparate outcomes in BCC, SCC, and melanoma for our patients with skin of color. This knowledge will inform the foundation for interventional efforts in prevention, early diagnosis, and treatments that may be specific to minority patients.

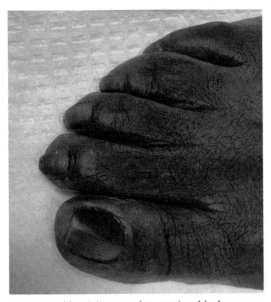

Fig. 4. Acral lentiginous melanoma in a black woman. (*Courtesy of* L. Strowd, MD, Winston Salem, NC.)

ACKNOWLEDGMENTS

Amy McMichael, MD, Christine Ahn, MD, Lindsay Strowd, MD.

REFERENCES

1. American Cancer Society. Facts & figures 2018. American Cancer Society; 2018.
2. Siegel RL, Miller KD, Jemal A. Cancer statistics, 2018. CA Cancer J Clin 2018;68(1):7–30.
3. Bradford PT. Skin cancer in skin of color. Dermatol Nurs 2009;21(4):170–7, 206; [quiz: 178].
4. Gloster HM Jr, Neal K. Skin cancer in skin of color. J Am Acad Dermatol 2006;55(5):741–60 [quiz: 761–4].
5. Corbie-Smith G, Henderson G, Blumenthal C, et al. Conceptualizing race in research. J Natl Med Assoc 2008;100(10):1235–43.
6. Pichon LC, Landrine H, Corral I, et al. Measuring skin cancer risk in African Americans: is the Fitzpatrick skin type classification scale culturally sensitive? Ethn Dis 2010;20(2):174–9.
7. Del Bino S, Bernerd F. Variations in skin colour and the biological consequences of ultraviolet radiation exposure. Br J Dermatol 2013;169(Suppl 3):33–40.
8. Agbai ON, Buster K, Sanchez M, et al. Skin cancer and photoprotection in people of color: a review and recommendations for physicians and the public. J Am Acad Dermatol 2014;70(4):748–62.
9. Battie C, Gohara M, Verschoore M, et al. Skin cancer in skin of color: an update on current facts, trends, and misconceptions. J Drugs Dermatol 2013;12(2):194–8.
10. Madronich S, de Gruijl FR. Skin cancer and UV radiation. Nature 1993;366(6450):23.
11. Watson M, Holman DM, Maguire-Eisen M. Ultraviolet radiation exposure and its impact on skin cancer risk. Semin Oncol Nurs 2016;32(3):241–54.
12. Sample A, Zhao B, Qiang L, et al. Adaptor protein p62 promotes skin tumor growth and metastasis and is induced by UVA radiation. J Biol Chem 2017;292(36):14786–95.
13. Langley RG, Sober AJ. A clinical review of the evidence for the role of ultraviolet radiation in the etiology of cutaneous melanoma. Cancer Invest 1997;15(6):561–7.
14. Gandini S, Sera F, Cattaruzza MS, et al. Meta-analysis of risk factors for cutaneous melanoma: III. Family history, actinic damage and phenotypic factors. Eur J Cancer 2005;41(14):2040–59.
15. Eide MJ, Weinstock MA. Association of UV index, latitude, and melanoma incidence in nonwhite populations—US Surveillance, Epidemiology, and End Results (SEER) Program, 1992 to 2001. Arch Dermatol 2005;141(4):477–81.
16. Hu S, Ma F, Collado-Mesa F, et al. UV radiation, latitude, and melanoma in US Hispanics and blacks. Arch Dermatol 2004;140(7):819–24.
17. Tadokoro T, Kobayashi N, Zmudzka BZ, et al. UV-induced DNA damage and melanin content in human skin differing in racial/ethnic origin. FASEB J 2003;17(9):1177–9.
18. Halder RM, Bridgeman-Shah S. Skin cancer in African Americans. Cancer 1995;75(2 Suppl):667–73.
19. Kim M, Boone SL, West DP, et al. Perception of skin cancer risk by those with ethnic skin. Arch Dermatol 2009;145(2):207–8.
20. Pichon LC, Corral I, Landrine H, et al. Perceived skin cancer risk and sunscreen use among African American adults. J Health Psychol 2010;15(8):1181–9.
21. Buster KJ, You Z, Fouad M, et al. Skin cancer risk perceptions: a comparison across ethnicity, age, education, gender, and income. J Am Acad Dermatol 2012;66(5):771–9.
22. Cestari T, Buster K. Photoprotection in specific populations: children and people of color. J Am Acad Dermatol 2017;76(3S1):S110–21.
23. Santiago-Rivas M, Wang C, Jandorf L. Sun protection beliefs among Hispanics in the US. J Skin Cancer 2014;2014:161960.
24. Friedman LC, Bruce S, Weinberg AD, et al. Early detection of skin cancer: racial/ethnic differences in behaviors and attitudes. J Cancer Educ 1994;9(2):105–10.
25. Summers P, Bena J, Arrigain S, et al. Sunscreen use: non-Hispanic Blacks compared with other racial and/or ethnic groups. Arch Dermatol 2011;147(7):863–4.
26. Hall HI, Rogers JD. Sun protection behaviors among African Americans. Ethn Dis 1999;9(1):126–31.
27. Briley JJ Jr, Lynfield YL, Chavda K. Sunscreen use and usefulness in African-Americans. J Drugs Dermatol 2007;6(1):19–22.
28. Taylor SC. Enhancing the care and treatment of skin of color, part 2: understanding skin physiology. Cutis 2005;76(5):302–6.
29. Korta DZ, Saggar V, Wu TP, et al. Racial differences in skin cancer awareness and surveillance practices at a public hospital dermatology clinic. J Am Acad Dermatol 2014;70(2):312–7.
30. Pourciau CY, Eide MJ, Mahan M, et al. Photoprotection counseling of non-white ethno-racial groups: a survey of the practice of expert dermatologists. Photodermatol Photoimmunol Photomed 2012;28(6):335–7.
31. Alam M, Ratner D. Cutaneous squamous-cell carcinoma. N Engl J Med 2001;344(13):975–83.
32. Rubin AI, Chen EH, Ratner D. Basal-cell carcinoma. N Engl J Med 2005;353(21):2262–9.
33. Higgins S, Nazemi A, Chow M, et al. Review of non-melanoma skin cancer in African Americans,

Hispanics, and Asians. Dermatol Surg 2018;44(7): 903–10.

34. Zhao H, Shu G, Wang S. The risk of non-melanoma skin cancer in HIV-infected patients: new data and meta-analysis. Int J STD AIDS 2016;27(7):568–75.

35. Burns JE, Eisenhauer ED, Jabaley ME, et al. Cellular immune deficiency in black patients with basal cell carcinoma. J Surg Oncol 1980;13(2):129–34.

36. Mora RG, Burris R. Cancer of the skin in blacks: a review of 128 patients with basal-cell carcinoma. Cancer 1981;47(6):1436–8.

37. Matsuoka LY, Schauer PK, Sordillo PP. Basal cell carcinoma in black patients. J Am Acad Dermatol 1981; 4(6):670–2.

38. Halder RM, Bang KM. Skin cancer in blacks in the United States. Dermatol Clin 1988;6(3):397–405.

39. McLeod MP, Ferris KM, Choudhary S, et al. Contralateral distribution of nonmelanoma skin cancer between older Hispanic/Latino and non-Hispanic/non-Latino individuals. Br J Dermatol 2013;168(1): 65–73.

40. Bigler C, Feldman J, Hall E, et al. Pigmented basal cell carcinoma in Hispanics. J Am Acad Dermatol 1996;34(5 Pt 1):751–2.

41. Loh TY, Ortiz A, Goldenberg A, et al. Prevalence and clinical characteristics of nonmelanoma skin cancers among Hispanic and Asian patients compared with white patients in the United States: a 5-year, single-institution retrospective review. Dermatol Surg 2016;42(5):639–45.

42. Mora RG, Perniciaro C. Cancer of the skin in blacks. I. A review of 163 black patients with cutaneous squamous cell carcinoma. J Am Acad Dermatol 1981;5(5):535–43.

43. Karagas MR, Nelson HH, Sehr P, et al. Human papillomavirus infection and incidence of squamous cell and basal cell carcinomas of the skin. J Natl Cancer Inst 2006;98(6):389–95.

44. Pritchett EN, Doyle A, Shaver CM, et al. Nonmelanoma skin cancer in nonwhite organ transplant recipients. JAMA Dermatol 2016;152(12):1348–53.

45. Halder RM, Ara CJ. Skin cancer and photoaging in ethnic skin. Dermatol Clin 2003;21(4):725–32, x.

46. McCall CO, Chen SC. Squamous cell carcinoma of the legs in African Americans. J Am Acad Dermatol 2002;47(4):524–9.

47. Cress RD, Holly EA. Incidence of cutaneous melanoma among non-Hispanic whites, Hispanics, Asians, and blacks: an analysis of California cancer registry data, 1988-93. Cancer Causes Control 1997;8(2):246–52.

48. Garnett E, Townsend J, Steele B, et al. Characteristics, rates, and trends of melanoma incidence among Hispanics in the USA. Cancer Causes Control 2016;27(5):647–59.

49. Clairwood M, Ricketts J, Grant-Kels J, et al. Melanoma in skin of color in Connecticut: an analysis of melanoma incidence and stage at diagnosis in non-Hispanic blacks, non-Hispanic whites, and Hispanics. Int J Dermatol 2014;53(4):425–33.

50. Cormier JN, Xing Y, Ding M, et al. Ethnic differences among patients with cutaneous melanoma. Arch Intern Med 2006;166(17):1907–14.

51. Hamilton EC, Nguyen HT, Chang YC, et al. Health disparities influence childhood melanoma stage at diagnosis and outcome. J Pediatr 2016;175: 182–7.

52. Hu S, Soza-Vento RM, Parker DF, et al. Comparison of stage at diagnosis of melanoma among Hispanic, black, and white patients in Miami-Dade County, Florida. Arch Dermatol 2006;142(6):704–8.

53. Damian DL, Halliday GM, Stc Barnetson R. Sun protection factor measurement of sunscreens is dependent on minimal erythema dose. Br J Dermatol 1999; 141(3):502–7.

Skin Cancer Detection Technology

Deborah N. Dorrell, MD[a], Lindsay C. Strowd, MD[b],*

KEYWORDS

- Skin cancer • Nonmelanoma skin cancer • Melanoma • Reflectance confocal microscopy
- Optical coherence tomography • Multispectral digital skin lesion analysis • Pigmented lesion assay

KEY POINTS

- Recently, many innovative skin cancer detection technologies have been developed to increase diagnostic accuracy for skin cancers.
- Such technologies include reflectance confocal microscopy, optical coherence tomography, high-frequency ultrasound, multispectral digital skin lesion analysis, electrical impedance spectroscopy, Raman spectroscopy, multiphoton tomography, and the pigmented skin lesion assay.
- The new technologies are beneficial because they are fast and noninvasive, provide comprehensive imaging of the lesion, allow for remote diagnosis, and provide high sensitivity.
- The new technologies are limited by high expense, the need for trained operators and interpreters, anatomic limitations, and low specificity.
- The use of newer skin cancer detection techniques is likely to increase as the technology and their diagnostic accuracies are better characterized by future research.

INTRODUCTION

Skin cancer is the most common malignancy in the United States.[1] Globally, it is estimated that more than 1 million new cases of nonmelanoma skin cancer (NMSC) were diagnosed in 2018 with 65,000 associated deaths, and more than 280,000 new cases of malignant melanoma (MM) were diagnosed, with 60,000 associated deaths.[2] These statistics represent a rapidly rising incidence of skin cancers over the past 30 years. Health care providers and patients alike are tasked with identifying and surveilling suspicious skin lesions in order to diagnose skin cancers early and treat them quickly. The earlier skin cancers are treated, the less likely they are to destruct local tissue, metastasize, and cause death. This is particularly true for MM because the 5-year relative survival rate decreases from 99% with local disease to 63% with regional disease and 20% with distant disease.[1] The normal pathway to skin cancer diagnosis is visual, with dermoscopic assessment of the lesion followed by biopsy and histopathologic evaluation. Concerns exist, however, about the diagnostic accuracy of each step of this pathway.

Dermoscopy is a quick and inexpensive method used by many dermatologists to evaluate lesions that appear suspicious to the naked eye because it allows for better visualization of lesional patterns and structures. Although visual assessment without magnification has a sensitivity of 71% and specificity of 81%, dermoscopy has been shown to have 90% sensitivity and specificity. The addition of dermoscopy also decreases the biopsy ratio from 15:1 (15 benign lesions for every 1 MM) to 5:1 and allows for diagnosis at earlier

Disclosure Statement: No conflicts of interest.
[a] Wake Forest School of Medicine, Medical Center Blvd, Winston-Salem, NC 27103, USA; [b] Department of Dermatology, Wake Forest School of Medicine, Medical Center Boulevard, Winston-Salem, NC 27157-1071, USA
* Corresponding author.
E-mail address: lchaney@wakehealth.edu

Dermatol Clin 37 (2019) 527–536
https://doi.org/10.1016/j.det.2019.05.010

stages of disease.[3] For these reasons, the use of dermoscopy among dermatologists increased by 56% between 2001 and 2015.[4] Dermoscopy is a subjective process, however, that requires extensive training to master, and it is still subject to the misidentification of lesions.

Although biopsy and histopathologic examination are the current gold standard for skin cancer diagnosis, this process has certain disadvantages. The biopsy procedure is invasive, and specimen interpretation may take several days to result. Sampling error also may be present because usually less than 2% of the total sample is viewed microscopically.[5] Despite being considered the gold standard, diagnosis with histopathology is not always clear. Discordance rates of 14% among dermatopathologists have been reported for pigmented skin lesions (PSLs).[6] The current system of visual assessment with biopsy and histologic evaluation has an estimated sensitivity of 84% and specificity of less than 30% for early-stage MMs.[7]

Recently, many innovative skin cancer detection technologies have been developed to increase diagnostic accuracy. Newer technologies are less invasive than biopsy and thus may be better options for lesions on cosmetically sensitive areas or in patients with history of hypertrophic scar formation. Some of these methods allow remote diagnosis by trained dermatologists, increasing accessibility. These new skin cancer detection techniques re reviewed in this article.

REFLECTANCE CONFOCAL MICROSCOPY

Reflectance confocal microscopy (RCM) was introduced to the field of dermatology in the 1990s and has been the focus of many studies evaluating its diagnostic accuracy for skin cancers, surgical mapping, and intraoperative ex vivo tissue assessment.[8] RCM has recently earned Food and Drug Administration (FDA) approval and has category I Current Procedural Terminology (CPT) reimbursement codes.[9] RCM uses a point laser light source to direct near-infrared light onto a tissue sample. The light is reflected back off the tissue into a pinhole-sized aperture that filters out any surrounding light not derived from the tissue sample. The signal created represents thin horizontal sections that can be stacked together vertically to create comprehensive images, which capture cellular structure on par with histologic evaluation.[10] Limitations of RCM include imaging time, which can take between 2 minutes and 45 minutes depending on the size and site of the lesion, and imaging depth of 250 μm.[8,11] RCM, however, can clearly visualize

highly refractive structures, including melanin, keratin, collagen, and hemoglobin.[10]

Two confocal microscopes are commercially available—the VivaScope 1500 and VivaScope 3000 (Caliber Imaging and Diagnostics, Rochester, NY, USA). The VivaScope 1500 is a portable standing machine with a single frame size of 0.5 mm^2. This device must be stationary to evaluate the skin of interest and is not freely moveable on the skin. Positioning the device can be difficult on contoured surfaces or fragile skin. The VivaScope 3000 is a handheld machine with a single frame size of 0.75 mm^2. This handheld version is beneficial because it can be used on small, contoured surfaces, captures images faster, and moves freely on the skin.[12]

Imaging of normal skin with RCM has been well defined. A characteristic honeycomb or cobblestone pattern describes uniform keratinocytes that form the spinous-granular layer of the epidermis. The dermal papillae are clearly demarcated by brightly pigmented keratinocytes and melanocytes and are termed, *edged papillae*. RCM cannot visualize past the papillary dermis or the upper reticular dermis due to its depth limitations. For this reason, RCM performs best on skin with thin epidermis, such as the face and photodamaged skin. Skin cancers disrupt the normal skin architecture and can be visualized with RCM.[13]

Although RCM is most often used to identify MMs, this technology can also play a role in the diagnosis of NMSCs. Basal cell carcinomas (BCCs) are characterized by sharply demarcated tumor islands with interspersed fibrous bundles, dilated blood vessels, and horizontal clefting of the epidermis on RCM imaging.[8] Guitera and colleagues[14] used these features to develop a diagnostic algorithm for identifying BCCs with a sensitivity of 100% and specificity of 88.5%. RCM even has the potential to differentiate between BCC subtypes, a benefit that can help make management decisions. Peppelman and colleagues[15] noted differences in the size, shape, and location of tumor nests, degree of fibrosis, and vascular diameter between superficial, nodular, and micronodular BCCs. The deeper dermal component of infiltrative BCCs, however, can escape RCM's limited depth parameters. A 2016 meta-analysis by Xiong and colleagues[11] reviewed 3 studies with 261 suspicious BCC lesions and reported sensitivity and specificity of 92% and 91%, respectively. RCM imaging for squamous cell carcinomas (SCCs) is more difficult due to the hyperkeratotic nature of these lesions, which restricts RCM views to the stratum corneum. Xiang and colleagues[13] were able to characterize features of SCC on RCM by débriding hyperkeratotic lesions before imaging. They found that SCCs often display an abnormal honeycomb pattern, nonedged dermal papillae, and atypical, disarranged keratinocytes. Ahlgrimm-Siess and colleagues'[8] review of the role of RCM in dermatology reported that this technology cannot reliably differentiate between actinic keratoses, SCCs in situ, and invasive SCCs.

The existing literature shows that RCM can reliably assist clinicians in diagnosing MM, which is the main role of RCM in clinical practice today. Because of the high reflective index of melanin, MMs make clear images with strong contrast on RCM.[8] Even lesions suspicious for amelanotic melanoma should be imaged with RCM because small amounts of melanin are still readily discernible.[11] MMs are typically characterized by nonedged papillae, atypical cells at the dermoepidermal junction (DEJ), and dendritic or pagetoid cells. At least 5 separate scoring systems have been created to recognize these features and diagnose MM. The Xiong and colleagues[11] meta-analysis calculated an RCM sensitivity of 93% and specificity of 78% for lentigo maligna. Furthermore, Cinotti and colleagues[16] reported that RCM had greater sensitivity for MM diagnosis and higher inter-investigator agreement than dermoscopy. Stevenson and colleagues[17] argue, however, that directly comparing dermoscopy and RCM is inconsequential because the time-intensive process of RCM will never replace the efficient practice of dermoscopy. Rather, RCM should be considered in addition to clinical assessment and dermoscopy for equivocal lesions suspicious for MM.

Studies have evaluated the utility of RCM for presurgical mapping and intraoperative ex vivo tissue imaging. The broad imaging field of RCT allows identification of the most abnormal areas within large lesions for biopsies, thus increasing diagnostic yield. Similarly, the technology can be used to outline lesion margins preoperatively to ensure the entire tumor is removed.[11,18] RCM of excised tissue may be used during Mohs procedures in place of frozen sections. Hartmann and colleagues[19] estimate that this method could decrease tissue processing time by two-thirds.

OPTICAL CONFOCAL TOMOGRAPHY

Optical confocal tomography (OCT) is another near-infrared technology used for skin imaging. OCT was first introduced to the field of dermatology in 1997 after becoming a popular tool for retinal imaging in ophthalmology.[10,20] OCT is FDA-approved to image biological tissues as a 510(k) class II regulatory device and recently received 2 of its own category III CPT codes.[21] OCT uses nonionizing, near-infrared light to generate 2-D cross-sectional images of tissue microstructure in real time. OCT divides light from an optical source into a probe beam directed at the tissue and a reference beam directed at the reference mirror. After reflecting off the tissue sample, the probe beam is reunited with the reference beam to create an interference signal, which is detected to generate the image.

Conventional OCT is limited to a depth of 470 μm and has a lateral resolution of 7.5 μm to 15 μm. Compared with RCM, OCT can capture deeper images but cannot show individual cellular structure. Various OCT modalities have been designed, however, to enhance OCT imaging ability. For example, high-definition OCT (HD-OCT) has an improved lateral resolution of 3 μm and is, therefore, able to provide greater cellular detail.[22] Dynamic OCT (D-OCT) or speckle-variance OCT can capture intricate vascular architecture by detecting the movement of blood through vessels.[23] OCT images of normal skin depict a clearly layered structure with visualization of the stratum corneum, epidermis, DEJ, papillary dermis, reticular dermis, hair follicles, eccrine sweat ducts, and sebaceous glands. Disruptions in this normal tissue pattern allow OCT to aid in the diagnosis of skin cancers.[24]

OCT is most useful for the diagnosis of BCCs, especially superficial BCCs. BCCs under OCT appear to have well-circumscribed, hyporeflective lobules that correspond to basaloid islands on histology, hyper-reflective peritumoural stroma, and dilated, branching vessels.[10,25] Ulrich and colleagues[26] analyzed 235 nonpigmented lesions suspicious for BCC with clinical assessment, dermoscopy, and OCT. Diagnostic accuracy was 66% for clinical assessment alone, 76% for clinical assessment plus dermoscopy, and 87% for clinical assessment and dermoscopy plus OCT. They reported the triple-assessment technique to have a sensitivity of 96% and specificity of 75%. Markowitz and colleagues[27] calculated similar diagnostic accuracies and concluded that 1 in 3 patients would avoid a diagnostic biopsy with the use of the triple assessment. Cheng and colleagues[28] assessed 168 lesions suspicious for superficial BCC and reported a strong correlation (Pearson coefficient $r = 0.86$) between OCT and biopsy for measuring tumor depth for superficial BCCs less than 0.4 mm. This correlation decreased for tumors extending deeper than 1 mm. For lesions with both high clinical suspicion and high OCT suspicion for BCCs, there was a 76% biopsy reduction rate with an error rate of

5%. The 2 most recent reviews of OCT for the diagnosis of BCC showed increased sensitivity and specificity. Xiong and colleagues[20] reported a sensitivity of 92% and specificity of 87% and noted that sensitivity was improved when the OCT images were read by experienced interpreters. Reddy and Nguyen[25] reported a sensitivity of 89% and specificity of 60% and found that frequency domain OCT had higher sensitivity and specificity than HD-OCT and time domain OCT. Although OCT is particularly useful in identifying superficial BCCs, the current technology is unable to differentiate between BCC subtypes.[20,22]

SCCs are not as easily identified on OCT because hyperkeratosis backscatters light and prevents imaging of deeper skin layers.[23] SCCs on OCT have a thickened stratum corneum, and infiltrative lesions obscure the DEJ, which is usually visualized as a dark line.[29] Despite challenges in reading these images and fewer clinical studies for SCC, Xiong and colleagues[20] reviewed 232 cases and reported a pooled OCT sensitivity and specificity of 92% and 99.5%, respectively. D-OCT may improve the ability to distinguish between AKs, SCCs in situ, and invasive SCCs based on differences in vasculature structure as characterized by Schuh and colleagues.[23] Further exploration of the D-OCT technology may enhance detection of SCCs.

D-OCT may also play a future role in MM detection. Conventional OCT is not a suitable technique for MM diagnosis because benign PSLs and malignant MM lesions have many overlapping features seen OCT images.[30] Xiong and colleagues reported an OCT sensitivity of 81% and specificity of 94% for MM, and Gambichler and colleagues[30] observed that 20% of malignant MMs showed no evidence of malignancy on OCT. A better way to differentiate between benign nevi, dysplastic nevi, and MM lies in their unique vascular structures, as characterized by Schuh and colleagues.[23]

OCT is not yet as commonplace as RCM, but the literature demonstrate reliable diagnosis of BCCs and measuring the depth of superficial BCCs. As OCT technology is refined, HD-OCT and D-OCT may allow for enhanced detection of SCCs and MM. The combination of RCM and OCT technology into 1 probe results in images with the resolution of RCM and the depth of OCT. Sahu and colleagues[31] tested a combined device and found that it was more sensitive for the detection of BCCs (100%) than RCM alone (93%). Both RCM and OCT have clinical utility in their own right, but their diagnostic power is enhanced when combined.

HIGH-FREQUENCY ULTRASOUND

Compared with the other technologies described in this article, most medical professionals are familiar with ultrasound (US) as an imaging modality. As advances in US technology continue, the applications of US have broadened. High-frequency US (HFUS) greater than 15 MHz has been applied to measurement of skin cancer depth, preoperative mapping of skin cancer margins, evaluation of metastases in local lymph nodes, and even skin cancer diagnosis. As the frequency of US sound waves increase, the image resolution improves, and skin can be imaged in greater detail. US can achieve depths of 60 mm with a single probe, allowing its images to visualize deeper structures compared with RCM and OCT. US can also access hard-to-reach areas of the skin, like the inner ear or interdigital spaces of the feet, thanks to compact linear probes. US is fast and cost-effective but requires a skilled technician to capture the images.[10,32]

Recent studies have characterized skin malignancies on US imaging. All skin cancers appear hypoechoic on US. BCCs and SCCs both appear as irregular hypoechoic lesions, but SCCs have a more prominent increased vascular pattern and high-grade BCCs have hyperechoic spots. MMs appear as fusiform structures that become less well-defined as they progress.[33] Crisan and colleagues[34] evaluated 23 nodular tumors with conventional US, HFUS, contrast elastography, and contrast-enhanced US to characterize distinguishing features between BCCs and benign growths. They found that BCCs were more likely to have central vasculature, a blood flow velocity greater than 2 cm/s, intense load of contrast agent, and quick contrast wash-out time. On the other hand, benign lesions were more likely to have peripheral circulation, blood flow velocity less than 2 cm/s, weak loading of the contrast agent, and slow contrast wash-out time.[34]

Although most studies regarding HFUS and skin cancers have investigated the role of HFUS in measuring tumor depth and presurgical mapping,[34,35] Wortsman and colleagues applied HFUS to the diagnosis of 4338 skin lesions before biopsy.[32] They found that clinical examination alone was 73% accurate for lesion diagnosis, whereas clinical examination plus HFUS was 97% accurate with an overall sensitivity of 99% and specificity of 100%. Although HFUS had a significant impact on the diagnosis of benign lesions and inflammatory skin diseases, however, it did not significantly improve malignant lesion diagnosis.[32] Maj and colleagues[35] later posited that cancer diagnosis is better left to other imaging modalities like dermoscopy and RCM and that HFUS should be reserved to evaluate the size and depth of tumors. HFUS needs further research to characterize is diagnostic ability.

MULTISPECTRAL DIGITAL SKIN LESION ANALYSIS

Multispectral digital skin lesion analysis (MSDSLA) uses visible and infrared light to image PSLs suspicious for MM along with computer algorithms that characterize the images and determine the likelihood of lesion malignancy. The 2 most studied MSDSLA techniques include MelaFind (MELA Sciences Inc, Irvington, New York) and SIAscopy (Spectrophotometric Intracutaneous Analysis) with SIAscope (Astron Clinica Limited, UK).

MelaFind is an FDA-approved handheld device that irradiates the skin with 10 spectral wavelengths ranging from 430 nm to 950 nm. The light reflected back from the skin creates 10 images with a depth of 2.5 mm that are segmented and analyzed by a computer algorithm. This algorithm recognizes changes in orientation, color, and texture to measure overall morphologic disorganization. The algorithm scores the lesion based on these features and advises for or against biopsy. This whole process takes 1 minute to 2 minutes per lesion. Studies have shown that MelaFind is a highly sensitive but poorly specific technique for MM detection.[36–38] Monheit and colleagues[39] used MelaFind to evaluate 1632 PSLs and reported a sensitivity and specificity of 98% and 11%, respectively. Rigel and colleagues[40] asked 179 dermatologists to evaluate 24 PSLs and decide whether or not to biopsy the lesion based on clinical history, clinical images, and dermoscopic images. Then, the providers were asked to make the same decision based on their prior assessment plus the MSDSLA results. The MSDSLA information increased the sensitivity of MM detection from 69% to 94% and decreased the specificity from 54% to 40%. A 2017 study of MelaFind in the evaluation of 360 PSLs resulted in a sensitivity of 100% and specificity of 5.5%.[36] The consequence of MelaFind's high sensitivity is that biopsy is almost always recommended.[37] Hauschild and colleagues[41] argue, however, that the low specificity and high biopsy number are justified by the improved detection of MM.

A second MSDSLA system is spectrophotometric intracutaneous analysis, also known as SIAscopy. SIAscopes are handheld devices that illuminate the skin with 400-nm to1000-nm wavelength light over a 1.2-cm^2 to 2.4-cm^2 region to form 8 high-resolution images. The associated computer algorithm analyzes the distribution and amount of tissue chromophores, including eumelanin, hemoglobin, and collagen.[37,38] The Moncrieff criteria are applied to the images in order to determine malignancy status. These criteria include the presence of dermal melanin, collagen holes (due to invasion of malignant cells into the papillary dermis), and erythematous blush with blood displacement (due to inflammatory vasodilation). Moncrieff and colleagues[42] determined the sensitivity and specificity of these criteria to be 82.7% and 80.1% for MM detection. A more recent review of SIAscopy in 2018 by Winkelmann and colleagues,[38] which included 5 studies with a total of 4669 PSLs, reported similar data with a pooled sensitivity of 85% and specificity of 81%. Emery and colleagues[43] modified the Moncrieff criteria to create the primary care scoring algorithm (PCSA), which was reported by its founders to have a sensitivity of 50% and specificity of 84% for the detection of suspicious lesions. The PCSA includes lesion diameter and patient age along with the Moncrieff factors. The PCSA was designed for use in the primary care setting and to distinguish PSLs from benign seborrheic keratoses and hemangiomas.[43] MoleMate, an FDA-approved SIAScope designed for primary care providers, uses the PCSA for lesion analysis.[38] Walter and colleagues,[44] however, found no evidence that using MoleMate in the primary care setting improved the appropriateness of referral for skin lesions. Nevertheless, primary care providers who used MoleMate earned higher patient satisfaction scores than providers who did not use this new technology.[44] Further investigation of SIAscopy is necessary to determine its role in dermatology and primary care.

ELECTRICAL IMPEDANCE SPECTROSCOPY

Electrical impedance spectroscopy (EIS) is based on the principle that malignant transformation of cells alters their electrical impedance. EIS systems like TransScan (TransScan Ltd., Migdal Haemek, Israel), SciBase (SciBase, Stockholm, Sweden), and the FDA-approved Nevisense (SciBase, Stockholm, Sweden) compare the electrical properties of normal skin to suspicious lesions. EIS is performed with a handheld probe that covers a 5-mm^2 × 5-mm^2 area of skin and contains an electrode. The probe applies an electrical current to the skin and subsequently receives the resulting current from the tissue. Two measurements must be performed — 1 at an unaffected area of skin for reference and 1 at the lesion of interest. Each measurement is painless and takes approximately 10 seconds. A computer algorithm then compares the data from the 2 sites to score the lesion on a scale of 0 to 10. Lesions that score 0 to 3 are designated as benign, and lesions that score 4 to 10 are designated as malignant.[36,37,45]

Studies have shown that EIS can play a helpful role in the diagnosis of both NMSCs and MM. Har-Shai and colleagues[46] compared the diagnostic accuracy of clinical assessment to that of clinical assessment plus EIS on 449 PSLs. The addition of EIS information increased sensitivity of MM diagnosis from 81% to 98% and decreased the specificity from 84% to 55%. They also noted that EIS had better diagnostic accuracy for PSLs located on the trunk and extremities than on the head or neck.[46] Mohr and colleagues[47] tested SciBase's ability to evaluate multiple cutaneous malignancies using 2 different algorithms. The first algorithm showed a sensitivity of 98% for MM, 100% for NMSCs and 84% for severely dysplastic nevi, with an overall specificity of 24%. The second algorithm resulted in a sensitivity of 99% for MM, 98% for NMSCs and 94% for severely dysplastic nevi, with an overall specificity of 25%.[47] A large study by Malvehy and colleagues[48] used Nevisense on 1946 skin lesions. This system was 97% sensitive and 34% specific for MM and 100% sensitive for NMSC. The sensitivity for MM increased with the thickness of the lesion and no invasive MMs were missed. A limitation of Nevisense was its inability to characterize seborrheic keratoses as benign.[48] Svoboda and colleagues[45] studied how EIS measurements affected dermatologists' decision to biopsy PSLs. The addition of EIS information changed 24.3% of biopsy decisions, caught 402 MMs that had been missed without EIS, and prevented 376 benign biopsies.[45] Between EIS' ease of use, fast processing time, and high diagnostic sensitivity for both NMSCs and MMs, EIS may find a role in the evaluation of various skin lesions.

RAMAN SPECTROSCOPY

The Raman effect is a physical principle that describes the minor change in energy between an incident photon and an inelastically scattered photon. This shift in energy corresponds to a slight color change in the scattered photon. Almost all skin molecules, including amino acids, lipids, and nucleic acids, cause inelastic optical scattering. Raman spectroscopy (RS) of the skin plots these transitions on a spectrum to create a molecular fingerprint of the tissue. Although the Raman spectra of all skin lesions appear very similar, small differences in signal intensity allow for the differentiation of benign and malignant lesions. The actual RS device is a handheld probe that covers a 3.5-mm diameter area of skin and emits a 758-nm laser. The device is also equipped with an internal algorithm that analyzes the Raman spectrum created for each skin lesion and generates a percentage predicted probability that the lesion is malignant.[36,49,50]

RS was originally limited to ex vivo tissue analysis due to its long acquisition time, but recent advances in the RS technology have allowed for faster in vivo evaluation of skin lesions. Lui and colleagues[50] performed 1 of the first studies of in vivo RS use on 518 skin lesions. They reported that RS was 90% sensitive and 68% specific for distinguishing skin cancers and precancers from benign lesions.[50] Zhao and colleagues[51] further modified the RS algorithm to increase the specificity to 75% at 90% sensitivity. The most recent review of RS was conducted by Zhang and colleagues[52] in 2018 and includes 12 studies with 2641 Raman spectra. Their results for in vivo skin lesions are as follows: 69% sensitive and 85% specific for BCC, 81% sensitive and 89% specific for SCC, and 93% sensitive and 96% specific for MM. They also noted that diagnostic accuracy for in vivo lesions was inferior to that of ex vivo lesions. RS technology needs continued research and refinement to be considered for regular in vivo use.

MULTIPHOTON TOMOGRAPHY

Multiphoton tomography (MLT) involves irradiating a skin lesion with near-infrared light and measuring the autofluorescence of naturally fluorescing molecules in the skin, which include NADPH, flavins, porphyrins, keratin, and melanin. Although collagen does not fluoresce, it can be also be imaged by MLT by inducing second harmonic generation. This technology can image to a depth of 200 μm and takes 10 minutes to 15 minutes to complete. DermaInspect (JenLab, Jena, Germany) is an MLT designed for in vivo evaluation of human skin.[36] DermaInspect includes a large standing console with a flexible arm attachment that contacts the skin. This structure limits the device's ability to image contoured surfaces.[53] Despite its acquisition time, depth, and surface restrictions, MLT has been used to characterize BCCs, SCCs, benign nevi, and MM.[54,55]

Few clinical trials have been performed to evaluate MLT's ability to diagnose skin lesions. Dimitrow and colleagues[53] conducted a small study of DermaInspect on 83 melanocytic lesions. They identified 6 characteristic features of MM on MLT: ascending melanocytes, architectural disarray, large intercellular distance, poorly defined keratinocyte cell borders, cell pleomorphism, and the presence of dendritic cells. DermaInspect was found to be 84% sensitive and 76% specific for MM in this study.[53] Seidenari and colleagues[55] subsequently studied MLT in combination with fluorescence lifetime imaging (FLIM) on 125 skin lesions, including benign nevi, BCCs, and MM. They reported a sensitivity of 100% and specificity of 98% for MM.[55] More research about MLT is needed before understanding its future role in dermatology, but MLT plus FLIM may be a promising technology for MM detection.

PIGMENTED LESION ASSAY

Unlike the other technologies addressed in this article, the pigmented lesion assay (PLA) analyzes the genetic makeup of lesions rather than their microscopic structure. PLA is performed through noninvasive biopsy with an adhesive patch. A circular patch is placed onto PSLs and collects a thin layer of stratum corneum tissue. This tissue contains genetic information from keratinocytes, melanocytes, and immune cells in the skin. Four patches are used on the same lesion, and the tissue collected from all 4 patches is combined for isolation of genetic material. Target gene expression analysis then evaluates the sample's expression of long intergenic noncoding RNA 518 (LINC) and preferentially expressed antigen in melanoma (PRAME), which are 2 genes associated with increased MM risk. The adhesive patch cannot be used on the palms of the hands, soles of the feet, nails, or mucous membranes.[5,56,57] The patch is also limited by the possibility of insufficient tissue collection, which occurred in 14% of PLA attempts in the recent study by Gerami and colleagues.[57]

Despite these technical limitations, PLA has displayed both high sensitivity and specificity for MM detection. Ferris and colleagues[58] studied how the addition of PLA results to clinical and dermoscopic images would change a dermatologist's decision to biopsy a PSL. They found that PLA improved biopsy sensitivity from 95% to 98.6% and specificity from 32.1% to 56.9%.[58] Gerami and colleagues[57] used PLA on 398 PSLs and reported a sensitivity and specificity of 91% and 69%, respectively. A more recent study by Ferris and colleagues[7] evaluated 381 PSLs with PLA and found a sensitivity of 95% and specificity of 91%. They estimated that unnecessary surgical procedures could be reduced by 88% with this new technology. They also noted that with PLA the number needed to biopsy was 2.7 and the biopsy ratio was 1.7.[7] This concept of noninvasive biopsy and genetic analysis is novel to the field of dermatology, but further investigation is needed to determine its clinical role in MM detection.

SUMMARY

This article presents technology currently being used and evaluated for skin cancer detection (**Table 1**). Although many of these technologies originated from other areas of science and medicine, some have been created specifically for skin evaluation. This list is not exhaustive because there are many other experimental methods, including quantitative dynamic infrared imaging, stepwise 2-photon laser spectroscopy, and deep learning convolutional neural networks for dermoscopic image analysis.[36,59] Although the growing and inventive field of skin cancer detection techniques is promising, translational issues remain. Cost is 1 barrier to widespread implementation. A single RCM machine can cost up to $100,000,

Table 1
Sensitivities and specificities of skin cancer detection techniques

Skin Cancer Detection Technology	Primary Type of Skin Cancer Evaluated	Sensitivity Range (%)	Specificity Range (%)
RCM[11]	MM	93	78
OCT[20,25,26]	BCC	89–96	60–87
HFUS[32]	NMSC and MM	99	100
MSDSLA	MM		
MelaFind[36,39,40]		94–100	6–40
SIAscopy[38,42]		83–85	80–81
EIS	NMSC[47,48]	98–100	34–55
	MM[46–48]	97–99	
RS	NMSC[52]	69–81	85–89
	MM[52]	93	96
MLT[53,55]	MM	84–100	76–98
PLA[7,57,58]	MM	91–99	57–91

and MelaFind costs $10,000 for installation plus annual fees.[37,60] Despite a large up-front expense, these machines could potentially save money in the long term by reducing the amount of unnecessary lesion surveillance and skin biopsies.[61,62] For example, Hornberger and Siegel[63] estimated a cost savings of $447 for every lesion evaluated with PLA despite the test costing $500. Another identified barrier is the requirement of some of the technology to use experienced trained professionals. Low specificity, lack of efficiency, and limitations on anatomic sites are additional issues to consider. As of 2015, only 11% of dermatologists incorporated newer technologies into their skin evaluation, but this number is likely to increase as the technologies, their diagnostic accuracy, and their limitations are better understood.[4]

REFERENCES

1. American Cancer Society. Cancer facts & figures 2018. Atlanta (GA): American Cancer Society; 2018.
2. Bray F, Ferlay J, Soerjomataram I, et al. Global cancer statistics 2018: GLOBOCAN estimates of incidence and mortality worldwide for 36 cancers in 185 countries. CA Cancer J Clin 2018;68(6):394–424.
3. Yélamos O, Braun RP, Liopyris K, et al. Usefulness of dermoscopy/dermatoscopy to improve the clinical and histopathologic diagnosis of skin cancers. J Am Acad Dermatol 2018;80(2):365–77.
4. Winkelmann RR, Rigel DS. Management of dysplastic nevi: a 14-year follow-up survey assessing practice trends among US dermatologists. J Am Acad Dermatol 2015;73(6):1056–9.
5. Rivers JK, Copley MR, Svoboda R, et al. Non-invasive gene expression testing to rule out melanoma. Skin Therapy Lett 2018;23(5):1–4.
6. Shoo BA, Sagebiel RW, Kashani-Sabet M. Discordance in the histopathologic diagnosis of melanoma at a melanoma referral center. J Am Acad Dermatol 2010;62(5):751–6.
7. Ferris LK, Gerami P, Skelsey MK, et al. Real-world performance and utility of a noninvasive gene expression assay to evaluate melanoma risk in pigmented lesions. Melanoma Res 2018;28(5):478–82.
8. Ahlgrimm-Siess V, Laimer M, Rabinovitz HS, et al. Confocal microscopy in skin cancer. Curr Dermatol Rep 2018;7:105.
9. Jain M, Pulijal SV, Rajadhyaksha M, et al. Evaluation of bedside diagnostic accuracy, learning curve, and challenges for a novice reflectance confocal microscopy reader for skin cancer detection in vivo. JAMA Dermatol 2018;154(8):962–5.
10. Halani S, Foster FS, Breslavets M, et al. Ultrasound and infrared-based imaging modalities for diagnosis and management of cutaneous diseases. Front Med (Lausanne) 2018;5:115.
11. Xiong YD, Ma S, Li X, et al. A meta-analysis of reflectance confocal microscopy for the diagnosis of malignant skin tumours. J Eur Acad Dermatol Venereol 2016;30(8):1295–302.
12. Waddell A, Star P, Guitera P. Advances in the use of reflectance confocal microscopy in melanoma. Melanoma Manag 2018;5(1):MMT04.
13. Xiang W, Peng J, Song X, et al. Analysis of debrided and non-debrided invasive squamous cell carcinoma skin lesions by in vivo reflectance confocal microscopy before and after therapy. Lasers Med Sci 2017;32(1):211–9.
14. Guitera P, Menzies SW, Longo C, et al. In vivo confocal microscopy for diagnosis of melanoma and basal cell carcinoma using a two-step method: analysis of 710 consecutive clinically equivocal cases. J Invest Dermatol 2012;132(10):2386–94.
15. Peppelman M, Wolberink EA, Blokx WA, et al. In vivo diagnosis of basal cell carcinoma subtype by reflectance confocal microscopy. Dermatology 2013;227(3):255–62.
16. Cinotti E, Labeille B, Debarbieux S, et al. Dermoscopy vs. reflectance confocal microscopy for the diagnosis of lentigo maligna. J Eur Acad Dermatol Venereol 2018;32(8):1284–91.
17. Stevenson AD, Mickan S, Mallett S, et al. Systematic review of diagnostic accuracy of reflectance confocal microscopy for melanoma diagnosis in patients with clinically equivocal skin lesions. Dermatol Pract Concept 2013;3(4):19–27.
18. Pellacani G, De Carvalho N, Ciardo S, et al. The smart approach: feasibility of lentigo maligna superficial margin assessment with hand-held reflectance confocal microscopy technology. J Eur Acad Dermatol Venereol 2018;32(10):1687–94.
19. Hartmann D, Krammer S, Vural S, et al. Immunofluorescence and confocal microscopy for ex-vivo diagnosis of melanocytic and non-melanocytic skin tumors: a pilot study. J Biophotonics 2018;11(3).
20. Xiong Y, Mo Y, Wen Y, et al. Optical coherence tomography for the diagnosis of malignant skin tumors: a meta-analysis. J Biomed Opt 2018;23:1–10.
21. Schwartz M, Levine A, Markowitz O. Optical coherence tomography in dermatology. Cutis 2017;100(3):163–6.
22. van Manen L, Dijkstra J, Boccara C, et al. The clinical usefulness of optical coherence tomography during cancer interventions. J Cancer Res Clin Oncol 2018;144(10):1967–90.
23. Schuh S, Holmes J, Ulrich M, et al. Imaging blood vessel morphology in skin: dynamic optical coherence tomography as a novel potential diagnostic tool in dermatology. Dermatol Ther (Heidelb) 2017;7(2):187–202.

24. Adabi S, Hosseinzadeh M, Noei S, et al. Universal in vivo textural model for human skin based on optical coherence tomograms. Sci Rep 2017;7:1–11.

25. Reddy N, Nguyen BT. The utility of optical coherence tomography for diagnosis of basal cell carcinoma: a quantitative review. Br J Dermatol 2018; 180(3):475–83.

26. Ulrich M, von Braunmuehl T, Kurzen H, et al. The sensitivity and specificity of optical coherence tomography for the assisted diagnosis of nonpigmented basal cell carcinoma: an observational study. Br J Dermatol 2015;173(2):428–35.

27. Markowitz O, Schwartz M, Feldman E, et al. Evaluation of optical coherence tomography as a means of identifying earlier stage basal cell carcinomas while reducing the use of diagnostic biopsy. J Clin Aesthet Dermatol 2015;8(10):14–20.

28. Cheng HM, Lo S, Scolyer R, et al. Accuracy of optical coherence tomography for the diagnosis of superficial basal cell carcinoma: a prospective, consecutive, cohort study of 168 cases. Br J Dermatol 2016;175(6):1290–300.

29. Sattler E, Kästle R, Welzel J. Optical coherence tomography in dermatology. J Biomed Opt 2013;18: 061224.

30. Gambichler T, Plura I, Schmid-Wendtner M, et al. High-definition optical coherence tomography of melanocytic skin lesions. J Biophotonics 2015;8: 681–6.

31. Sahu A, Yélamos O, Iftimia N, et al. Evaluation of a combined reflectance confocal microscopy-optical coherence tomography device for detection and depth assessment of basal cell carcinoma. JAMA Dermatol 2018;154(10):1175–83.

32. Wortsman X, Wortsman J. Clinical usefulness of variable-frequency ultrasound in localized lesions of the skin. J Am Acad Dermatol 2010;62: 247–56.

33. Bard RL. High-frequency ultrasound examination in the diagnosis of skin cancer. Dermatol Clin 2017; 35(4):505–11.

34. Crişan D, Badea AF, Crişan M, et al. Integrative analysis of cutaneous skin tumours using ultrasonographic criteria. Preliminary results. Med Ultrason 2014;16:285–90.

35. Maj M, Warszawik-Hendzel O, Szymanska E, et al. High frequency ultrasonography: a complementary diagnostic method in evaluation of primary cutaneous melanoma. G Ital Dermatol Venereol 2015; 150:595–601.

36. Fink C, Haenssle HA. Non-invasive tools for the diagnosis of cutaneous melanoma. Skin Res Technol 2017;23(3):261–71.

37. March J, Hand M, Grossman D. Practical application of new technologies for melanoma diagnosis: Part I. Noninvasive approaches. J Am Acad Dermatol 2015;72(6):929–41.

38. Winkelmann RR, Farberg AS, Glazer AM, et al. Noninvasive technologies for the diagnosis of cutaneous melanoma. Dermatol Clin 2017;35(4):453–6.

39. Monheit G, Cognetta AB, Ferris L, et al. The performance of MelaFind: a prospective multicenter study. Arch Dermatol 2011;147:188–94.

40. Rigel DS, Roy M, Yoo J, et al. Impact of guidance from a computer-aided multispectral digital skin lesion analysis device on decision to biopsy lesions clinically suggestive of melanoma. Arch Dermatol 2012;148:541–3.

41. Hauschild A, Chen SC, Weichenthal M, et al. To excise or not: impact of MelaFind on German dermatologists' decisions to biopsy atypical lesions. J Dtsch Dermatol Ges 2014;12:606–14.

42. Moncrieff M, Cotton S, Claridge E, et al. Spectrophotometric intracutaneous analysis: a new technique for imaging pigmented skin lesions. Br J Dermatol 2002;146:448–57.

43. Emery JD, Hunter J, Hall PN, et al. Accuracy of SIAscopy for pigmented skin lesions encountered in primary care: development and validation of a new diagnostic algorithm. BMC Dermatol 2010; 10:9.

44. Walter FM, Morris HC, Humphrys E, et al. Effect of adding a diagnostic aid to best practice to manage suspicious pigmented lesions in primary care: randomised controlled trial. BMJ 2012;345:e4110.

45. Svoboda RM, Prado G, Mirsky RS, et al. Assessment of clinician accuracy for diagnosing melanoma based on electrical impedance spectroscopy score plus morphology versus lesion morphology alone. J Am Acad Dermatol 2018;80(1):285–7.

46. Har-Shai Y, Glickman YA, Siller G, et al. Electrical impedance scanning for melanoma diagnosis: a validation study. Plast Reconstr Surg 2005;116: 782–90.

47. Mohr P, Birgersson U, Berking C, et al. Electrical impedance spectroscopy as a potential adjunct diagnostic tool for cutaneous melanoma. Skin Res Technol 2013;19:75–83.

48. Malvehy J, Hauschild A, Curiel-Lewandrowski C, et al. Clinical performance of the Nevisense system in cutaneous melanoma detection: an international, multicentre, prospective and blinded clinical trial on efficacy and safety. Br J Dermatol 2014;171(5): 1099–107.

49. Zhao J, Zeng H, Kalia S, et al. Using raman spectroscopy to detect and diagnose skin cancer in vivo. Dermatol Clin 2017;35(4):495–504.

50. Lui H, Zhao J, McLean D, et al. Real-time Raman spectroscopy for in vivo skin cancer diagnosis. Cancer Res 2012;72:2491–500.

51. Zhao J, Zeng H, Kalia S, et al. Wavenumber selection based analysis in Raman spectroscopy improves skin cancer diagnostic specificity. Analyst 2016;141:1034–43.

52. Zhang J, Fan Y, Song Y, et al. Accuracy of Raman spectroscopy for differentiating skin cancer from normal tissue. Medicine (Baltimore) 2018;97(34): e12022.

53. Dimitrow E, Ziemer M, Koehler MJ, et al. Sensitivity and specificity of multiphoton laser tomography for in vivo and ex vivo diagnosis of malignant melanoma. J Invest Dermatol 2009;129(7):1752–8.

54. Klemp M, Meinke MC, Weinigel M, et al. Comparison of morphologic criteria for actinic keratosis and squamous cell carcinoma using in vivo multiphoton tomography. Exp Dermatol 2016;25(3):218–22.

55. Seidenari S, Arginelli F, Dunsby C, et al. Multiphoton laser tomography and fluorescence lifetime imaging of melanoma: morphologic features and quantitative data for sensitive and specific non-invasive diagnostics. PLoS One 2013;8:e70682.

56. Yao Z, Moy R, Allen T, et al. An adhesive patch-based skin biopsy device for molecular diagnostics and skin microbiome studies. J Drugs Dermatol 2017;16:979–86.

57. Gerami P, Yao Z, Polsky D, et al. Development and validation of a noninvasive 2-gene molecular assay for cutaneous melanoma. J Am Acad Dermatol 2017;76:114–20.

58. Ferris LK, Jansen B, Ho J, et al. Utility of a noninvasive 2-gene molecular assay for cutaneous melanoma and effect on the decision to biopsy. JAMA Dermatol 2017;153:675–80.

59. Haenssle HA, Fink C, Schneiderbauer R, et al. Man against machine: diagnostic performance of a deep learning convolutional neural network for dermoscopic melanoma recognition in comparison to 58 dermatologists. Ann Oncol 2018;29(8): 1836–42.

60. Cameron MC, Lee E, Hibler B, et al. Basal cell carcinoma, PART II: contemporary approaches to diagnosis, treatment, and prevention. J Am Acad Dermatol 2018;80(2):321–9.

61. Pellacani G, Pepe P, Casari A, et al. Reflectance confocal microscopy as a second-level examination in skin oncology improves diagnostic accuracy and saves unnecessary excisions: a longitudinal prospective study. Br J Dermatol 2014;171(5):1044–51.

62. Wilson EC, Emery JD, Kinmonth AL, et al. The cost-effectiveness of a novel SIAscopic diagnostic aid for the management of pigmented skin lesions in primary care: a decision-analytic model. Value Health 2013;16(2):356–66.

63. Hornberger J, Siegel DM. Economic analysis of a noninvasive molecular pathologic assay for pigmented skin lesions. JAMA Dermatol 2018;154(9): 1025–31.

Dermatology in the Diagnosis of Noncutaneous Malignancy
Paraneoplastic Diseases

Jesse J. Keller, MD*, Nicole M. Fett, MD, Lynne H. Morrison, MD

KEYWORDS

• Paraneoplastic • Dermatology • Sweet syndrome • Dermatomyositis • Pemphigus

KEY POINTS

• Dermatologists may encounter cutaneous syndromes indicating an underlying malignancy.
• Paraneoplastic conditions share a common onset and parallel course with an underlying malignancy, and often resolve with treatment of the malignancy.
• The type of skin eruption can indicate which organs are likely to be the site of malignancy and accelerate a search for the responsible tumor.

INTRODUCTION

A paraneoplastic process is when a malignancy is linked to a specific cutaneous syndrome via concurrent onset and parallel course. The syndrome generally subsides with resolution of the underlying neoplasm. These paraneoplastic conditions offer an opportunity for prompt workup and decreased time to cancer detection.

COMMON PARANEOPLASTIC CONDITIONS
Sweet Syndrome

Sweet syndrome classically presents as tender, juicy red plaques on the face and upper body (**Fig. 1**). Patients with Sweet syndrome often also present with fever, arthralgias, malaise, and leukocytosis. Sweet syndrome is characterized histologically by a dense neutrophilic infiltrate with papillary dermal edema. It may be elicited by medications, systemic inflammatory conditions, and hematologic malignancies, most often leukemia and myelodysplastic syndrome. Three large retrospective studies have reported malignancy as the cause in 7% to 35% of cases.[1]

Myeloproliferative and myelodysplastic disorders predominated, although solid organ malignancies were also reported. It is estimated that 1% of patients with acute myeloid leukemia (AML) will develop Sweet syndrome.[2] AML patients with SS are more likely to have −5/del(5q) karyotype, FLT3 mutations, and AML with myelodysplasia-related features than AML patients without Sweet syndrome.[2]

Dermatomyositis

Dermatomyositis, defined as characteristic skin manifestations with accompanying myositis, has been recognized as a paraneoplastic condition since the early 1900s. Large retrospective reviews have reported incidences ranging from 9.4% to 42%,[3–5] with the relative risk of malignancy ranging from 2.4 (1.6–3.6) for males and 3.4 (2.4–4.7) for females.[3] The risk of concurrent malignancy seems to be highest within first year after diagnosis of dermatomyositis, but remains elevated for more than 5 years after diagnosis.[4,5]

By the late 1990s, clinically amyopathic dermatomyositis (CADM), defined as characteristic skin

Disclosure Statement: The author has no relevant financial disclosures.
Oregon Health & Science University, 3303 Southwest Bond Avenue CH16D, Portland, OR 97239, USA
* Corresponding author.
E-mail address: kellerje@ohsu.edu

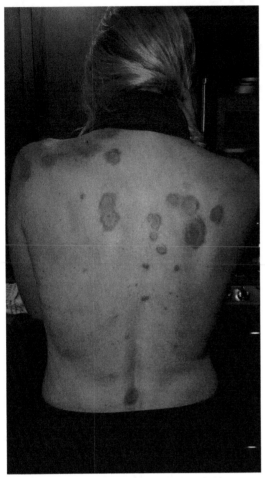

Fig. 1. Edematous truncal plaques representing Sweet syndrome.

manifestations without myositis, was recognized as a clinical entity. The risk of malignancy in patients with CADM appears to be similar to that of classic dermatomyositis. Three meta-analyses were carried out to assess the risk of malignancy in patients with dermatomyositis and CADM. Standardized incident ratios of 4.79 (3.71–5.87)[6] and 5.5 (4.31–6.7)[7] were calculated in these meta-analyses. The risk of malignancy increased with age, male sex, cutaneous necrosis, dysphagia, and during the first year after diagnosis.[6–8]

In an effort to limit screening to only those patients at the highest risk of cancer, the malignant correlation with specific dermatomyositis-associated antibodies has been extensively studied. Serum level of transcription intermediary factor 1γ (TIF-1γ) is highly associated with malignancy in patients with dermatomyositis and CADM. A recent meta-analysis found a 27-fold increased risk of cancer in patients with dermatomyositis and CADM who also had TIF-1γ antibodies.[9] In addition, patients with dermatomyositis or CADM and TIF-1γ antibodies have more advanced cancer at the time of diagnosis.[10] Patients with TIF-1γ antibodies and dermatomyositis or CADM and malignancy have been found to have increased genetic mutations and loss of heterozygosity in TIF1 genes within their tumors.[11] These patients have high expression of TIF-1γ in their tumors, muscle, and skin, which suggests a possible pathogenic mechanism.[12]

Nuclear matrix protein 2 (NXP-2) is another antibody that may be associated with an increased risk of malignancy in a subset of patients with dermatomyositis/CADM.[12–14] Men with NXP-2 antibodies seem to be the most at risk for malignancy.[14]

High serum levels (>16.1 ng/mL) of programmed death ligand 1 (sPD-L1) have also been associated with malignancy in patients with dermatomyositis and CADM.[15] When high sPD-L1 levels were combined with the presence or absence of TIF-1γ antibodies, the positive predictive value of a malignancy was 70%, and the negative predictive value was 92%.[15]

Based on the known increased risk of underlying malignancy in patients with dermatomyositis and CADM, screening for malignancy is recommended. However, there is no consensus on what types of screening should occur and how frequently. There is consensus that a full history and physical examination should be performed, as well as basic laboratory evaluation (complete blood count [CBC], comprehensive metabolic panel [CMP], and urinalysis) and age-appropriate malignancy screening.[16] Most experts in the field also recommend a computed tomography (CT) scan of the chest, abdomen, and pelvis based on 2 studies assessing screening for malignancy in asymptomatic patients. In a recent retrospective review, 13% of cancers were found after a CT scan of the chest, abdomen, and pelvis in asymptomatic dermatomyositis and CADM patients.[17] Further supporting these data, Leatham and colleagues[18] found that 23% of the malignancies detected in dermatomyositis and CADM patients were detected in asymptomatic patients with "blind" screening. Additional testing that has been recommended, but is not evidence based, includes traditional serum malignancy markers, mammograms at an earlier age than recommended for the general population, transvaginal ultrasonography, PET/CT scanning, and full-body MRI.[16,19,20] Although early detection of malignancy in patients with dermatomyositis and CADM is thought to increase survival, to date there are no data supporting this hypothesis.

LEUKEMIA AND LYMPHOMA
Paraneoplastic Pemphigus

Paraneoplastic pemphigus (PNP) is a rare, autoimmune, mucocutaneous blistering disease also termed paraneoplastic autoimmune multiorgan syndrome to reflect the potential for pulmonary involvement. The disease most often affects adults aged 45 to 70 years but has been reported in children.[21]

PNP is almost universally associated with an underlying neoplasm, most often hematologic malignancies. The conditions most often associated with PNP are non-Hodgkin lymphoma (40%), chronic lymphocytic leukemia (18%), Castleman disease (18%), thymoma (6%), carcinoma (9%), sarcoma (6%), and Waldenstrom macroglobulinemia (%).[22] Castleman disease is the most commonly found tumor in children and adolescents with PNP.[21]

Clinically PNP is characterized by severe erosive stomatitis, a polymorphic skin eruption, and occasional pulmonary involvement with features of bronchiolitis obliterans. The most constant clinical feature of PNP is severe, intractable stomatitis. The variable skin manifestations may include features of pemphigus vulgaris, bullous pemphigoid, erythema multiforme, lichen planus, or toxic epidermal necrolysis, reflecting the proposed pathophysiology involving neoplastic induction of both humoral and cellular arms of the immune system.

Bronchiolitis obliterans may occur more commonly in those with underlying Castleman disease. It is hypothesized that antibody deposition in bronchial epithelium causes acantholysis, resulting in accumulation of epithelial cells that occlude the distal alveolar sacs.[23]

Diagnosis rests on correlation of clinical features, histopathology, and direct immunofluorescent and serologic findings. The histopathologic changes most often show a combination of suprabasal acantholysis, lichenoid interface changes, and keratinocyte necrosis. Histopathology may also show changes similar to lichen planus, bullous pemphigoid, or erythema multiforme. Direct immunofluorescent studies may reveal the presence of immunoglobulin G deposited on the epidermal cell surface as well as deposition along the basement membrane zone. Indirect immunofluorescence (IIF) studies done on rodent bladder are important in establishing a diagnosis of PNP. These studies are typically available through laboratories performing IIF and are approximately 80% sensitive and specific.[24] If the diagnosis is made in a patient with no pre-existing malignancy, a CBC, CMP, serum protein electrophoresis, and CT scan of the chest, abdomen, and pelvis should be obtained.

Treatment of the underlying thymoma or Castleman disease often induces disease remission, but unfortunately treatment of other underlying malignancies is not as beneficial. Prognosis of PNP is guarded, and although improved from past decades, 5-year survival was found to be 38% in a French multicenter study.[25]

Acquired Ichthyosis

Acquired ichthyosis is reported most commonly in association with Hodgkin lymphoma.[26] Other causes include non-Hodgkin lymphoma, leiomyosarcoma, Kaposi sarcoma, multiple myeloma, cutaneous T cell lymphoma, and carcinomas of the ovary, breast, lung, and cervix.[27] The etiology is thought to involve production of transforming growth factor α.[28]

PULMONARY MALIGNANCIES
Hypertrichosis Lanuginosa

Acquired hypertrichosis lanuginosa describes an eruption of long fine nonpigmented (lanugo) hairs on the face, most commonly in women,[29,30] and in association with an underlying, usually metastatic,[31] solid organ neoplasm. The most commonly reported associations are lung and colon, at 27% and 24%, respectively.[30,32,33] It has also been reported in tumors of the pancreas, uterus, ovary, kidney, bladder, and gallbladder in addition to leukemia and Ewing sarcoma. The mechanism is thought to involve prolongation of the anagen phase of vellus hair follicles.[29,34]

Erythema Gyratum Repens

Erythema gyratum repens is described as a dermatosis with a "whorled," "wood-grain" appearance that may expand as quickly as 1 cm per day across the skin. Histology is generally nonspecific. The mechanism is unknown. More than 80% of cases are paraneoplastic. The most common underlying neoplasms are pulmonary, although esophageal and breast cancers have also been reported.[35]

GASTROINTESTINAL MALIGNANCIES
Bazex Syndrome

Acrokeratosis paraneoplastica, also known as Bazex syndrome, is a rare paraneoplastic condition in which psoriasiform changes affect the hands, feet, ears, and nose. Bazex syndrome is classically associated with squamous cell carcinoma of the upper aerodigestive tract. Additional associations include distant lymph node metastasis to the head and neck, pulmonary squamous cell and adenocarcinomas, and gastric or colon adenocarcinomas. It may also occur with genitourinary tumors, lymphomas, and neuroendocrine tumors. There is a male predominance, and the mean age is 64 years.[36] Initial workup should include chest radiography, laryngoscopy, and esophageal endoscopy in addition to a CBC and fecal occult blood testing. A handful of case reports suggest improvement with prednisone,[37,38] dexamethasone,[39] etretinate,[40,41] and PUVA (psoralen and ultraviolet A) therapy.[42]

Malignant Acanthosis Nigricans

Acanthosis nigricans is a common entity composed of textured, velvety, hyperpigmented plaques in flexural areas such as the neck and axillae in the setting of traditional risk factors such as obesity and diabetes mellitus. Malignant acanthosis nigricans occurs more suddenly, in older individuals, and more widespread in distribution, including unusual areas such as the trunk, oral mucosa, and perianal area.[43] Fifty-five percent to 61% of associated malignancies are identified as gastric adenocarcinoma.[44] Other associated neoplasms include lung, ovary, breast, and genitourinary.[44–46] Tumor necrosis factor α is thought to play a prominent role in keratinocyte overstimulation.[47–50]

Tripe Palms

This particular finding frequently coexists with malignant acanthosis nigricans and refers to exaggeration of the palmar ridge pattern resembling that of the bovine intestinal tract, hence the term "tripe." Ninety percent are associated with an underlying neoplasm. When coexistent with acanthosis nigricans and/or eruptive seborrheic keratoses, gastric adenocarcinoma is the most common neoplasm. When in isolation, pulmonary neoplasms are most common.[51]

OTHER
Glucagonoma (Necrolytic Migratory Erythema)

Necrolytic migratory erythema (NME) consists of flaccid vesicles and bullae progressing to widespread erosions and crusting, most predominantly in the groin, perianal area, and legs. Biopsy may show necrolysis and vacuolated keratinocytes in the upper epidermis.[52] Seventy percent present with NME as an early sign of disease.[53] Glucagonoma is a rare malignancy of pancreatic islet cells, with annual incidence of 1 in 20 million, and represents 1.3% of pancreatic

cancers.[54] Prevalence is equal in men and women. It usually presents in the sixth decade and metastasis, usually hepatic, is present at diagnosis in half of the cases.[55] Other symptoms and signs of glucagonoma include new-onset diabetes, diarrhea, weight loss, anemia, thromboembolism, and neuropsychiatric changes. The mechanism involves deficiency of amino acids, zinc, and fatty acids induced by high levels of glucagon. Diagnosis is by confirmation of significantly elevated serum glucagon. Glucagonomas grow slowly; median survival is 3 to 7 years.[56,57] Case reports demonstrate clearance with cyclosporine,[58] amino acid infusion,[59] and octreotide.[60–62]

Multicentric Reticulohistiocytosis

Multicentric reticulohistiocytosis (MRH) is a destructive arthritis most commonly affecting distal interphalangeal joints with skin-colored to red-brown papules and nodules over the dorsal hands, extensor joints, and face (Fig. 2). Associated malignancies occur in 25% of cases and include nearly all solid organ and hematologic malignancies (Fig. 3).[63] MRH has also been reported to co-occur with autoimmune and infectious conditions. Histopathologically, MRH presents with osteoclast-like multinucleated giant cells. Treatment includes steroids, disease-modifying antirheumatics, bisphosphonates, and biologics. Facial lesions may be treated with carbon dioxide laser.

PLASMA CELL DISORDERS
POEMS Syndrome

POEMS syndrome (ie, polyneuropathy, organomegaly, endocrinopathy, monoclonal protein, skin changes) is a rare multisystem disease

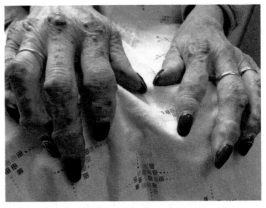

Fig. 2. Papules and nodules on dorsal hands representing multicentric reticulohistiocytosis.

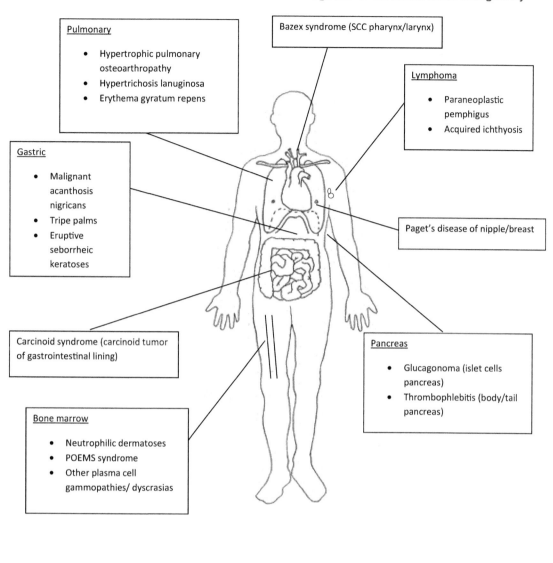

Pulmonary

- Hypertrophic pulmonary osteoarthropathy
- Hypertrichosis lanuginosa
- Erythema gyratum repens

Bazex syndrome (SCC pharynx/larynx)

Lymphoma

- Paraneoplastic pemphigus
- Acquired ichthyosis

Gastric

- Malignant acanthosis nigricans
- Tripe palms
- Eruptive seborrheic keratoses

Paget's disease of nipple/breast

Carcinoid syndrome (carcinoid tumor of gastrointestinal lining)

Pancreas

- Glucagonoma (islet cells pancreas)
- Thrombophlebitis (body/tail pancreas)

Bone marrow

- Neutrophilic dermatoses
- POEMS syndrome
- Other plasma cell gammopathies/ dyscrasias

Wide range of malignancies

- Dermatomyositis
- Multicentric reticulohistiocytosis

Fig. 3. Paraneoplastic syndromes presented visually in association with commonly involved internal organ malignancy.

of peripheral demyelinating polyneuropathy, λ-restricted plasma cell dyscrasia, Castleman disease, and sclerotic bone lesions. Associated skin findings include hyperpigmentation, hypertrichosis, glomeruloid hemangioma, plethora, acrocyanosis, flushing, and white nails. Glomeruloid hemangiomas are highly suggestive of POEMS syndrome, as is thrombocytosis. Markedly elevated vascular endothelial growth factor levels are confirmatory.[64]

Gammopathies

These conditions, marked by a characteristic skin eruption usually linked to an underlying gammopathy, are detailed in **Table 1**.

Table 1
Cutaneous syndromes associated with underlying gammopathies

Name	Cutaneous Findings	Hematologic Disorder	Other Associated Conditions
Scleromyxedema	Widespread firm waxy papules, sclerodermoid induration, "doughnut sign" over proximal interphalangeal joints, Shar-Pei sign of the trunk	IgG-λ; multiple myeloma	Dermato-neuro syndrome
Necrobiotic xanthogranuloma	Necrotic ulcerated xanthomatous plaques in periorbital area and upper chest	Immunoglobulin (Ig)G-κ; multiple myeloma, lymphoma	
Primary systemic amyloidosis	Periorbital purpura, waxy translucent papules, macroglossia	Ig light chain; multiple myeloma	
Cryoglobulinemia (type I)	Acral retiform purpura, livedo reticularis, digital necrosis	Monoclonal Ig (usually IgM); Waldenstrom macroglobulinemia, lymphoma	
Normolipemic plane xanthoma	Yellow thin plaques in periorbital location, intertriginous areas, upper trunk	Multiple myeloma; IgG-κ; lymphoma	
Schnitzler syndrome	Chronic urticaria	IgM-κ; lymphoma	Associated with fevers, arthralgias, bone pain

Data from Bolognia J, Jorizzo J, Schaffer J, eds. Dermatology, 3rd ed. Philadelphia, PA: Elsevier Saunders, 2012.

SUMMARY

There are numerous paraneoplastic conditions with characteristic cutaneous findings. This article guides their recognition and discusses epidemiology, prognosis, and data supporting the most common underlying associations for each syndrome.

REFERENCES

1. Casarin Costa J, Virgens A, deOliveira Mestre L, et al. Sweet syndrome: clinical features, histopathology, and associations of 83 cases. J Cutan Med Surg 2017;21(3):211–6.
2. Kazmi S, Pemmaraju N, Patel K, et al. Characteristics of Sweet syndrome in patients with acute myeloid leukemia. Clin Lymphoma Myeloma Leuk 2015;15(6):358–63.
3. Sigurgeirsson B, Lindelof B, Edhag O, et al. Risk of cancer in patients with dermatomyositis or polymyositis. A population-based study. N Engl J Med 1992;326:363–7.
4. Buchbinder R, Forbes A, Hall S, et al. Incidence of malignant disease in biopsy-proven inflammatory myopathy. A population-based cohort study. Ann Intern Med 2001;134:1087–95.
5. Chen YJ, Wu CY, Huang YL, et al. Cancer risks of dermatomyositis and polymyositis: a nationwide cohort study in Taiwan. Arthritis Res Ther 2010;12:R70.
6. Olazagasti JM, Baez PJ, Wetter DA, et al. Cancer risk in dermatomyositis: a meta-analysis of cohort studies. Am J Clin Dermatol 2015;16:89–98.
7. Yang Z, Lin F, Qin B, et al. Polymyositis/dermatomyositis and malignancy risk: a metaanalysis study. J Rheumatol 2015;42:282–91.
8. Wang J, Guo G, Chen G, et al. Meta-analysis of the association of dermatomyositis and polymyositis with cancer. Br J Dermatol 2013;169:838–47.
9. Trallero-Araguas E, Rodrigo-Pendas JA, Selva-O'Callaghan A, et al. Usefulness of anti-p155 autoantibody for diagnosing cancer-associated dermatomyositis: a systematic review and meta-analysis. Arthritis Rheum 2012;64:523–32.
10. Ogawa-Momohara M, Muro Y, Mitsuma T, et al. Strong correlation between cancer progression and anti-transcription intermediary factor 1gamma antibodies in dermatomyositis patients. Clin Exp Rheumatol 2018;36(6):990–5.

11. Pinal-Fernandez I, Ferrer-Fabregas B, Trallero-Araguas E, et al. Tumour TIF1 mutations and loss of heterozygosity related to cancer-associated myositis. Rheumatology 2018;57:388–96.

12. Ichimura Y, Matsushita T, Hamaguchi Y, et al. Anti-NXP2 autoantibodies in adult patients with idiopathic inflammatory myopathies: possible association with malignancy. Ann Rheum Dis 2012;71:710–3.

13. Rogers A, Chung L, Li S, et al. Cutaneous and systemic findings associated with nuclear matrix protein 2 antibodies in adult dermatomyositis patients. Arthritis Care Res 2017;69:1909–14.

14. Fiorentino DF, Chung LS, Christopher-Stine L, et al. Most patients with cancer-associated dermatomyositis have antibodies to nuclear matrix protein NXP-2 or transcription intermediary factor 1gamma. Arthritis Rheum 2013;65:2954–62.

15. Chen H, Peng Q, Yang H, et al. Increased levels of soluble programmed death ligand 1 associate with malignancy in patients with dermatomyositis. J Rheumatol 2018;45:835–40.

16. Selva-O'Callaghan A, Martinez-Gomez X, Trallero-Araguas E, et al. The diagnostic work-up of cancer-associated myositis. Curr Opin Rheumatol 2018. https://doi.org/10.1097/BOR.0000000000000535.

17. Sparsa A, Liozon E, Herrmann F, et al. Routine vs extensive malignancy search for adult dermatomyositis and polymyositis: a study of 40 patients. Arch Dermatol 2002;138:885–90.

18. Leatham H, Schadt C, Chisolm S, et al. Evidence supports blind screening for internal malignancy in dermatomyositis: data from 2 large US dermatology cohorts. Medicine 2018;97:e9639.

19. Selva-O'Callaghan A, Grau JM, Gamez-Cenzano C, et al. Conventional cancer screening versus PET/CT in dermatomyositis/polymyositis. Am J Med 2010; 123:558–62.

20. Huang ZG, Gao BX, Chen H, et al. An efficacy analysis of whole-body magnetic resonance imaging in the diagnosis and follow-up of polymyositis and dermatomyositis. PLoS One 2017; 12:e0181069.

21. Mimouni D, Anhalt GJ, Lazarova Z, et al. Paraneoplastic pemphigus in children and adolescents. Br J Dermatol 2002;147:725–32.

22. Anhalt GJ. Paraneoplastic pemphigus. J Investig Dermatol Symp Proc 2004;9:29–33.

23. Maldonado F, Pittelkow MR, Rya JH. Constrictive bronchiolitis associated with paraneoplastic autoimmune multi-organ syndrome. Respirology 2009;14: 129–33.

24. Czernik A, Camilleri M, Pittelkow MR, et al. Paraneoplastic autoimmune multi-organ syndrome: 20 years after. Int J Dermatol 2011;50:905–14.

25. Leger S, Picard D, Ingen-Houz-Oro S, et al. Prognostic factors of paraneoplastic pemphigus. Arch Dermatol 2012;148:1165–72.

26. Patel N, Spencer L, English J, et al. Acquired ichthyosis. J Am Acad Dermatol 2006;55(4):647–56.

27. Flint G, Flam M, Soter N. Acquired ichthyosis—a sign of nonlymphoproliferative malignant disorders. Arch Dermatol 1975;111:1446–7.

28. Rizos E, Milionis H, Pavlidis N, et al. Acquired ichthyosis: a paraneoplastic skin manifestation of Hodgkin's disease. Lancet Oncol 2002;3:727.

29. Perez-Losada E, Pujol RM, Domingo P, et al. Hypertrichosis lanuginosa acquisita preceding extraskeletal Ewing's sarcoma. Clin Exp Dermatol 2001;26: 182–3.

30. Farina M, Tarin N, Grilli R, et al. Acquired hypertrichosis lanuginosa: case report and review of the literature. J Surg Oncol 1998;68:199–203.

31. Hovenden A. Acquired hypertrichosis lanuginosa associated with malignancy. Arch Intern Med 1987; 147:2013–8.

32. Weismann K. Skin disorders as markers of internal disease: paraneoplastic dermatoses. Ugeskr Laeger 2000;162:6834–9.

33. Bauer H, Kaatz M, Elsner P. Circumscribed hypertrichosis lanuginosa in acute myeloid leukemia. Dtsch Med Wochenschr 2001;126:845–6.

34. Wendelin D, Pope D, Mallory S. Hypertrichosis. J Am Acad Dermatol 2003;48:161–79.

35. Boyd A, Neldner K, Menter A. Erythema gyratum repens: a paraneoplastic eruption. J Am Acad Dermatol 1992;26(5):757–62.

36. RaBler F, Goetze S, Elsner P. Acrokeratosis paraneoplastica (Bazex syndrome)—a systematic review on risk factors, diagnosis, prognosis and management. J Eur Acad Dermatol Venereol 2017;31(7):1119–36.

37. Medenica L, Gajic-Veljic M, Skiljevic D, et al. Acrokeratosis paraneoplastica Bazex syndrome associated with esophageal squamocellular carcinoma. Vojnosanit Pregl 2008;65:485–7.

38. Abreu Velez A, Howard M. Diagnosis and treatment of cutaneous paraneoplastic disorders. Dermatol Ther 2010;23:662–75.

39. Driessen C, van Rossum M, Blokx W, et al. Skin lesions in a patient with head and neck cancer. Neth J Med 2013;71:481–5.

40. Wishart J. Bazex paraneoplastic acrokeratosis: a case report and response to Tigason. Br J Dermatol 1986;115:595–9.

41. Esteve E, Serpier H, Cambie M, et al. Bazex paraneoplastic acrokeratosis. Treatment with acitretin. Ann Dermatol Venereol 1995;122:26–9.

42. Gill D, Fergin P, Kelly J. Bullous lesions in Bazex syndrome and successful treatment with oral psoralen phototherapy. Australas J Dermatol 2001;42: 278–80.

43. Kubicka-Wolkowska J, Debska-Szmich S, Lisik-Habib M, et al. Malignant acanthosis nigricans associated with prostate cancer: a case report. BMC Urol 2014;14:88.

44. Rigel D, Jacobs M. Malignant acanthosis nigricans: a review. J Dermatol Surg Oncol 1980;11:923–7.

45. Kamińska-Winciorek G, Brzezińska-Wcisło L, Lis-Swiety A, et al. Paraneoplastic type of acanthosis nigricans in patient with hepatocellular carcinoma. Adv Med Sci 2007;52:254–6.

46. Lenzner U, Ramsauer J, Petzoldt W, et al. Acanthosis nigricans maligna. Case report and review of the literature. Hautarzt 1998;49:41–7.

47. Ellis D, Kafka S, Chow J, et al. Melanoma, growth factors, acanthosis nigricans, the sign of Leser-Trelat, and multiple acrochordons. A possible role for alpha-transforming growth factor in cutaneous paraneoplastic syndromes. N Engl J Med 1987; 317:1582–7.

48. Koyama S, Ikeda K, Sato M, et al. Transforming growth factor alpha (TGF-alpha)-producing gastric carcinoma with acanthosis nigricans: an endocrine effect of TGF-alpha in the pathogenesis of cutaneous paraneoplastic syndrome and epithelial hyperplasia of the esophagus. J Gastroenterol 1997; 32:71–7.

49. Torley D, Bellus G, Munro C. Genes, growth factors and acanthosis nigricans. Br J Dermatol 2002;147: 1096–101.

50. Wilgenbus K, Lentner A, Kuckelkorn R, et al. Further evidence that acanthosis nigricans maligna is linked to enhanced secretion by the tumour of transforming growth factor alpha. Arch Dermatol Res 1992;284: 266–70.

51. Chung V, Moschella S, Zembowicz A, et al. Clinical and pathologic findings of paraneoplastic dermatoses. J Am Acad Dermatol 2006;54:745–62.

52. van Beek A, de Haas E, van Vloten WA, et al. The glucagonoma syndrome and necrolytic migratory erythema: a clinical review. Eur J Endocrinol 2004;151: 531–7.

53. Stavropoulos P, Papafragkaki D, Averginou G, et al. Necrolytic migratory erythema: a common cutaneous clue of uncommon syndromes. Cutis 2013; 92(5):e1–4.

54. Chastain MA. The glucagonoma syndrome: a review of its features and discussion of new perspectives. Am J Med Sci 2001;321:306–20.

55. Mallinson C, Bloom S, Warin A. A glucagonoma syndrome. Lancet 1974;6:1–5.

56. John A, Schwartz R. Glucagonoma syndrome: a review and update on treatment. J Eur Acad Dermatol Venereol 2016;30(12):2016–22.

57. Mendoza-Guil F, Hernandez-Jurado I, Burkhardt P, et al. Necrolytic migratory erythema associated with glucagonoma. Actas Dermosifiliogr 2005; 96(3):175–8.

58. Jimenez-Gall D, Ossorio-Garcia L, de la Varga-Martinez R, et al. Necrolytic migratory erythema associated with glucagonoma treated successfully with cyclosporine. Dermatol Ther 2017;30(4). https://doi.org/10.1111/dth.12498.

59. Thomaidou E, Nahmias A, Gilead L, et al. Rapid clearance of necrolytic migratory erythema following intravenous administration of amino acids. JAMA Dermatol 2016;152(3):345–6.

60. Kimbara S, Fujiwara Y, Toyoda M, et al. Rapid improvement of glucagonoma-related necrolytic migratory erythema with octreotide. Clin J Gastroenterol 2014;7(3):255–9.

61. Lo C, Ho C, Shih Y. Glucagonoma with necrolytic migratory erythema exhibiting responsiveness to subcutaneous octreotide injections. QJM 2014; 107(2):157–8.

62. Virani S, Prajapati V, Devani A, et al. Octreotide-responsive necrolytic migratory erythema in a patient with pseudoglucagonoma syndrome. J Am Acad Dermatol 2013;68(2):e44–6.

63. Selmi C, Greenspan A, Huntley A, et al. Multicentric reticulohistiocytosis: a critical review. Curr Rheumatol Rep 2015;17(6):511.

64. Dispenzieri A, Kourelis T, Buadi F. POEMS syndrome: diagnosis and investigative work-up. Hematol Oncol Clin North Am 2018;32(1):119–39.

Cutaneous Metastasis of Internal Tumors

Evan Alexander Choate, BA[a], Alexander Nobori, MD[b], Scott Worswick, MD[c],*

KEYWORDS

• Cutaneous • Metastasis • Malignancy • Internal tumor • Histopathology • Dermatopathology

KEY POINTS

• Cutaneous metastasis portends a poor prognosis and should necessitate a thorough work-up including skin biopsy with appropriate histologic stains.
• Frequent clinical manifestations of cutaneous metastasis include red nodules or less commonly plaques. Ulcers and pink papules are less common.
• Unique presentations exist for individual cancers, including alopecia (breast, colorectal), blue color (liver, renal, neuroblastoma), vesicles (breast, colorectal, gastric, prostate), and acrochordon-like (colorectal).
• Most cancers metastasize to the trunk, head, and neck. When a tumor presents in the perineum, pelvic region or umbilicus, suspect a gastrointestinal or genitourinary origin.
• Immunostain panels to assess for breast, lung, colorectal, and prostate metastases alongside primary adnexal tumors may guide histologic evaluation in morphologically ambiguous cases.

INTRODUCTION

Although primary skin cancers comprise most cancerous lesions of the skin, secondary metastases from internal malignancies remain an often overlooked yet highly relevant contributor, particularly as total cancer incidence increases and more cancer survivors require surveillance for relapse.[1] The purpose of this review is to aid the presenting clinician in developing a differential diagnosis for cutaneous metastases that considers epidemiologic trends, anatomic location, and morphologic appearance before performing a skin biopsy. Similarly, the authors hope to elaborate for the dermatopathologist the process by which immunohistochemical techniques can identify the source of malignancy in these often clinically ambiguous lesions.

Epidemiology

The skin remains a relatively uncommon destination for internal tumor metastasis considering its massive surface area. Older studies suggest that the prevalence in patients with cancer stands around 5%[2,3] but could be as high as 10.4%.[4] More recent data point to a prevalence of 1% to 4.3%,[5–7] with other studies observing even lower rates.[8,9] There also exists heterogeneity in the affinity each respective primary cancer has toward the skin. For instance, Lookingbill and colleagues[3] note that cancers of the breast (23.9% of cases), oral cavity (5.3%), and ovary (3%) more commonly metastasize to the skin, whereas those of the endometrium (0.6%), uterine cervix (0.3%), and prostate (0.3%) were much rarer culprits. A more

Disclosure Statement: The authors have nothing to disclose.
[a] David Geffen School of Medicine, University of California, Los Angeles, Los Angeles, CA, USA; [b] Department of Pathology and Laboratory Medicine, David Geffen School of Medicine, University of California, Los Angeles, 10833 Le Conte Avenue, Los Angeles, CA 90095, USA; [c] Department of Dermatology, Keck School of Medicine, University of Southern California, 1441 Eastlake Avenue, Ezralow Tower, Suite 5301, Los Angeles, CA 90033-9174, USA
* Corresponding author.
E-mail address: scott.worswick@med.usc.edu

Dermatol Clin 37 (2019) 545–554
https://doi.org/10.1016/j.det.2019.05.012
0733-8635/19/© 2019 Elsevier Inc. All rights reserved.

recent retrospective study in Taiwan attests to a similar distribution.[6]

Overall, when considering skin metastasis, breast, lung, oral cavity-pharynx-larynx, and colorectum, respectively, encompass the most common underlying solid malignancies, although hematologic-lymphatic malignancies share a comparably elevated incidence (**Table 1**).[3,5,7–24] Other investigations that further trace prevalence by sex find that for women, breast cancer was the overwhelming leader (46%–69%), although hematologic-lymphatic, colorectal, ovarian, and gallbladder cancers were implicated fairly often. In men, hematologic-lymphatic cancers tend to occur most frequently (32%–36%), with lung and colorectal cancer not far behind.[10,11,25]

Maintaining a high index of suspicion for cancer in evaluating these lesions is particularly consequential, as a cutaneous metastasis may be the initial symptom that prompts workup for malignancy. Around 16% to 21% of cutaneous metastases are discovered before the underlying primary tumor, with newer data suggesting a prevalence as high as 26.8%.[3,11,26] Of note, this phenomenon is more common in men than women, which may be reflective of the different distribution of cancer types by sex.[13,25]

Clinical Presentation

Cutaneous metastases regularly present as single or multiple nodules with firm consistency and flesh- or red-pink coloration; additional defining features and atypical manifestations are highlighted in **Table 1**. Notable common unique morphologic presentations include sessile acrochordon-type lesions with metastatic colon cancer; kidney, liver, and neuroblastoma can present as bluish nodules; and oral cavity metastases can present as ulcers. Less common but unique manifestations include associated alopecia with breast and colon cancer metastases; papulovesicles or a zosteriform distribution again with colon and breast cancer, but also with gastric and prostate cancer; flushing or a pellagra-like presentation with carcinoid tumors; and lastly larynx and breast cancers present as sclerodermoid plaques.

These lesions have the potential to invade nearly every segment of the skin. Taken together, they have a predilection for the chest, followed by the abdomen-umbilicus and head-neck. In contrast, the back, buttock, pelvis-perineum, and extremities are each involved in less than 10% of metastases.[11,12,25] As summarized in **Table 2**,[3–5,7–9,16,27] a preliminary differential diagnosis can be proposed based on the anatomic location of the lesion, which can be useful in such instances where underlying malignancy is suspected but workup not yet commenced. Notably, when a clinician does encounter a cutaneous metastasis to either the pelvic-perineal region or the umbilicus, it is highly likely that the primary tumor is of gastrointestinal or genitourinary origin. Internal tumor affinities for particular sites are driven by factors including contiguity, pattern of hematogenous and/or lymphatic spread, and iatrogenic manipulation.[13]

Prognosis

In general, discovery of a cutaneous metastasis often portends a poor prognosis. In a review of 77 patients, primarily men, Saeed and colleagues[28] observe a mean survival time of 7.5 months, with a 75% mortality by 1 year. A 76.6% of these individuals already had widespread metastases to other organs as well. Another analysis, which excluded skin metastases originating from hematologic primary cancers or spread via direct extension, found there to be a mean survival time of 9.4 months and 67% mortality, with a mean follow-up of 13.3 months.[14] Most patients (43/51) had known stage IV cancer. In an article by Kovács and colleagues,[15] 38 of 80 patients with skin metastasis from nonhematologic or nonbreast sources had inoperable primaries.

Approach to Therapy

Although targeting the underlying primary malignancy remains of utmost prognostic and therapeutic importance, interventions focused at the level of the skin represent increasingly relevant priorities for managing pain, tumor burden, and quality of life. Of note, adjunctive electrochemotherapy, whereby electric pulses delivered to the tumor to increase absorption of intralesional chemotherapeutics (eg, bleomycin), induced complete regression of 58% to 64% of metastatic cutaneous breast cancer lesions[29,30]; this echoes the findings of an earlier meta-analysis studying primary and secondary skin cancers alike.[31] Imiquimod, a toll-like receptor-7 agonist applied topically as a 5% cream, has been linked to regression of tumor size and surrounding pain in extramammary Paget disease[32,33] and in case reports of metastatic ductal carcinoma[34] and highly vascular cancers including renal cell carcinoma (RCC).[35,36] Certainly, conventional techniques such as excision and radiation remain mainstays of therapy for such lesions. The immunomodulatory therapies used in advanced visceral and primary skin cancers treatment likely have a role in treating cutaneous metastases; however, they are yet to be investigated expressly by systematic studies.

Table 1
Presentation of new cutaneous lesion in patients with primary malignancy

Primary Cancer	% of Skin Mets (2014)[72]	% of Skin Mets (1993)[4]	Presenting Location		Presenting Qualities	
			Common	Less Common	Common	Less Common
Adrenal	–	0.7%	Head-neck	Back	Nodules Erythematous	Subcutaneous
Bile Duct	0.5%[a]	0.48%	Abdomen *Umbilicus*	Head-neck Surgical scar	Nodules Subcutaneous	Erythematous plaque Ulcer Papules
Bladder	0.2%	1.7%	Abdomen *Pelvis-perineum*	Extremities	Nodules Red Violaceous	Erythematous plaque Induration Pruritus
Breast	32.7%	50.4%	Chest Abdomen	Head-neck Back Extremities Surgical scar	Nodules Flesh-color Pink-red	*Sclerodermoid-* or erythematous *plaque* *Alopecia* Ulcer *Papulovesicles*
Bronchus-Lung	13.2%	5%	Head-neck Chest Back	Abdomen Extremities	Nodules Red-pink Violaceous	Erythematous plaque Ulcer Telangiectasia
Carcinoid	–	–	Chest *Umbilicus*	Abdomen	Nodules	Painful *Flushing* *Pellagra*
Cervix-vagina	1.0%	0.48%	Chest Abdomen *Pelvis-perineum*	*Umbilicus* Extremities	Nodules Red Violaceous Flesh-color	Erythematous plaque Induration Pruritus
CNS	–	–	Head-neck	Surgical scar	Nodules	Ulcer
Colon-Rectum	4.2%	4.3%	Abdomen *Umbilicus*	Head-neck Chest *Pelvis-perineum* Surgical scar	Nodules *Sessile* *Pedunculated* Red Whitish	Erythematous plaque Ulcer *Alopecia* *Zosteriform*

(continued on next page)

Table 1
(continued)

Primary Cancer	% of Skin Mets (2014)[72]	% of Skin Mets (1993)[4]	Presenting Location		Presenting Qualities	
			Common	Less Common	Common	Less Common
Esophagus	1.2%	0.7%	Head-neck, Abdomen	Chest, Extremities	Nodules, Plaques	Erythematous, Indurated
Gallbladder	0.2%	–	Abdomen, *Umbilicus*	Chest, Surgical scar	Nodules	Swelling
Gastric	2.2%	0.7%	Chest, Abdomen, *Umbilicus*	Head-neck	Nodules	Erythematous plaque, Induration, *Zosteriform*
Heme-Lymph	13.0%	–	Head-neck, Chest, Abdomen, Extremities	Back, Buttock	Nodules, Papules, Violaceous, Flesh-color	Plaque, Ulcer, Swelling, Hemorrhagic
Kidney	2.7%	1.4%	Head-neck, Chest	Back, Extremities, Surgical scar	Nodules, Black-brown, *Blue-purple*, Vascular	Plaque, Ulcer, Pulsation
Larynx	6.2%[b]	1.9%	Head-neck, Chest	Extremities	Nodules	*Erythema sclerodermoid plaque*
Liver	0.5%[a]	0.24%	Head-neck, Chest	Back, Extremities	Nodules, *Red-blue*, Vascular	Telangiectasia, Papules
Neuroblastoma	–	–	Head-neck	Chest, Extremities	Nodules, *Blue*	Erythematous, Blanching
Oral Cavity	6.2%[b]	4.3%	Head-neck	Chest, Back	Nodules, Ulcers	Plaque
Ovary	0.5%	2.4%	Chest, Abdomen, *Umbilicus*	*Pelvis-perineum* Surgical scar	Nodules, Plaques	Erythematous, Scarring
Pancreas	1.7%	0.48%	Abdomen, *Umbilicus*	Back, Buttock, Chest	Nodules, Plaques	Erythematous, Subcutaneous

Pharynx	6.2%[b]	—	Head-neck Chest	Extremities	Nodules	Plaque Ulcer Swelling
Prostate	0.5%	0%	Abdomen *Umbilicus*	*Pelvis-perineum* Extremities	Nodules Violaceous	Erythematous plaque Ulcer *Zosteriform*
Salivary	0.7%	—	Head-neck	Chest	Nodules	Erythematous plaque Ulcer
Soft Tissue	1.9%	—	Head-neck Back Extremities	Chest Abdomen Buttock	Nodules Plaque	Skin-color Erythema Hemorrhagic Swelling
Testes	0.5%	0%	Head-neck Chest *Pelvis-perineum*	Back	Nodules Red Violaceous	Induration
Thyroid	—	—	Head-neck Chest	Abdomen Surgical scar	Nodules Red Violaceous	Erythematous plaque Flesh-color Telangiectasias
Uterus	1.2%	0.95%	Head-neck Chest Extremities	Abdomen Umbilicus Surgical scar	Nodules	Ulcer Pruritus

Primary skin cancers excluded. Columns 2 and 3 list the reported percent of cutaneous metastases caused by each primary malignancy.
Abbreviation: CNS, central nervous system.
[a] The percent of cutaneous metastases caused by liver and bile duct primaries reported as a combined value.
[b] The percent of cutaneous metastases caused by oral cavity, pharynx, and larynx primaries reported as a combined value.

Table 2
Differential diagnosis of causative internal malignancy by anatomic location of skin lesion

Location	Common Primary Malignancies	Less Common Primary Malignancies
Head-neck	Breast, heme-lymph, lung	Colorectum, kidney, larynx, oral cavity, stomach
Chest	Breast, lung	Colorectum, heme-lymph, kidney, larynx, stomach
Abdomen	Breast, colorectum, gastric	Gallbladder, heme-lymph, lung, ovary
Umbilicus	Ovary, gastric	Colorectum
Pelvis-perineum	Colorectum	Cervix-vagina, ovary
Back and buttock	Breast, lung	Heme-lymph, kidney, liver
Extremities	Heme-lymph, lung	Breast, colorectum, kidney, liver, soft tissue
Surgical scar	Breast, ovary, uterus	Colorectum, kidney, larynx, thyroid

Primary skin cancers excluded.

SPOTLIGHT ON NOTABLE PRIMARY MALIGNANCIES
Breast Cancer

Cutaneous breast cancer metastases exhibit a diverse assortment of pigmentation, texture, and secondary skin findings. The most common presentation is that of skin-toned or pink nodules, either solitary or in multiples.[13] These malignancies, typically ductal or lobular carcinoma, frequently access the skin via direct extension, thereby grossly explaining their proclivity for the chest and abdomen.[3,37] In contrast, lesions may occasionally appear as indurated erythematous plaques (carcinoma en cuirasse or sclerodermoid carcinoma), erythematous patches with overlying telangiectasias (telangiectatic carcinoma), violaceous papulovesicles, or as pink-red plaques presenting as well-demarcated zones of alopecia (alopecia neoplastica).[13,26,37,38] With inflammatory breast cancers, erythematous patches and plaques resembling erysipelas (carcinoma erysipeloides) extend over a large surface area and may infiltrate lymphatics to create its peau d'orange appearance. Likewise, Paget disease of the breast, representing lactiferous duct invasion, produces erythematous plaques over the breast. However, these sharply demarcated rashes localize to the nipple and areola and may express scale or bloody discharge.[13,39,40]

Separately, skin tumors from underlying breast cancer are known to mimic numerous dermatologic ailments, including erythema annulare centrifugum,[41] herpes zoster,[37] angiosarcoma,[42] folliculitis,[43] and malignant melanoma.[44,45] Rare case reports describe lesions emerging from distant surgical scars or presenting as cryptic dermal nodules without overlying epidermal texture changes or pigmentation.[46,47] Importantly, continued surveillance of patients with breast cancer is critical, as 23% of metastatic breast cancer cases involve the skin.[2] Similarly, identifying cutaneous metastases from breast cancer adds valuable diagnostic and prognostic information; in previous retrospective studies, 3% to 3.5% of breast cancer diagnoses presented initially as a cutaneous lesion[3,25] and was associated with a mean survival time of 31 months.[4]

Lung Cancer

As with breast cancer metastases, those from lung cancer present as red, pink, or violaceous nodules that may be accompanied by ulceration or pain.[13,48] Less commonplace are variants with zosteriform pattern,[49] inflammatory carcinoma,[39] or telangiectasia.[50] In addition, lesions may mimic keratoacanthoma with prominent keratin plugs or imitate a vasculitic nodule.[51] Lung cancer metastases have been known to erupt within previous incision sites and scars.[52–54]

Meta-analysis suggests 3.4% of lung cancer cases ultimately involve the skin at autopsy; another study of exclusively non–small cell lung carcinoma cites a comparable 2.8% rate.[2,55] Different lung cancer subtypes have separate metastatic tendencies, with large cell carcinoma or adenocarcinoma the most likely to reach the skin.[56,57] Cutaneous metastases have been documented for rarer histologic subtypes including carcinoid,[58] mesothelioma,[59] and sarcomatoid carcinoma.[60] Unsurprisingly, men older than 40 years of age have a much greater likelihood of their cutaneous metastases deriving from the lung than their younger counterparts (27% vs 10%).[25] Once diagnosed, these patients have a particularly poor prognosis, with mean survival of less than 5 months.[4,55]

Renal Cell Carcinoma

Dermal spread of RCC typically presents as a single nodule with a predilection for the head, particularly the scalp.[4,15,25,61] As highly vascularized tumors, they tend to express bluish-purple pigmentation, with possible black-brown hue from hemosiderin deposition. For these reasons, they invoke comparable appearances to Kaposi sarcoma,[62] pyogenic granuloma,[63,64] angioma,[65] and abscess.[66] Additional case reports corroborate that RCC presentation is more variable than previously thought, including multiple ulcerative nodules[67] and extensive dermal plaques with diffuse nodules.[68]

Although RCC seemingly comprises a small subset of total cutaneous metastases, one Hungarian institution[15] found that by correcting for its prevalence at autopsy, RCC was the most likely to metastasize to the skin (relative prevalence of 1.5). Cumulatively, approximately 4% of renal cancer cases develop secondary skin tumors.[2] Because RCC tends to develop asymptomatically, skin lesions are often the first indication of disease.[69] For instance, Brownstein and Helwig[25] once noted that a skin lesion presented before RCC diagnosis in 53% of consultations. Advanced disease at discovery in these individuals contributes to a mean survival of 7 to 21 months.[4,61]

HISTOPATHOLOGY

Morphologically, cutaneous metastases are often characterized by involvement of the deep dermis or subcutaneous tissue. Common architectural patterns include a nodular, cellular proliferation with minimal intervening stroma or strands of tumor cells infiltrating a fibrotic dermis. Well-differentiated metastases may show characteristic morphologic features of the primary tumor, such as infiltrative glands with intraluminal necrotic debris in colorectal carcinoma metastases.[70] In a series of cutaneous metastases, Guanrizoli and colleagues reported that 34/45 (75%) cases showed typical morphologic features of the primary tumor, and only 7% demonstrated poorly differentiated morphology. Traditionally, cutaneous metastases are thought to more frequently demonstrate lymphovascular invasion, although several reports describe the range from 5% to 25%.[14,15] In addition, cutaneous metastases should lack features that suggest a primary skin neoplasm, including continuity with the epidermis, growth into skin appendages, and the presence of a benign counterpart within the lesion.

Immunohistochemical studies are frequently used to characterize metastatic tumor origin and distinguish it from its main histologic differential diagnosis, a primary adnexal tumor. In the appropriate morphologic and clinical context, an initial panel of immunostains may include cytokeratins 7 and 20, mammaglobin and estrogen receptor for breast cancer, thyroid transcription factor 1 and p40 for lung cancer, CDX-2 for colorectal cancer, and prostate specific antigen for prostatic cancer.[15,70,71] Immunostains for adnexal tumors may also be performed to distinguish primary skin from metastatic tumors. p63 positivity has been shown to have a 96% sensitivity for adnexal tumors and 96% negative predictive value for metastases. The addition of calretinin; cytokeratin 5/6, typically positive in adnexal tumors; and B72.3, typically negative, increases the diagnostic yield.[14]

SUMMARY

Internal malignancies metastasizing to the skin are highly prevalent phenomena, with an estimated 1% to 4.3% ultimately causing cutaneous disease.[5-7] Breast, lung, hematologic-lymphatic, and colorectum remain the predominant offenders, with lesions commonly presenting as flesh-colored, pink-red, or violaceous nodules or plaques that may mimic other dermatologic conditions.

There are some important clinical clues that can be used to raise a clinician's suspicion of a particular tumor even before a biopsy is done. When a patient presents with a sessile acrochordon-type lesion, a metastatic colon cancer can be suspected. Likewise, the presence of blue, blue-purple, or blue-red lesions suggests a highly vascularized primary cancer, most commonly kidney, liver, and neuroblastoma. When an associated alopecia is noted, or when vesicles or papulovesicles are found, breast and colon cancer metastasis is most likely.

Histologically, cutaneous metastases are typically centered in the deep dermis or subcutaneous tissues and may demonstrate a nodular or infiltrative architecture. An initial panel of immunostains may include markers for lung, colorectal, breast, and prostate metastases as well as primary adnexal tumors.

Our conception of cutaneous metastases defers heavily to case reports and single institution studies; larger systematic studies predate our modern tools and informatics for early cancer diagnosis and use nonuniform inclusion criteria. Fully informed clinical acumen awaits future investigations that build on existing evidence and appropriately address these limitations.

REFERENCES

1. U.S. Cancer Statistics Working Group. U.S. Cancer Statistics Data Visualizations Tool, based on November 2017 submission data (1999-2015). U.S. Department of Health and Human Services, Centers for Disease Control and Prevention and National Cancer Institute. Available at: www.cdc.gov/cancer/dataviz. Accessed November 17, 2018.

2. Krathen RA, Orengo IF, Rosen T. Cutaneous metastasis: a meta-analysis of data. South Med J 2003; 96(2):164–7.

3. Lookingbill DP, Spangler N, Sexton FM. Skin involvement as the presenting sign of internal carcinoma. A retrospective study of 7316 cancer patients. J Am Acad Dermatol 1990;22(1):19–26.

4. Lookingbill DP, Spangler N, Helm KF. Cutaneous metastases in patients with metastatic carcinoma: a retrospective study of 4020 patients. J Am Acad Dermatol 1993;29(2):228–36.

5. Gül U, Kiliç A, Gönül M, et al. Spectrum of cutaneous metastases in 1287 cases of internal malignancies: a study from Turkey. Acta Derm Venereol 2007; 87(2):160–2.

6. Hu SC, Chen GS, Wu CS, et al. Rates of cutaneous metastases from different internal malignancies: experience from a Taiwanese medical center. J Am Acad Dermatol 2009;60(3):379–87.

7. Chopra R, Chhabra S, Samra SG, et al. Cutaneous metastases of internal malignancies: a clinicopathologic study. Indian J Dermatol Venereol Leprol 2010; 76(2):125–31.

8. Benmously R, Souissi A, Badri T, et al. Cutaneous metastases from internal cancers. Acta Dermatovenerol Alp Pannonica Adriat 2008; 17(4):167–70.

9. Oualla K, Arifi S. Cutaneous metastases of internal cancers: a retrospective study about 12 cases. J Cancer Sci Ther 2012;4:155–7.

10. Fernandez-Flores A. Cutaneous metastases: a study of 78 biopsies from 69 patients. Am J Dermatopathol 2010;32(3):222–39.

11. Handa U, Kundu R, Dimri K. Cutaneous metastasis: a study of 138 cases diagnosed by fine-needle aspiration cytology. Acta Cytol 2017;61(1):47–54.

12. El Khoury J, Khalifeh I, Kibbi AG, et al. Cutaneous metastasis: clinicopathological study of 72 patients from a tertiary care center in Lebanon. Int J Dermatol 2014;53(2):147–58.

13. Alcaraz I, Cerroni L, Rütten A, et al. Cutaneous metastases from internal malignancies: a clinicopathologic and immunohistochemical review. Am J Dermatopathol 2012;34(4):347–93.

14. Sariya D, Ruth K, Adams-McDonnell R, et al. Clinicopathologic correlation of cutaneous metastases: experience from a cancer center. Arch Dermatol 2007;143(5):613–20.

15. Kovács KA, Kenessey I, Tímár J. Skin metastasis of internal cancers: a single institution experience. Pathol Oncol Res 2013;19(3):515–20.

16. Ayyamperumal A, Tharini G, Ravindran V, et al. Cutaneous manifestations of internal malignancy. Indian J Dermatol 2012;57(4):260–4.

17. Piette WW. Metastatic disease. In: Bonnett C, editor. Dermatological signs of internal disease. 4th edition. Philadelphia: Elsevier Health Sciences; 2009. p. 117–23.

18. Piette WW. Cutaneous manifestations of leukemias, myelodysplastic and myeloproliferative syndromes, and systemic lymphomas. In: Bonnett C, editor. Dermatological signs of internal disease. 4th edition. Philadelphia: Elsevier Health Sciences; 2009. p. 125–33.

19. Koller EA, Tourtelot JB, Pak HS, et al. Papillary and follicular thyroid carcinoma metastatic to the skin: a case report and review of the literature. Thyroid 1998;8(11):1045–50.

20. Liu M, Liu BL, Liu B, et al. Cutaneous metastasis of cholangiocarcinoma. World J Gastroenterol 2015; 21(10):3066–71.

21. Satter EK, Barnette DJ. Adrenocortical carcinoma with delayed cutaneous metastasis. J Cutan Pathol 2008;35(7):677–80.

22. Duquia RP, de Almeida HL, Traesel M, et al. Cutaneous metastasis of pheochromocytoma in multiple endocrine neoplasia IIB. J Am Acad Dermatol 2006;55(2):341–4.

23. Royer MC, Rush WL, Lupton GP. Hepatocellular carcinoma presenting as a precocious cutaneous metastasis. Am J Dermatopathol 2008;30(1):77–80.

24. Maher-Wiese VL, Wenner NP, Grant-Kels JM. Metastatic cutaneous lesions in children and adolescents with a case report of metastatic neuroblastoma. J Am Acad Dermatol 1992;26(4):620–8.

25. Brownstein MH, Helwig EB. Patterns of cutaneous metastasis. Arch Dermatol 1972;105(6):862–8.

26. Brownstein MH, Helwig EB. Spread of tumors to the skin. Arch Dermatol 1973;107(1):80–6.

27. Gan EY, Chio MT, Tan WP. A retrospective review of cutaneous metastases at the National Skin Centre Singapore. Australas J Dermatol 2015;56(1):1–6.

28. Saeed S, Keehn CA, Morgan MB. Cutaneous metastasis: a clinical, pathological, and immunohistochemical appraisal. J Cutan Pathol 2004;31(6): 419–30.

29. Cabula C, Campana LG, Grilz G, et al. Electrochemotherapy in the treatment of cutaneous metastases from breast cancer: a multicenter cohort analysis. Ann Surg Oncol 2015;22(Suppl 3):S442–50.

30. Bourke MG, Salwa SP, Sadadcharam M, et al. Effective treatment of intractable cutaneous metastases of breast cancer with electrochemotherapy: ten-year audit of single centre experience. Breast Cancer Res Treat 2017;161(2):289–97.

31. Spratt DE, Gordon Spratt EA, Wu S, et al. Efficacy of skin-directed therapy for cutaneous metastases from advanced cancer: a meta-analysis. J Clin Oncol 2014;32(28):3144–55.

32. Sanderson P, Innamaa A, Palmer J, et al. Imiquimod therapy for extramammary Paget's disease of the vulva: a viable non-surgical alternative. J Obstet Gynaecol 2013;33(5):479–83.

33. Luyten A, Sörgel P, Clad A, et al. Treatment of extramammary Paget disease of the vulva with imiquimod: a retrospective, multicenter study by the German Colposcopy Network. J Am Acad Dermatol 2014;70(4):644–50.

34. Henriques L, Palumbo M, Guay MP, et al. Imiquimod in the treatment of breast cancer skin metastasis. J Clin Oncol 2014;32(8):e22–5.

35. Asakura M, Miura H. Imiquimod 5% cream for the treatment of nasal lesion of metastatic renal cell carcinoma. Dermatol Ther 2011;24(3):375–7.

36. Okino T, Fujioka A, Nakajima H, et al. Effective treatment of metastatic renal cell carcinoma with topical imiquimod therapy. J Dtsch Dermatol Ges 2014; 12(2):155–7.

37. Mordenti C, Peris K, Concetta Fargnoli M, et al. Cutaneous metastatic breast carcinoma: a study of 164 patients. Acta Dermatovenerol Alp Pannonica Adriat 2000;9(4):143–8.

38. Conner KB, Cohen PR. Cutaneous metastasis of breast carcinoma presenting as alopecia neoplastica. South Med J 2009;102(4):385–9.

39. Hazelrigg DE, Rudolph AH. Inflammatory metastic carcinoma. Carcinoma erysipelatoides. Arch Dermatol 1977;113(1):69–70.

40. Al Ameer A, Imran M, Kaliyadan F, et al. Carcinoma erysipeloides as a presenting feature of breast carcinoma: a case report and brief review of literature. Indian Dermatol Online J 2015;6(6):396–8.

41. Sabater V, Ferrando F, Morera A, et al. Cutaneous metastasis of inflammatory breast carcinoma mimicking an erythema annulare centrifugum: a sign of locally recurrent cancer. Clin Exp Dermatol 2016;41(8):906–10.

42. Dobson CM, Tagor V, Myint AS, et al. Telangiectatic metastatic breast carcinoma in face and scalp mimicking cutaneous angiosarcoma. J Am Acad Dermatol 2003;48(4):635–6.

43. Paolino G, Panetta C, Didona D, et al. Folliculotropic cutaneous metastases and lymphangitis carcinomatosa: when cutaneous metastases of breast carcinoma are mistaken for cutaneous infections. Acta Dermatovenerol Croat 2016;24(2):154–7.

44. Requena L, Sangueza M, Sangueza OP, et al. Pigmented mammary Paget disease and pigmented epidermotropic metastases from breast carcinoma. Am J Dermatopathol 2002;24(3):189–98.

45. Kitamura S, Hata H, Homma E, et al. Pigmented skin metastasis of breast cancer showing dermoscopic features of malignant melanoma. J Eur Acad Dermatol Venereol 2015;29(5):1034–6.

46. Chen SX, Lum N, Chen SY, et al. An unusual case of metastatic breast carcinoma metastasizing to an antecedent rhytidectomy procedural scar. JAAD Case Rep 2018;4(4):392–5.

47. Mayer JE, Maurer MA, Nguyen HT. Diffuse cutaneous breast cancer metastases resembling subcutaneous nodules with no surface changes. Cutis 2018;101(3):219–23.

48. Alkhayat H, Hong CH. Cutaneous metastases from non-small cell lung cancer. J Cutan Med Surg 2006;10(6):304–7.

49. Matarasso SL, Rosen T. Zosteriform metastases: case presentation and review of the literature. J Dermatol Surg Oncol 1988;14:774–8.

50. Park JJ, Choi YD, Lee JB, et al. Telangiectatic cutaneous metastasis from lung adenocarcinoma. J Am Acad Dermatol 2011;64:798–9.

51. Babacan NA, Kiliçkap S, Sene S, et al. A case of multifocal skin metastases from lung cancer presenting with vasculitic-type cutaneous nodule. Indian J Dermatol 2015;60(2):213.

52. Dunn PT, Bigler CF. Metastasis in an electrodesiccation and curettage scar. J Am Acad Dermatol 1997; 36(1):117–8.

53. Shieh S, Grassi M, Schwarz JK, et al. Pleural mesothelioma with cutaneous extension to chest wall scars. J Cutan Pathol 2004;31:497–501.

54. Sabater-Marco V, García-García JA, Roig-Vila JV. Basaloid large cell lung carcinoma presenting as cutaneous metastasis at the colostomy site after abdominoperineal resection for rectal carcinoma. J Cutan Pathol 2013;40(8):758–64.

55. Song Z, Lin B, Shao L, et al. Cutaneous metastasis as a initial presentation in advanced non-small cell lung cancer and its poor survival prognosis. J Cancer Res Clin Oncol 2012;138(10):1613–7.

56. Hidaka T, Ishii Y, Kitamura S. Clinical features of skin metastasis from lung cancer. Intern Med 1996;35(6): 459–62.

57. Marcoval J, Penín RM, Llatjós R, et al. Cutaneous metastasis from lung cancer: retrospective analysis of 30 patients. Australas J Dermatol 2012;53(4):288–90.

58. Falto-Aizpurua L, Seyfer S, Krishnan B, et al. Cutaneous metastasis of a pulmonary carcinoid tumor. Cutis 2017;99(5):E13–5.

59. Elbahaie AM, Kamel DE, Lawrence J, et al. Late cutaneous metastases to the face from malignant pleural mesothelioma: a case report and review of the literature. World J Surg Oncol 2009;7:84.

60. Terada T. Sarcomatoid carcinoma of the lung presenting as a cutaneous metastasis. J Cutan Pathol 2010;37(4):482–5.

61. Dorairajan LN, Hemal AK, Aron M, et al. Cutaneous metastases in renal cell carcinoma. Urol Int 1999; 63(3):164–7.

62. Rogow L, Rotman M, Roussis K. Renal metastases simulating Kaposi sarcoma. Arch Dermatol 1975; 111:717–9.

63. Batres E, Knox JM, Wolf JE. Metastatic renal cell carcinoma resembling a pyogenic granuloma. Arch Dermatol 1978;114(7):1082–3.

64. Estrada-Chavez G, Vega-Memije ME, Lacy-Niebla RM, et al. Scalp metastases of a renal cell carcinoma. Skinmed 2006;5(3):148–50.

65. Arrabal-Polo MA, Arias-Santiago SA, Aneiros-Fernandez J, et al. Cutaneous metastases in renal cell carcinoma: a case report. Cases J 2009;2:7948.

66. Porter NA, Anderson HL, Al-Dujaily S. Renal cell carcinoma presenting as a solitary cutaneous facial metastasis: case report and review of the literature. Int Semin Surg Oncol 2006;3(1):27–30.

67. Errami M, Margulis V, Huerta S. Renal cell carcinoma metastatic to the scalp. Rare Tumors 2016;8(4):6400.

68. Sheth N, Petrof G, Greenblatt D, et al. Unusual presentation of cutaneous metastases in renal cell carcinoma. Clin Exp Dermatol 2008;33(4): 538–9.

69. Schwartz RA. Cutaneous metastatic disease. J Am Acad Dermatol 1995;33(2):161–82.

70. Guanziroli E, Coggi A, Del Gobbo A, et al. Cutaneous metastases of internal malignancies: an experience from a single institution. Eur J Dermatol 2017; 27(6):609–14.

71. Lin F, Liu H. Immunohistochemistry in undifferentiated neoplasm/tumor of uncertain origin. Arch Pathol Lab Med 2014;138(12):1583–610.

72. Wong CY, Helm MA, Helm TN, et al. Patterns of skin metastases: a review of 25 years' experience at a single cancer center. Int J Dermatol 2014;53(1): 56–60.

Cutaneous Adverse Reactions of Anticancer Agents

Subuhi Kaul, MBBS, MD[a], Benjamin H. Kaffenberger, MD[b],
Jennifer N. Choi, MD[c], Shawn G. Kwatra, MD[d],*

KEYWORDS

- Skin • Drugs • Cutaneous adverse effects • Anticancer • Chemotherapy • Immunotherapy

KEY POINTS

- Traditional anticancer drugs tend to result in alopecia, mucositis, and nail changes due to cell death/injury and have significant systemic adverse effects.
- Targeted agents tend to have more cutaneous adverse effects when compared with systemic involvement. Several agents have characteristic adverse effects, such as epidermal growth factor receptor inhibitors frequently causing papulopustular reactions.
- Immunotherapeutic agents (anti–programmed cell death 1 (PD-1)/programmed cell death ligand 1 and cytotoxic T-lymphocyte–associated protein 4) most commonly cause immune activation–related adverse effects.
- Need for treatment depends on the type and severity of adverse effect, with discontinuation of drug being the last resort in most cases.

INTRODUCTION

Conventional anticancer agents target rapidly dividing cells, which explains the common adverse effects (AEs) seen in organ systems with a dominant population of proliferative cells, such as the hair follicle, mucosae, and bone marrow.[1] Targeted agents work on molecular mechanisms responsible for cancer occurrence and progression. These include epidermal growth factor receptor inhibitors (EGFRi), BRAF inhibitors (BRAFi), MEK inhibitors (MEKi), mammalian target of rapamycin inhibitors (mTORi), and Multikinase inhibitors (MKIs). These agents frequently give rise to cutaneous adverse reactions (CARs) with relatively less systemic involvement.[2] Similarly, oncoimmunotherapeutic agents such as programmed cell death protein 1 (PD-1) and cytotoxic T-lymphocyte–associated protein 4 (CTLA-4) inhibitors are commonly associated with dermatologic reactions and immune-related adverse events.[3] Comprehensive cancer care requires treating oncologists and dermatologists to understand these adverse events and provide effective management. This review discusses the cutaneous adverse effects of anticancer agents.

CONTENT
Eruptions/Rashes

Palmar-plantar erythrodysesthesia
Palmar-plantar erythrodysesthesia (PPE), hand-foot syndrome, acral erythema, and Burgdorf

Disclosure Statement: The authors have nothing to disclose.
[a] Department of Dermatology, All India Institute of Medical Sciences, Ansari Nagar, New Delhi 110029, India;
[b] Ohio State Dermatology, 1328 Dublin Road, Suite 100, Columbus, OH 43212, USA; [c] Department of Dermatology, Division of Oncodermatology, Robert H. Lurie Comprehensive Cancer Center, Northwestern University Feinberg School of Medicine, 676 North Street Clair, Suite 1600, Chicago, IL 60611, USA; [d] Johns Hopkins University School of Medicine, 1550 Orleans Street, CRB II Suite 206, Baltimore, MD 21231, USA
* Corresponding author.
E-mail address: skwatra1@jhmi.edu

Dermatol Clin 37 (2019) 555–568
https://doi.org/10.1016/j.det.2019.05.013

reaction are the various terms used for chemotherapy associated acral changes (**Fig. 1**).[1,4] Bolognia and colleagues[5] proposed an umbrella term, "toxic erythema of chemotherapy," that incorporates the abovementioned terms, along with chemotherapy-associated neutrophilic eccrine hidradenitis (NEH) and intertrigo-like reactions. Although some experts still use individualized terms based on clinical distribution and histologic findings, others prefer to use the term "toxic erythema of chemotherapy" to refer to any of these clinical diagnoses. PPE begins as a burning sensation of the palms and soles, followed by well-defined erythematous macules, with or without edema. These may occasionally be followed by blistering and desquamation.[4] Onset is 2 to 3 weeks after chemotherapy but can be delayed up to several months.[1,5–7] Histopathology usually shows a mild spongiotic tissue reaction.[4,8] Graft-versus-host disease is an important differential and has near-identical clinical and histopathologic features. A history of preceding allogenic bone marrow transplantation and progression of erythema to non-acral sites may help recognize the latter.[9] Although the exact mechanism is unknown, the most accepted theory is that of direct toxicity to skin. Other hypotheses put forth to explain palmoplantar predilection are microtrauma to capillaries by antiangiogenic MKIs, drug excretion by eccrine glands with resultant local drug concentration, and higher palmoplantar activity of dihydropyrimidine dehydrogenase, which breaks down 5-fluorouracil (5-FU) and capecitabine into toxic byproducts.[10] The most commonly implicated drugs are liposomal doxorubicin, cytarabine, capecitabine, taxanes, and 5-FU.[4]

MKIs are also reported to cause changes similar to PPE caused by conventional drugs.[7,11] However, important clinical differences warrant a separate term—hand-foot skin reaction (HFSR). It is characterized by an inflammatory phase with focal blistering and perilesional erythema on pressure points followed by a hyperkeratotic phase, with tender keratoderma-like plaques (**Fig. 2**).[11] The incidence of PPE varies with drug dosage and duration of administration. Drugs or formulations with longer plasma half-lives confer greater risk, exemplified by an incidence of 50% in patients receiving liposomal doxorubicin versus 26% with the nonliposomal formulation. Another risk factor is certain drug combinations—doxorubicin with continuous 5-FU has a reported incidence of 89%.[10] HFSR is reported in 10% to 60% cases receiving MKIs, with a higher incidence with a combination of bevacizumab and sorafenib (79%). Renal cell carcinoma and female gender also increase the risk of HFSR.[7] Drugs reported to cause PPE and HFSR are in **Table 1**.

Treatment is generally directed at symptom control, and resolution occurs with drug discontinuation or dose reduction.[4,7] Various preventive measures have been proposed; however, no single method is entirely effective. Indeed, most evidence is based on case reports and series or expert opinion.[12,13] Nevertheless, there are recent controlled studies that have demonstrated the effectiveness of several strategies. Regional cooling using frozen gloves and socks just prior, during, and for 15 minutes after each chemotherapy session has been shown to be effective in a recent study.[14] A randomized controlled trial (RCT) found bidaily application of urea-based creams useful in the prevention of MKI-triggered HFSR.[15] A double-blind placebo-controlled study demonstrated decreased rates of PPE with the use of a topical antiperspirant.[16] Systemic medications such as oral pyridoxine, dexamethasone, and celecoxib have also been used.[7,17] However, a systematic review found only celecoxib to effectively prevent HFS when compared with oral pyridoxine, topical urea, and antiperspirants.[18]

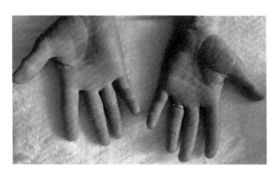

Fig. 1. Cytarabine-induced palmoplantar erythrodysesthesia.

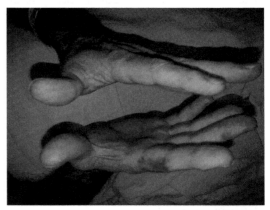

Fig. 2. Hand-foot skin reaction—erythema and callosities in a patient who received sunitinib for metastatic renal cell cancer.

Table 1 Drugs associated with palmoplantar dysesthesia and hand-foot skin reaction	
Palmar-Plantar Erythrodysesthesia	Hand-Foot Skin Reaction
Capecitabine	Sorafenib
Docetaxel	Sunitinib
Epirubicin	Vemurafenib
5-FU	Axitinib
Gemcitabine	Pazopanib
Doxorubicin	Regorafenib
	Cabozantinib

Data from Refs.[4,7,9–11,18,19]

Table 2 Drugs associated with neutrophilic eccrine hidradenitis	
Anthracyclines	5-Fluorouracil
Bleomycin	Imatinib
Cetuximab	Methotrexate
Cyclophosphamide	Mitoxantrone
Cytarabine	Vemurafenib
Dabrafenib	Vinca alkaloids

Data from Refs.[20–23]

Neutrophilic eccrine hidradenitis

Chemotherapy-induced NEH is a rare dermatosis, first described in association with acute myeloid leukemia treated with cytarabine.[19] It presents with painful erythematous papules, pustules, or plaques on the extremities, head, neck, and trunk (Fig. 3).[4] Fever often accompanies rash onset and occurs in 1 to 2 weeks of drug initiation.[4,20] Rash resolves without sequelae over several days to weeks after drug discontinuation. Histopathology is characterized by neutrophilic infiltration of the eccrine glands and vacuolar degeneration with spared acrosyringium.[4,20] Sweet syndrome and infections such as cellulitis are clinical differentials and a skin biopsy may help determine the diagnosis in challenging cases. NEH is thought to result from excretion of the drug by eccrine glands with consequent local toxicity.[4] Cytarabine is the most frequently associated chemotherapeutic agent. The BRAFi, dabrafenib, and vemurafenib were associated with cases with an earlier onset (within 3–4 days, of commencing therapy) that resolved in a few days after discontinuation.[21] Others are listed in Table 2. Spontaneous resolution is common and there is seldom need for active management.[4,22] However, recurrence is known with readministration of the drugs.[23] Systemic steroids and dapsone have been used successfully in the past; however, steroids must be used cautiously in immunosuppressed patients.[4,20] NEH due to BRAFi does not seem to recur on switching to an alternative BRAFi, and this can be used to manage NEH without compromising the chemotherapy regimen.[21]

Eccrine squamous syringometaplasia

Eccrine squamous syringometaplasia (ESS) is an uncommon cutaneous eruption characterized by erythematous macules, papules, and plaques that appear about 2 to 30 days after starting chemotherapy.[24,25] A case series observed the bilaterally symmetric intertriginous pattern to be the most common presentation. Sites affected were axillae, groin, and sides of neck, in descending order of frequency.[26] Resolution occurs in about 2 to 4 weeks with fine desquamation and occasional postinflammatory hyperpigmentation.[4,26] Similar to NEH, it is thought that secretion and subsequent concentration of drugs in the eccrine apparatus results in injury.[25] Histopathologically, keratinized squamous cells replace the normal ductal and glandular cuboidal epithelium.[4,25,26] It is most commonly associated with liposomal doxorubicin and the combination cytostatic drugs administered in autologous hematopoietic stem cell transplant regimens.[26,27] Other drugs associated with ESS have been included in Table 3. Expected self-resolution after drug cessation eliminates the need for specific therapy; indeed, topical or short course oral corticosteroids are used only to augment patient comfort. Recurrence with reinstitution of the same chemotherapy regimen is known and may be prevented with a 15% dose reduction.[26,28,29]

Hypersensitivity reactions

Several conventional chemotherapeutic as well as targeted agents are associated with hypersensitivity reactions (HSRs), most commonly Gell and

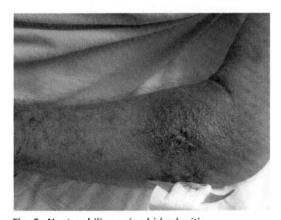

Fig. 3. Neutrophilic eccrine hidradenitis.

Table 3 Drugs associated with eccrine squamous syringometaplasia	
Busulfan	5-Fluorouracil
Bleomycin	Imatinib
Carmustine	Melphalan
Cisplatin	Methotrexate
Cyclophosphamide	Mitoxantrone
Cytarabine	Pemextrexed
dabrafenib	Suramin
Daunorubicin	Sunitinib
Doxorubicin	Thiotepa
Etoposide	Vemurafenib

Data from Refs.[24–29]

Coombs Type I.[4] Clinically, type I reactions induced by chemotherapeutics can manifest along the spectrum of urticaria to anaphylaxis and can be due to the drug itself or the vehicle. It is common with asparaginase, taxanes, platins, doxorubicin, and epipodophyllotoxins (etoposide/teniposide).[30] The incidence and time from first dose vary widely—20% to 63% with oxaliplatin after an average of 5 cycles, to about 41% with paclitaxel, in which case the reactions are more likely to occur in the first cycle itself.[30,31] In the case of platins, the most important risk factor for development of HSRs is the total number of cycles.[30] With taxanes HSRs are most likely to occur with the first few exposures, suggesting underlying direct mast cell and/or basophil activation. Asparaginase is highly immunogenic, and the pegylated form decreases its immunogenic potential. In contrast, use of the liposomal formulation of doxorubicin has a higher rate of HSRs hinting at complement activation by the liposome fraction.[30] Most reactions to monoclonal antibodies present as infusion reactions and skin involvement (pruritus, flushing, and urticaria) are uncommon fever, chills, and rigors and occur in up to 85% with rituximab.[31,32] Pretreatment with antihistamines, both anti-H1 and H2, with or without corticosteroids is advised for patients receiving asparaginase, taxanes, or cetuximab.[4,31,33] Rapid drug desensitization for type I HSRs allows safe readministration and continuation of first-line chemotherapy. This is done for several drugs—taxanes, platins, doxorubicin, and biologics such as rituximab, cetuximab, trastuzumab, and infliximab.[34,35]

Other idiosyncratic CARs such as toxic epidermal necrolysis (TEN), Steven-Johnson syndrome (SJS), and erythema multiforme are also known to occur. Thalidomide, asparaginase, methotrexate, bleomycin, cladribine, chlorambucil, cytarabine, doxorubicin, and topical nitrogen mustard have all been associated with the SJS/TEN spectrum. Targeted agents most often causing SJS/TEN are imatinib, EGFRi, vemurafenib, nivolumab, and cetuximab.[36–39] Immediate discontinuation of the suspected drugs and acute and supportive management by a multidisciplinary team are necessary in SJS/TEN. Dexamethasone, intravenous immunoglobulin, and cyclosporine are commonly used; nevertheless, management differs in various centers for want of a standard treatment protocol.

Allergic contact dermatitis has been observed with topical use of chemotherapeutic agents such as mechlorethamine, 5-FU, cisplatin, daunorubicin, and doxorubicin.[32] Cessation of drug use followed by emollient and topical corticosteroids ameliorate the dermatitis.

Papulopustular eruption

An aseptic papulopustular eruption in a seborrheic distribution is the characteristic CAR observed with EGFRi. A similar eruption also occurs with MEKi, mTORi, and vandetanib. The incidence with either class is greater than 75% in patients.[3,40] After 1 to 2 weeks of therapy, a sensory disturbance arises, followed by erythema and papules and/or pustules that can rupture and crust over. Unlike acne, there are no comedones or cysts (**Fig. 4**).[41]

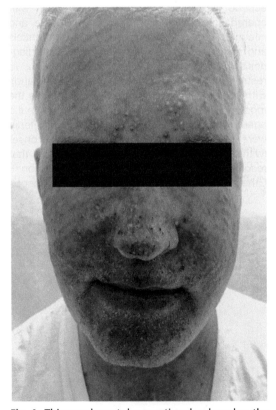

Fig. 4. This papulopustular eruption developed on the face, neck, and upper chest after EGFR inhibitor use.

Telangiectasias and hyperpigmentation are occasional sequelae.[42] Exacerbation with photoexposure is recognized and sun protection is recommended prophylactically.[2] Approximately 10% develop a severe rash (>30% body surface area involvement) adversely affecting quality of life.[43] The rash is dose dependent and associated with favorable tumor response.[2] Histopathologically, there is T-cell infiltration around the follicular infundibulum evolving into granulomas and a destructive folliculitis.[42]

Preventive measures recommended are use of neutral pH cleansers, regular hydrophilic cream application, sunscreen use, and oral tetracyclines started simultaneously with chemotherapy.[44] Management depends on the severity of rash, which is graded 1 to 5 based on body surface area (BSA) involved and impairment of activities of daily living.[44] Mild rashes (grade 1, <10% BSA) can be treated with topical antibiotics or topical low potency corticosteroids. Moderate involvement (grade 2, 10%–30% BSA with pain/pruritus/superinfection) necessitate administration of oral antibiotics, most commonly doxycycline or minocycline, with more potent topical steroids. Severe rashes (grade 3 and above, >30% BSA) or nonresponsive moderate grades require dose reduction; a trial of isotretinoin or low-dose acitretin may also be considered.[44] Systemic steroids can be used in rare severe cases but are generally avoided because they may share this same adverse effect.[2] Whenever pustules are present, it is prudent to get bacterial and/or fungal cultures, as superinfections are common and culture results can direct the use of appropriate antimicrobials.

Generalized eruptions

Typical drug rashes can result from traditional chemotherapy drugs that present as blanchable erythematous macules and plaques on the trunk and limbs. Resolution occurs with fine desquamation 1 to 2 weeks after drug withdrawal. Gemcitabine, etoposide, estramustine, and cytarabine are commonly associated with a morbilliform drug rash.[6] cKIT and Bcr-abl inhibitors are associated with a diffuse pruritic morbilliform eruption that begins around 9 weeks after treatment initiation. Imatinib and female sex are independent risk factors for this rash.[2] The rash affects nearly half of the treated patients and preferentially occurs on the trunk and extremities.[40] A pruritic erythematous rash with small hyperkeratotic keratosis pilaris–like papules, predominantly affecting the trunk and limbs, affects up to 75% of the patients treated with BRAFi.[40] Antiangiogenic tyrosine kinase inhibitor use is associated with a generalized erythematous maculopapular rash that appears within days of treatment initiation. In descending order, sorafenib (50% incidence), sunitinib, regorafenib, axitinib, and pazopanib (less than 10%) are implicated. Rash is usually mild and spontaneously resolves despite treatment continuation.[40] A maculopapular pruritic rash is the most frequent immune-related cutaneous AE seen with PD-1, programmed cell death ligand 1 (PD-L1), and CTLA-4i. It affects up to 68% of the patients treated with ipilimumab.[45] However, the risk of this rash is lower with other immune checkpoint inhibitors, being less than 10% with use of PD-L1 inhibitors.[46]

Lichenoid dermatitis

Lichenoid reactions are one of the most common skin reactions seen with the PD-1 inhibitors, pembrolizumab and nivolumab (**Fig. 5**).[47] The incidence is approximately 25% and onset tends to be delayed, occurring on an average of 8 months after initiation of therapy. The rash is pruritic and predominantly affects the trunk. A similar reaction may be seen with CTLA-4 agents, although the incidence is lower.[47] Reactivation of previous hypertrophic lichen planus with nivolumab use has been noted.[48] Histologically, a lichenoid pattern is seen in the majority, with about 10% cases showing basal vacuolar change.[45] A granulomatous pattern admixed with lichenoid infiltrate was reported with nivolumab use.[49] In most cases, application of emollients and topical steroids is sufficient therapy, and modification of cancer regimen is not required. Antihistamines, GABA antagonists, antidepressants, or neurokinin 1 receptor inhibitors can be used to alleviate troublesome pruritus.[45] Recent reports of cutaneous growths resembling keratoacanthomas and squamous cell carcinomas, with lichenoid histologic changes, and hypertrophic lichen planus mimicking squamous cell carcinomas have emerged in the setting of PD-1 inhibitor therapy.[50] In such a scenario, nonsurgical management, including topical steroids, intralesional steroids, cryotherapy, and/or imiquimod, should be strongly considered in lieu of surgical excision.

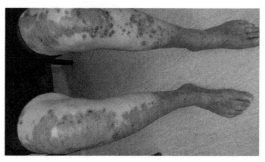

Fig. 5. Lichenoid dermatitis after starting nivolumab.

Pigmentary changes

Hyperpigmentation is the most common pigmentary change experienced with several cytotoxic agents, most commonly cyclophosphamide, cisplatin, bleomycin, anthracyclines, and antimetabolites (**Fig. 6**).[4,32] The mechanism is postulated to be either melanocyte stimulation or postinflammatory hyperpigmentation. Various patterns of hyperpigmentation are reported—diffuse, localized, or figurate.[32] Cyclophosphamide, hydroxyurea, procarbazine, and busulfan are associated with a generalized increase in pigmentation (see **Fig. 5**).[4,32] 5-FU can cause diffuse, irregular patchy, as well as localized hyperpigmentation over infused veins.[4,6] A unique patterned "flagellate" pigmentation, thought to correspond to linear excoriated areas, is seen with bleomycin. Pigmentation can also be diffuse or occur on pressure sites such as elbows.[4,6] Docetaxel is associated with 2 peculiar forms of hyperpigmentation—a reticulate pigmentation and a supravenous erythematous reaction, which evolves into a pigmented band at the infusion site. Hyperpigmentation gradually fades with drug withdrawal; however, repeat exposure is associated with recurrence.[4] Photoprotective measures and topical retinoids can help facilitate disappearance; however, no specific intervention is warranted.[44]

In contrast to traditional drugs, certain targeted agents are associated with skin hypo- or depigmentation. A meta-analysis revealed Bcr-abl inhibitors (imatinib, dasatinib), EGFRi (gefitinib), vascular endothelial growth factor inhibitor (VEGFi) (sunitinib, pazopanib), BRAFi (vemurafenib), and PD-1 inhibitor (pembrolizumab) to be most commonly associated with cutaneous hypopigmentation. Downstream inhibition of tyrosinase activity is hypothesized to be responsible for this reversible loss of pigmentation; conversely, paradoxical hyperpigmentation has also been reported with imatinib.[51,52]

Inflammatory and immune-related dermatoses

A higher risk of developing de novo bullous pemphigoid (BP) is reported with anti-PD-1 (pembrolizumab, nivolumab) and anti-PD-L1 (atezolizumab, durvalumab) agents (**Fig. 7**).[46,53] Flare of preexisting BP has been noted with anti-CTLA-4 therapy.[46] The onset can be immediate or delayed and mucosal involvement is seldom seen. Management is individualized based on severity and topical or systemic corticosteroids form the mainstay of treatment. Treatment interruption may be required to facilitate healing.[46] Immune check point inhibitors, most commonly ipilimumab, are reported to be associated with development of classic cutaneous features of dermatomyositis, Sjogren syndrome, and subacute cutaneous lupus erythematosus.[46,53] Vasculitis presenting with livedo and digit necrosis has been rarely reported with anti-PD-1 use.[46] Vitiligo like depigmentation is reported with immune check point inhibitors and is resultant of immune system activation. This clinical change acts as a surrogate marker of favorable tumor response to therapy. This occurs in about a quarter of patients treated with anti-PD-1 agents, pembrolizumab and nivolumab, and overwhelmingly in patients being treated for melanoma, with isolated case reports in patients being treated for other cancers, such as lung cancer.[51] Occasional reports of Grover disease with ipilimumab and anti-PD-1 therapy are present. Clinically, a polymorphic pruritic vesicular or papulokeratotic eruption is observed and diagnosis needs histopathologic confirmation.[46] Psoriasis may be triggered, or preexisting psoriasis can be exacerbated by anti-PD-1/PD-L1 and anti-CTLA-4 agents (**Fig. 8**). Management needs to be tailored to the individual—mild cases can be treated with topical steroids or vitamin D analogues, whereas extensive psoriasis may need

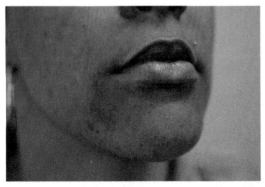

Fig. 6. Perioral pigmentation with cyclophosphamide use.

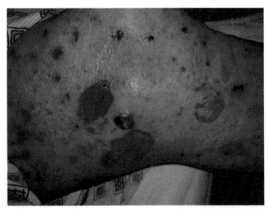

Fig. 7. Keratoacanthoma and bullous pemphigoid developed in a patient with melanoma after administration of pembrolizumab.

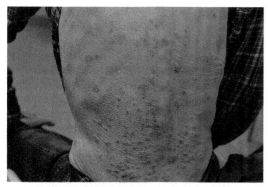

Fig. 8. Psoriasis in a patient on pembrolizumab for oral squamous cell carcinoma.

additional treatment, such as narrowband ultraviolet B (UVB) phototherapy or oral acitretin.[46] BRAFi are associated with a painful panniculitis of the extremities along with arthralgias. Nonsteroidal anti-inflammatory drugs provide effective symptom control; however, a short course of oral steroids may be required in some cases.[3] Cellulitis-like aseptic inflammatory plaques have been noted with selumetinib use.[40]

Extravasation

Inadvertent escape of chemotherapeutic agents into surrounding extravascular tissue during infusion leads to extravasation injury. Chemotherapeutic agents are classified as irritants, if they cause an inflammatory reaction with erythema and/or edema without necrosis and, vesicants, if they lead to necrosis and ulceration.[1] Immediate cessation of infusion, aspiration of extravasated drug through the catheter if possible, and limb elevation are required in all cases. This is followed by cooling of the affected area with ice packs in all cases except those due to vinca alkaloids (vincristine and vinblastine) and epipodophyllotoxins (etoposide).[1,4]

Photosensitivity or radiation sensitivity

Cutaneous recall reactions are inflammatory chemotherapy-induced skin eruptions occurring at a site of previous radiation- or sun-induced damage. These skin effects are thought to result from a superimposed drug toxicity on a previously damaged section of the skin.[4] There is production of a well-defined area of erythematous skin localized to previously irradiated areas and can be generalized in those with past full-body irradiation.[4] Drugs frequently associated with radiation recall reactions are methotrexate, gemcitabine, capecitabine, docetaxel, etoposide, and doxorubicin. Newer drugs such as pemetrexed, gefitinib, and combinations of bevacizumab with

gemcitabine and of trastuzumab with vinorelbine also result in similar reactions.[41]

Of the traditional drugs, sun sensitivity has been reported with use of 5-FU, dacarbazine, and vinblastine most commonly.[4] UVA photosensitivity is noted in up to 50% of patients administered vemurafenib and presents with erythema and edema in sun-exposed sites.[40,54] EGFRi are also associated with a photosensitive rash with postinflammatory hyperpigmentation.[2] Management includes strict photoprotection with use of broad-spectrum sunscreens and protective clothing to prevent painful disfiguring burns. Bleaching agents and camouflage may provide cosmetic relief.[2]

Benign and malignant neoplasms

The most common CAR with BRAFi (vemurafenib, dabrafenib) are hyperproliferative epidermal neoplasms. Verrucous keratoses occur in up to 72% and 66% with vemurafenib and dabrafenib use, respectively.[54] These skin papillomas can have various clinical appearances and can mimic seborrheic keratosis, viral warts, or cutaneous horns and generally develop in 6 to 12 weeks of commencing therapy.[40,54] Plantar keratoses occur in about 39% and actinic keratoses occur in about 30% with either agent. Cutaneous squamous cell carcinoma (cSCC) incidence with their use is reported to be 36% and 26%, respectively.[54] The cSCCs are usually well differentiated, occur within 3 months of BRAFi therapy, and are usually eruptive papules with a hyperkeratotic rim. They mimic keratoacanthomas clinically and histologically, which are also known to occur with these agents (see **Fig. 7**). Eruptive keratoacanthomas were reported with pembrolizumab use.[55] The proposed mechanism is a paradoxic activation of mitogen-activated protein kinase pathway in cells not carrying a BRAF mutation.[56] The risk of cSCC development may be compounded by photodamage and papillomavirus infection.[40,54] A full-body skin examination is recommended before initiating BRAFi therapy, followed by monthly checks throughout therapy.[54] Actinic keratoses (AKs) should be preemptively treated at the initial visit by cryotherapy, electrodessication, or curettage. For numerous lesions, topical field therapy with 5-FU, imiquimod, or tretinoin can be done.[54] Treatment options for cSCCs include saucerization followed by electrodessication and curettage, full fusiform excisions, or aggressive cryotherapy.[54] Eruptive nevi, change in preexisting melanocytic nevi, dysplastic nevi, and primary melanoma are associated with BRAFi use.[54] The incidence for new and changed nevi is about 10% on clinical examination and increases to 50% with dermoscopic evaluation; in addition, incidence of new melanomas is 1% to 2% with their use.[40,54] Thus, close dermatologic monitoring should be carried out throughout the treatment period. Inflammation of preexisting AKs occurs with 5-FU, doxorubicin, and sorafenib and could be attributed to toxic effects on the actively replicating cells. Topical steroid application generally mitigates symptoms.[4]

Hair changes

Chemotherapy-induced alopecia, with an incidence of 65%, is one of the most common and apparent AEs of chemotherapy.[57] There are 2 major types: anagen effluvium and telogen effluvium (TE). TE is less common, presents as thinning of hair, and is most noticeable 3 to 4 months after chemotherapy. Agents that often cause TE are retinoids, methotrexate, and 5-FU.[58] Anagen effluvium begins within 1 to 3 weeks of commencing therapy and is complete by 2 months. Direct insult to the rapidly dividing anagen follicle cells leads to interruption of mitosis. The resultant hair loss is substantial because at any given time about 90% of the hair follicles on the scalp are in the anagen phase.[4,57] Traditional chemotherapeutic agents such as taxanes, topoisomerase inhibitors, alkylating agents, and antimetabolites cause varying degrees of alopecia in up to 50% to 100% of cases.[57] Among the newer drugs, sorafenib has resulted in mild non-scarring alopecia in about half of the patients.[40] Although thought to be reversible with cessation of chemotherapy, a cohort study found rates of permanent partial hair loss to be as high as 42% at the 3-year post-chemotherapy follow-up. Risk was higher with taxane-based regimens (**Fig. 9**).[59,60] Others

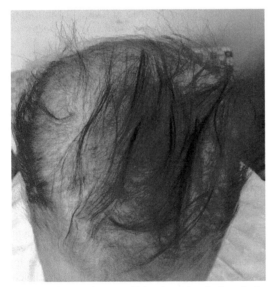

Fig. 9. Permanent partial alopecia induced by chemotherapy.

causing persistent alopecia are cyclophosphamide, busulfan, melphalan, etoposide, docetaxel, carboplatin, and paclitaxel.[59] Cicatricial alopecia has also been reported with gefitinib and erlotinib.[61,62] Alopecia is one of the most traumatic effects of chemotherapy and is even a cause for refusal of chemotherapy.[58] The best studied method of preventing it is scalp cooling, which is hypothesized to decrease drug delivery to the scalp by regional vasoconstriction.[58,63,64] An RCT found improved hair preservation in half of those treated with taxanes and/or along with use of a scalp cooling device.[64] Other effective measures aim at accelerating regrowth, primarily with bidaily topical application of 2% minoxidil.[58,65] Once daily topical application of 0.03% bimatoprost to upper eyelids was safe and effective in patients with lash hypotrichosis.[66]

Eyelash trichomegaly is common with EGFRi, occurring a few months after initiating treatment. Lashes become thick, long, and curly, and inward growing lashes may cause mechanical conjunctivitis.[40] Hypertrichosis of the face, particularly involving the upper lip, cheek, and brows can also occur and is troublesome in women. Trichomegaly can be managed by regularly cutting the lashes.[2] Temporary hair removal or topical eflornithine are useful options for distressing facial hypertrichosis.[40]

Changes in hair texture and color have been noted with MKIs.[2] Hair becomes curly and difficult to manage after 3 to 6 months in about 50% of patients treated with sorafenib and sunitinib.[40] Reversibly decreased hair pigmentation is reported with sunitinib (7%–14%) and pazopanib (44%).[2]

Nail changes

Chemotherapy-induced nail changes involve several or all nails and occur weeks after treatment initiation. The clinical features vary with the part of the nail unit affected and the causative drug.[67] Various mechanisms explain nail changes; direct drug toxicity to nail epithelia resulting in an abrupt halt of mitosis accounts for Beau lines (**Fig. 10**). Stimulation of matrical melanocytes and drug accumulation in nail plate both can lead to discoloration. Interruption of nail bed vessels is a suggested cause for Raynaud phenomenon and splinter hemorrhages.[67–69] Pyogenic granuloma-like lesions are thought to result from downstream EGFR inhibition, leading to keratinocyte apoptosis and a thinned trauma-prone periungual epidermis, whereas retinoids are believed to have antiangiogenic properties and cause decreased attachment between nail keratinocytes leading to cell retention under the proximal nail

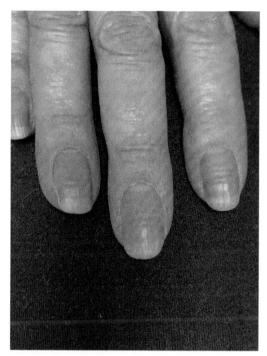

Fig. 10. Beau lines lining up with chemotherapy cycles.

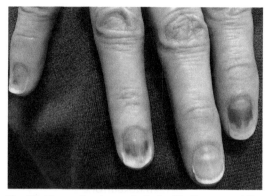

Fig. 12. Hemorrhagic onycholysis affecting several fingernails in a patient on chemotherapy.

plate and periungual inflammation.[67] In general, nail plate and bed changes are more commonly induced by cytotoxic therapy, whereas periungual tissue is affected adversely by targeted therapy (Figs. 11 and 12).[68] The commonly encountered nail changes with causative drugs are presented in Table 4.

Most of the chemotherapy-induced nail changes are reversible and do not need specific treatment. However, paronychia and pyogenic granulomas require appropriate care. In case of paronychia, daily antiseptic soaks are a judicious preventive measure, with additional topical steroid application

when inflammation is evident.[2] Regular use of emollients and protective gloves during work involving irritants and cushioned well-fitting shoes can help decrease nail fold damage. Superinfection, if present, requires systemic antibiotics or antifungals.[2] A recent study found daily autologous platelet-rich plasma application to be beneficial in paronychia.[70] Frozen gloves and socks in patients receiving taxanes were found to be effective in the prevention of taxane-induced onycholysis.[71] Camouflaging nail plate discoloration with nail varnish is a good option for those disturbed by nail pigmentation.

Mucosal changes

Stomatitis is a common dose-limiting AE of virtually all cytotoxic agents. It is either due to direct toxicity or due to secondary chemotherapy-induced neutropenia.[32] It occurs in about 20% to 40% of patients undergoing chemotherapy.[72] The initial symptoms are a burning pain and mucosal erythema followed by oral ulceration, which often develop superimposed fungal or viral infection. The ulcers typically develop in 3 to 4 days of starting therapy and heal without scarring 2 to 3 weeks after discontinuation of chemotherapy.[72] Agents most frequently associated with stomatitis are 5-FU, methotrexate, taxanes, bleomycin, and anthracyclines.[32] Newer agents associated with mucositis are mTORi and EGFRi.[2,3] Management should focus on prevention/elimination of infections along with symptom control. Maintenance of oral hygiene and antiseptic mouthwashes are important preventive measures and reduce the risk of ulceration.[72] Topical anesthetic rinses or gels and semiliquid nutrition will help maintain intake and avoid pain.[32] Potent topical corticosteroids for symptom relief have been recommended by some investogators.[1,3] However, the only approved

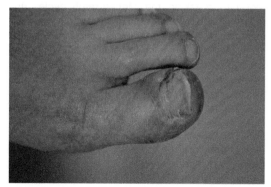

Fig. 11. Paronychia of the great toe in a patient on cetuximab.

Table 4
Nail changes observed with anticancer drugs

Nail Alteration	Drugs	Features
Melanonychia	Cyclophosphamide, doxorubicin, hydroxyurea, imatinib	There may be alternating bands of melanonychia and normal nail, corresponding to chemotherapy cycles and intervening drug-free intervals. This pigmentation usually resolves in 6–8 wk after drug cessation.
Hemorrhagic onycholysis	Taxanes	It is painful and more commonly associated with docetaxel.
Onycholysis	Capecitabine, etoposide, mitoxantrone	Affects several digits simultaneously.
Beau lines	5-FU, bleomycin, melphalan	Can occur with most cytotoxic agents.
Elkonyxis	Retinoids	Full-thickness variant of a pit.
Paronychia	Taxanes, retinoids, EGFRi, capecitabine	Mimics acute paronychia.
Pyogenic granuloma	EGFRi, retinoids	Simultaneous involvement of several finger and/or toe nails and onset within 1–2 mo of therapy points to a drug-induced pathology.
Splinter hemorrhages	Sorafenib, sunitinib	More common with sorafenib, these are asymptomatic and affect several digits simultaneously.

Data from Refs.[4,40,67–69]

pharmacologic agent is keratinocyte growth factor 1, palifermin, for mucositis with conditioning regimens in hematologic malignancies.[73]

Xerostomia has been noted with both anti-PD1 (4%–7% patients) and anti PD-L1 (3%) therapy and is uncommon with CTLA-4 inhibitors.[46] Oral lichenoid reactions characterized by white lacy patterns on the buccal mucosa, multiple ulcers, and dysgeusia are also associated with immunotherapy.[46,74]

Mucocutaneous bleeding is reported with bevacizumab and ranibizumab (selective VEGFi). Epistaxis is the most common presentation and occurs in about one-third of patients taking bevacizumab. Continuation or initiation of VEGFi is not recommended in the presence of any mucocutaneous bleeding.[2]

Xerosis
Xerosis is a common AE with EGFRi and mTORi, affecting about one-third of the patients treated.[2,40,41] MEKi and c-KITi are also noted to cause dryness.[40] It occurs within the first 3 months of treatment and is most pronounced on the extremities. Xerosis can be associated with pruritus, fissuring, and secondary staphylococcal or herpetic infection. Treatment includes frequent application of a bland emollient and avoidance of dehydrating behaviors such as hot showers and use of harsh soaps.[2]

Pruritus
Pruritus is a frequent AE with an often unanticipated negative impact on patient's quality of life.[75] A metanalysis demonstrated that targeted agent use was associated with a significant risk of developing pruritus. The overall incidence of pruritus was about 17% and 2 classes—anti-CTLA4 agents (31%) and EGFRi (23%–55%)—were found to be most commonly associated with pruritus.[76] Gerber and colleagues described periadnexal mast cell clustering in patients treated with EGFRi, providing an explanation for itch in these cases. Management of pruritus requires an integrative approach that includes patient education, maintenance of skin barrier, and topical and systemic therapies. Adequate emollient use is integral to breaking the "itch-scratch cycle" and may in itself be enough in patients with xerosis-associated itch. Other topical options include corticosteroids, calcineurin inhibitors, capsaicin, anesthetics, salicylic acid, and menthol.[76,77] For severe itch systemic antihistamines, anticonvulsants, aprepitant, antidepressants, and mu antagonists have shown benefit.[76]

Miscellaneous
Long-term hydroxyurea is associated with a dermatomyositis-like cutaneous eruption without systemic involvement. Also referred to as pseudodermatomyositis or hydroxyurea dermopathy, the onset varies from 1 to 10 years

from use. It manifests as a linear scaly erythema with telangiectasias and atrophic lesions on the upper limbs. Resolution on drug cessation is usual; however atrophic plaques may persist.[78] Characteristic painful bilateral perimalleolar ulcers are also associated with hydroxyurea and drug withdrawal leads to spontaneous healing.[79] Prolonged healing time is reported with everolimus and selective VEGFi and their use should be avoided in the perioperative period.[2,40] Imatinib-induced periorbital edema is noted in 60% to 85% of patients. A diffuse involvement of the face, limbs, and even pleural/peritoneal effusions are possible.[40] Salt restriction and diuretics are required in severe cases.[2] Extremity edema is reported with mTORi, sunitinib, and pazopanib use in about 35%, is usually mild, and does not require treatment.[40]

SUMMARY

This review discusses the common adverse effects observed with the traditional chemotherapeutic agents as well as the newer targeted agents. The classic side effects of cytotoxics include alopecia, stomatitis, and nail changes. However, newer agents have cutaneous reactions related to each molecule's mechanism of action. Dermatologists need to be aware of effective preventive as well as treatment strategies to facilitate essential cancer therapy.

REFERENCES

1. Shi VJ, Levy LL, Choi JN. Cutaneous manifestations of nontargeted and targeted chemotherapies. Semin Oncol 2016;43:419–25.

2. Macdonald JB, Macdonald B, Golitz LE, et al. Cutaneous adverse effects of targeted therapies: part I: inhibitors of the cellular membrane. J Am Acad Dermatol 2015;72:203–18.

3. Macdonald JB, Macdonald B, Golitz LE, et al. Cutaneous adverse effects of targeted therapies: part II: inhibitors of intracellular molecular signaling pathways. J Am Acad Dermatol 2015;72:221–36.

4. Sanborn RE, Sauer DA. Cutaneous reactions to chemotherapy: commonly seen, less described, little understood. Dermatol Clin 2008;26:103–19.

5. Bolognia JL, Cooper DL, Glusac EJ. Toxic erythema of chemotherapy: a useful clinical term. J Am Acad Dermatol 2008;59:524–9.

6. Remlinger KA. Cutaneous reactions to chemotherapy drugs. Arch Dermatol 2006;139:45–63.

7. Miller KK, Gorcey L, McLellan BN. Chemotherapy-induced hand-foot syndrome and nail changes: a review of clinical presentation, etiology, pathogenesis,

8. Patterson JW. The spongiotic reaction pattern. In: Weedon's skin pathology. 4th edition. Beijing (China): Churchill Livingstone Elsevier; 2016. p. 128–9.

9. Johnson ML, Farmer ER. Graft-versus-host reactions in dermatology. J Am Acad Dermatol 1998;38: 369–92.

10. Degen A, Alter M, Schenck F, et al. The hand-foot-syndrome associated with medical tumor therapy - classification and management. J Dtsch Dermatol Ges 2010;8:652–61.

11. Belum VR, Serna-Tamayo C, Wu S, et al. Incidence and risk of hand-foot skin reaction with cabozantinib, a novel multikinase inhibitor: a meta-analysis. Clin Exp Dermatol 2016;41:8–15.

12. Anderson R, Jatoi A, Robert C, et al. Search for evidence-based approaches for the prevention and palliation of hand-foot skin reaction (HFSR) caused by the multikinase inhibitors (MKIs). Oncologist 2009;14:291–302.

13. Chanprapaph K, Rutnin S, Vachiramon V. Multikinase inhibitor-induced hand–foot skin reaction: a review of clinical presentation, pathogenesis, and management. Am J Clin Dermatol 2016;17: 387–402.

14. Bun S, Yunokawa M, Tamaki Y, et al. Symptom management: the utility of regional cooling for hand-foot syndrome induced by pegylated liposomal doxorubicin in ovarian cancer. Support Care Cancer 2018;26:2161–6.

15. Ren Z, Zhu K, Kang H, et al. Randomized controlled trial of the prophylactic effect of urea-based cream on sorafenib-associated hand-foot skin reactions in patients with advanced hepatocellular carcinoma. J Clin Oncol 2015;33:894–900.

16. Templeton AJ, Ribi K, Surber C, et al. Prevention of palmar–plantar erythrodysesthesia with an antiperspirant in breast cancer patients treated with pegylated liposomal doxorubicin (SAKK 92/08). Breast 2014;23:244–9.

17. Zhang RX, Wu XJ, Wan DS, et al. Celecoxib can prevent capecitabine-related hand-foot syndrome in stage II and III colorectal cancer patients: result of a single-center, prospective randomized phase III trial. Ann Oncol 2012;23:1348–53.

18. Macedo LT, Lima JPN, dos Santos LV, et al. Prevention strategies for chemotherapy-induced hand–foot syndrome: a systematic review and meta-analysis of prospective randomised trials. Support Care Cancer 2014;22:1585–93.

19. Wong GC, Lee LH, Chong YY. A case report of neutrophilic eccrine hidradenitis in a patient receiving chemotherapy for acute myeloid leukaemia. Ann Acad Med Singapore 1998;27: 860–3.

20. Miller JL. Diseases of the eccrine and apocrine sweat glands. In: Bolognia JL, Jorizzo JL, Schaffer JV, editors. Dermatology. 3rd edition. Beijing (China): Elsevier Saunders; 2012. p. 599–600.

21. Herms F, Franck N, Kramkimel N, et al. Neutrophilic eccrine hidradenitis in two patients treated with *BRAF* inhibitors: a new cutaneous adverse event. Br J Dermatol 2017;176:1645–8.

22. Harrist TJ, Fine JD, Berman RS, et al. Neutrophilic eccrine hidradenitis. A distinctive type of neutrophilic dermatosis associated with myelogenous leukemia and chemotherapy. Arch Dermatol 1982;118:263–6.

23. Brehler R, Reimann S, Bonsmann G, et al. Neutrophilic hidradenitis induced by chemotherapy involves eccrine and apocrine glands. Am J Dermatopathol 1997;19:73–8.

24. Liuti F, Martín PA, Montenegro Damaso T, et al. Eccrine squamous syringometaplasia associated with dabrafenib therapy. J Am Acad Dermatol 2013;69:273–4.

25. Abbas O, Bhawan J. Syringometaplasia: variants and underlying mechanisms. Int J Dermatol 2016;55:142–8.

26. Martorell-Calatayud A, Sanmartín O, Botella-Estrada R, et al. Chemotherapy-related bilateral dermatitis associated with eccrine squamous syringometaplasia: reappraisal of epidemiological, clinical, and pathological features. J Am Acad Dermatol 2011;64:1092–103.

27. Nethers K, Messina J, Seminario-Vidal L. Eccrine squamous syringometaplasia in an allogenic stem cell transplant patient undergoing chemotherapy. Dermatol Online J 2017;23.

28. Story SG, Beschloss JK, Dolan CK, et al. Eccrine squamous syringometaplasia associated with vemurafenib therapy. J Am Acad Dermatol 2012;67:208–10.

29. Santosa A, Liau MM, Tan KB, et al. Pemetrexed-induced eccrine squamous syringometaplasia manifesting as pseudocellulitis (in a patient with non-small cell lung cancer). JAAD Case Rep 2017;3:64–6.

30. Castells MC. Anaphylaxis to chemotherapy and monoclonal antibodies. Immunol Allergy Clin North Am 2015;35:335–48.

31. Kang SP, Saif MW. Infusion-related and hypersensitivity reactions of monoclonal antibodies used to treat colorectal cancer–identification, prevention, and management. J Support Oncol 2007;5:451–7.

32. Guillot B, Bessis D, Dereure O. Mucocutaneous side effects of antineoplastic chemotherapy. Expert Opin Drug Saf 2004;3:579–87.

33. Jeerakornpassawat D, Suprasert P. Randomized, controlled trial of dexamethasone versus dexamethasone plus hydrocortisone as prophylaxis for hypersensitivity reactions due to paclitaxel treatment for gynecologic cancer. Int J Gynecol Cancer 2017;27:1794–801.

34. Bavbek S, Kendirlinan R, Çerçi P, et al. Rapid drug desensitization with biologics: a single-center experience with four biologics. Int Arch Allergy Immunol 2016;171:227–33.

35. Castells M. Rapid desensitization of hypersensitivity reactions to chemotherapy agents. Curr Drug Saf 2006;1:243–51.

36. Ng CY, Chen C-B, Wu M-Y, et al. Anticancer drugs induced severe adverse cutaneous drug reactions: an updated review on the risks associated with anticancer targeted therapy or immunotherapies. J Immunol Res 2018;2018:5376476.

37. Shah KM, Rancour EA, Al-Omari A, et al. Striking enhancement at the site of radiation for nivolumab-induced Stevens-Johnson syndrome. Dermatol Online J 2018;24 [pii:13030/qt97g3t63v].

38. Tahseen AI, Patel NB. Successful dabrafenib transition after vemurafenib-induced toxic epidermal necrolysis in a patient with metastatic melanoma. JAAD Case Rep 2018;4:930–3.

39. Lerch M, Mainetti C, Terziroli Beretta-Piccoli B, et al. Current perspectives on stevens-johnson syndrome and toxic epidermal necrolysis. Clin Rev Allergy Immunol 2018;54:147–76.

40. Peuvrel L, Dréno B. Dermatological toxicity associated with targeted therapies in cancer: optimal management. Am J Clin Dermatol 2014;15:425–44.

41. Owczarek W, Slowinska M, Lesiak A, et al. The incidence and management of cutaneous adverse events of the epidermal growth factor receptor inhibitors. Postepy Dermatol Alergol 2017;34:418–28.

42. Heidary N, Naik H, Burgin S. Chemotherapeutic agents and the skin: an update. J Am Acad Dermatol 2008;58:545–70.

43. Qi W-X, Sun Y-J, Shen Z, et al. Risk of anti-EGFR monoclonal antibody-related skin rash: an up-to-date meta-analysis of 25 randomized controlled trials. J Chemother 2014;26:359–68.

44. Hofheinz R-D, Deplanque G, Komatsu Y, et al. Recommendations for the prophylactic management of skin reactions induced by epidermal growth factor receptor inhibitors in patients with solid tumors. Oncologist 2016;21:1483–91.

45. Hwang SJE, Fernández-Peñas P. Adverse reactions to biologics: melanoma (Ipilimumab, Nivolumab, Pembrolizumab). Curr Probl Dermatol 2018;53:82–92.

46. Sibaud V. Dermatologic reactions to immune checkpoint inhibitors : skin toxicities and immunotherapy. Am J Clin Dermatol 2018;19:345–61.

47. Collins LK, Chapman MS, Carter JB, et al. Cutaneous adverse effects of the immune checkpoint inhibitors. Curr Probl Cancer 2017;41:125–8.

48. Maarouf M, Alexander C, Shi VY. Nivolumab reactivation of hypertrophic lichen planus, a case report and review of published literature. Dermatol Online J 2018;24 [pii:13030/qt4xf465w6].

49. Diaz-Perez JA, Beveridge MG, Victor TA, et al. Granulomatous and lichenoid dermatitis after IgG4 anti-PD-1 monoclonal antibody therapy for advanced cancer. J Cutan Pathol 2018;45:434–8.

50. Feldstein SI, Patel F, Larsen L, et al. Eruptive keratoacanthomas arising in the setting of lichenoid toxicity after programmed cell death 1 inhibition with nivolumab. J Eur Acad Dermatol Venereol 2018;32:58–9.

51. Dai J, Belum VR, Wu S, et al. Pigmentary changes in patients treated with targeted anticancer agents: a systematic review and meta-analysis. J Am Acad Dermatol 2017;77:902–10.

52. Di Tullio F, Mandel VD, Scotti R, et al. Imatinib-induced diffuse hyperpigmentation of the oral mucosa, the skin, and the nails in a patient affected by chronic myeloid leukemia: report of a case and review of the literature. Int J Dermatol 2018;57:784–90.

53. Marano AL, Clarke JM, Morse MA, et al. Subacute cutaneous lupus erythematosus and dermatomyositis associated with anti-programmed cell death (PD)-1 therapy. Br J Dermatol 2018. [Epub ahead of print].

54. de Golian E, Kwong BY, Swetter SM, et al. Cutaneous complications of targeted melanoma therapy. Curr Treat Options Oncol 2016;17:57.

55. Freites-Martinez A, Kwong BY, Rieger KE, et al. Eruptive keratoacanthomas associated with pembrolizumab therapy. JAMA Dermatol 2017;153:694–7.

56. Manousaridis I, Mavridou S, Goerdt S, et al. Cutaneous side effects of inhibitors of the RAS/RAF/MEK/ERK signalling pathway and their management. J Eur Acad Dermatol Venereol 2013;27:11–8.

57. Trüeb RM. Chemotherapy-induced alopecia. Semin Cutan Med Surg 2009;28:11–4.

58. Yeager CE, Olsen EA. Treatment of chemotherapy-induced alopecia. Dermatol Ther 2011;24:432–42.

59. Kang D, Kim IR, Choi EK, et al. Permanent chemotherapy-induced alopecia in patients with breast Cancer: a 3-year prospective cohort study. Oncologist 2019;24(3):414–20.

60. Kim GM, Kim S, Park HS, et al. Chemotherapy-induced irreversible alopecia in early breast cancer patients. Breast Cancer Res Treat 2017;163:527–33.

61. Donovan JC, Ghazarian DM, Shaw JC. Scarring alopecia associated with use of the epidermal growth factor receptor inhibitor gefitinib. Arch Dermatol 2008;144:1524–5.

62. Hepper DM, Wu P, Anadkat MJ. Scarring alopecia associated with the epidermal growth factor receptor inhibitor erlotinib. J Am Acad Dermatol 2011;64:996–8.

63. Vasconcelos I, Wiesske A, Schoenegg W. Scalp cooling successfully prevents alopecia in breast cancer patients undergoing anthracycline/taxane-based chemotherapy. Breast 2018;40:1–3.

64. Nangia J, Wang T, Osborne C, et al. Effect of a scalp cooling device on alopecia in women undergoing chemotherapy for breast cancer. JAMA 2017;317:596.

65. Sikora M, Rudnicka L. Chemotherapy-induced alopecia - the urgent need for treatment options. J Eur Acad Dermatol Venereol 2019;33(2):e69–70.

66. Glaser DA, Hossain P, Perkins W, et al. Long-term safety and efficacy of bimatoprost solution 0·03% application to the eyelid margin for the treatment of idiopathic and chemotherapy-induced eyelash hypotrichosis: a randomized controlled trial. Br J Dermatol 2015;172:1384–94.

67. Piraccini BM, Alessandrini A. Drug-related nail disease. Clin Dermatol 2013;31:618–26.

68. Robert C, Sibaud V, Mateus C, et al. Review nail toxicities induced by systemic anticancer treatments. Lancet Oncol 2015;16:181–9.

69. Baran R, Fouilloux B, Robert C. Drug-induced nail changes. In: Baran R, de Berker DAR, Holzberg M, et al, editors. Baran and Dawber's diseases of the nails and their management. 4th edition. Singapore: Wiley-Blackwell; 2012. p. 413–35.

70. Kwon S-H, Choi J-W, Hong J-S, et al. Gefitinib-induced paronychia: response to autologous platelet-rich plasma. Arch Dermatol 2012;148:1399–402.

71. Scotté F, Banu E, Medioni J, et al. Matched case-control phase 2 study to evaluate the use of a frozen sock to prevent docetaxel-induced onycholysis and cutaneous toxicity of the foot. Cancer 2008;112:1625–31.

72. Villa A, Sonis ST. Pharmacotherapy for the management of cancer regimen-related oral mucositis. Expert Opin Pharmacother 2016;17:1801–7.

73. Sonis ST, Villa A. Phase II investigational oral drugs for the treatment of radio/chemotherapy induced oral mucositis. Expert Opin Investig Drugs 2018;27:147–54.

74. Obara K, Masuzawa M, Amoh Y. Oral lichenoid reaction showing multiple ulcers associated with anti-programmed death cell receptor-1 treatment: a report of two cases and published work review. J Dermatol 2018;45:587–91.

75. Gandhi M, Oishi K, Zubal B, et al. Unanticipated toxicities from anticancer therapies: survivors' perspectives. Support Care Cancer 2010;18:1461–8.

76. Ensslin CJ, Rosen AC, Wu S, et al. Pruritus in patients treated with targeted cancer therapies:

systematic review and meta-analysis. J Am Acad Dermatol 2013;69:708–20.

77. Gerber PA, Buhren BA, Cevikbas F, et al. Preliminary evidence for a role of mast cells in epidermal growth factor receptor inhibitor–induced pruritus. J Am Acad Dermatol 2010;63:163–5.

78. Dacey MJ, Callen JP. Hydroxyurea-induced dermatomyositis-like eruption. J Am Acad Dermatol 2003;48:439–41.

79. Quattrone F, Dini V, Barbanera S, et al. Cutaneous ulcers associated with hydroxyurea therapy. J Tissue Viability 2013;22:112–21.

Review of Graft-Versus-Host Disease

Vignesh Ramachandran, BS[a], Sree S. Kolli, BA[b],*, Lindsay C. Strowd, MD[b]

KEYWORDS

- Acute • Chronic • Graft-versus-host disease • Management • Systemic • Topicals • Trials
- Treatment

KEY POINTS

- Graft-versus-host disease (GVHD) is a life-threatening condition commonly encountered in hematopoietic stem cell transplant patients.
- Dermatologists play an integral role in diagnosing and treating GVHD because cutaneous manifestations are an early and common presentation.
- Current treatments available are effective, including corticosteroids, but many emerging treatments, including monoclonal antibodies and adoptive cell transfer of T cells, are currently being investigated.

INTRODUCTION

Graft-versus-host disease (GVHD) is an adverse immunologic phenomenon observed after allogenic hematopoietic stem cell transplant (HSCT).[1] It is rarely observed after blood product transfusion, solid organ transplants, or autologous HSCT.[2–4] GVHD can be viewed as an exaggerated and undesirable manifestation of normal inflammation, wherein donor lymphocytes interact with foreign antigens in a background that promotes inflammation.[5] The incidence of GVHD is as high as 40% to 60% of patients receiving HSCTs.[6,7] In this potentially lethal disease, the mortality may approach 15%.[6] GVHD is a complex disease with acute and chronic presentations, multiorgan involvement, multispecialty management, and many therapeutic options. Cutaneous GVHD, the earliest and most common presentation, may portend worse prognosis in some patients.[8]

Dermatologists play an integral role in the diagnosis and management of GVHD. Lifesaving treatment options for patients with cutaneous T-cell lymphoma can include allogeneic HSCT.[9] More commonly, dermatology may be called on to help diagnose and manage GVHD in oncology patients with history of other lymphoproliferative disorders. This article provides an overview of the pathophysiology, clinical manifestations, histology, diagnostic criteria, and treatment options for acute and chronic GVHD (cGVHD).

METHODS

A PubMed search was conducted using the search terms "graft versus host disease," "acute GVHD," "chronic GVHD," "pathophysiology," "diagnosis," and "treatment." Selection of articles focused on most recent guidelines for the treatment of GVHD, and other articles were chosen for citation frequency and relevance. One-hundred and nineteen articles were chosen.

Disclosure Statement: Dr L.C. Strowd has received grant support from Pfizer, consulting support from Sanofi Regeneron Granzyme, and is a speaker for Actelion. V. Ramachandran and S.S. Kolli have no conflicts to disclose.
[a] Baylor College of Medicine, 1 Baylor Plaza, Houston, TX 77030, USA; [b] Department of Dermatology, Wake Forest School of Medicine, 1 Medical Center Boulevard, Winston-Salem, NC 27157-1071, USA
* Corresponding author.
E-mail address: skolli@wakehealth.edu

RESULTS
Pathophysiology

Acute
In acute GVHD (aGVHD), 3 processes occur that lead to this disease.[5] First, chemotherapy and radiotherapy during the conditioning phase before graft infusion trigger tissue damage and subsequent release of numerous exogenous (eg, lipopolysaccharides) and endogenous (eg, tumor necrosis factor-α) molecular activators of the immune response.[10] This process leads to increased expression of major histocompatibility complex (MHC) antigens and adhesion molecules, resulting in heightened recognition of host alloantigens by donor T cells.[11] In the next step, donor T cells interact with host antigen-presenting cells (APCs) in the early post-HSCT phase (and donor APCs later), which provide costimulatory signals leading to donor T-cell activation and expansion into T-helper (Th) 1, T-cytotoxic (Tc), and Th17/Tc17 subtypes.[12,13] In the final step, cytotoxic effector T cells reach target organs (eg, skin) through molecular attractants and receptor interactions, causing tissue damage. In addition, mononuclear phagocytes are activated by lipopolysaccharides released during the first step (tissue damage), resulting in a feedback loop amplifying aGVHD response.[11,14]

Chronic
The pathophysiology of cGVHD can be described by 3 phases. In phase I, tissue injury from cytotoxic injury, infections, and aGVHD activates innate immune cells as well as nonhematopoietic cells such as endothelial cells and fibroblasts.[15] Inflammatory mediators, including damage-associated molecular patterns such as interleukin (IL)-33 and pathogen-associated molecular patterns such as lipopolysaccharide are released into circulation and the extracellular space.[15] Th17 cells are also implicated because an IL-12 blockade suppressing Th17 cells reduces skin, liver, and salivary gland manifestations of cGVHD.[15] The IL-1 superfamily is released in response to tissue damage associated with aGVHD and its receptor is increased in the blood of patients with cGVHD.[15] Phase II is characterized by hyperresponsiveness of the adaptive immune system and reduction of immune cell regulators.[15] There is an immune response to host foreign MHC proteins, resulting in an upregulation of Th1, Th2, and Th17 cells with a reduction in regulatory immune cells such as regulatory T cells (Tregs).[15] Phase III involves abnormal tissue repair promoted by activated macrophages that produce transforming factor-β and platelet-derived growth factor leading to

fibroblast activation.[15] The activated fibroblasts produce extracellular matrix collagen and biglycan, which cross-links collagen, contributing to tissue stiffness.[15] This process is reinforced by Th17 cells that were upregulated during phase II. Because of the profound immunosuppression in cGVHD, recurrent infections are a key factor in contributing to the morbidity and mortality of patients with cGVHD.[15]

Clinical Manifestations

Affected organs
GVHD is a multisystemic disorder that may implicate several organs, including the lungs, hepatobiliary system, musculoskeletal system, gastrointestinal (GI) tract, and skin. Internal organ manifestations are typically managed by respective specialists.[16] Cutaneous manifestations are the most common (and earliest) presentation.[7] As such, an understanding of the acute and chronic cutaneous presentations may aid diagnosis and assess clinical response to treatment.

Acute graft-versus-host disease skin changes
aGVHD commonly occurs in the early posttransplant period. Previous definitions of aGVHD required onset of symptoms within 100 days after transplant; however, the current National Institutes of Health (NIH) consensus criteria uses clinical findings to differentiate between aGVHD and cGVHD rather than a 100-day cutoff (**Table 1**).[17]

Chronic graft-versus-host disease skin findings
In 2014, the NIH Working Group report for diagnosis and staging of cGVHD established criteria for diagnosis by various clinical manifestoes, including cutaneous ones (**Table 2**).[17]

Diagnosis

Criteria
The diagnosis of aGVHD is made by clinical manifestations that develop in patients who have undergone allogeneic HSCT. Classically, patients present with a maculopapular rash, abdominal cramps with diarrhea, and increasing serum bilirubin level usually within the first 100 days.[18] Histologic confirmation with a skin or GI tract biopsy can help support diagnosis of aGVHD and rule out other possible causes, including drug eruptions and infections. The NIH consensus criteria classify 2 categories of aGVHD that occur without diagnostic or distinctive features of cGVHD: (1) classic aGVHD, involving clinical features of aGVHD occurring within 100 days of HCT; (2) persistent, recurrent, late-onset aGVHD, involving clinical features of aGVHD after 100 days.[17]

Table 1
Cutaneous and mucosal manifestations in acute graft-versus-host disease

Location	Clinical Manifestations	Severity
Skin[18]	Maculopapular rash, follicular erythema, epidermolysis, pruritus	Stage 1: maculopapular rash over <25% of body area Stage 2: maculopapular rash over 25%–50% of body area Stage 3: generalized erythroderma Stage 4: generalized erythroderma with bullous formation, often with desquamation
Oral cavity[19]	Erythema, erosions, ulcers, lichenoid lesions, xerostomia and pain	NA

Abbreviation: NA, not available.

Overlap syndrome has features of both aGVHD and cGVHD.[17]

The diagnosis of cGVHD requires the presence of at least 1 diagnostic manifestation or 1 distinctive feature confirmed by biopsy, laboratory tests, or radiology in the same or a separate organ (see **Table 2**).[13,16]

Histopathology
In GVHD, biopsy can be instrumental in differentiating this condition from drug rash or other causes.[20] In aGVHD, histologic changes include focal/diffuse vacuolar degeneration of basal cells, spongiosis, subepidermal clefts, mononuclear perivascular infiltrate by cluster of differentiation (CD) 4 and CD8 T lymphocytes, and even complete loss of the epidermis in severe cases.[18,21] Epidermal damage may occur at the tips of rete ridges and hair follicles.[22] Findings in cGVHD may include lichenoid lesions with acanthosis and wedge-shaped hypergranulosis similar to idiopathic lichen sclerosis. Hyperparakeratosis and dermal sclerosis may also be apparent.[23]

Grading
Grading of aGVHD is based on the degree of skin, liver, and GI tract involvement. There are 2 systems for grading: the Glucksberg grade (I–IV) and the International Bone Marrow Transplant Registry grading system (A–D)[24,25] (**Table 3**).

Grading of cGVHD is based NIH consensus criteria and is based on the number of organs or sites involved and the severity within the affected organ[26] (**Table 4**).

Biomarkers
Biomarkers have been investigated as a means to aid clinical and histopathologic diagnosis. Biomarkers may also play a role in assessing response to treatment. Biomarkers studied in clinical trials are elafin, B cell–activating factor, chemokine receptors such as CXCL10 and CXCL11, T-cell immunoglobulin and mucin-domain-containing-3, IL-6, soluble tumor necrosis factor receptor-1, and many others.[27–29] Although these have some efficacy, the evidence for their use in routine clinical practice is limited.[18]

Prevention of Acute Graft-Versus-Host Disease

Prophylaxis of aGVHD involves immunosuppression of donor cells. There is no standard approach and it often varies by institution. The European Group for Blood and Marrow Transplantation (EBMT) and European LeukemiaNet (ELN) guidelines propose various prophylactic pharmacologic regimens and T-cell depletion.[30]

Methotrexate and cyclosporine
Numerous clinical trials support the combination of methotrexate (MTX) and cyclosporine (CSA) compared with either drug alone in reducing the incidence of aGVHD and is commonly used in patients receiving a myeloablative conditioning regimen. In a clinical trial of recipients receiving marrow from donors other than human leukocyte antigen (HLA)–identical siblings, those receiving MTX or CSA had a 73% incidence of GVHD compared with 34% receiving the combination treatment.[31]

Methotrexate and tacrolimus
A combination of MTX and tacrolimus is as effective as MTX plus CSA, with no difference in patient survival or relapse. In a phase III randomized trial, the incidence of grade II to IV aGVHD was lower in patients who received tacrolimus and MTX than in patients receiving CSA and MTX (31.9% vs 44.4%, respectively; $P = .01$).[32] There was no difference in incidence of grade III to IV aGVHD and cGVHD between groups.[32]

Table 2
Cutaneous and mucosal manifestations in chronic graft-versus-host disease

Location Affected	Diagnostic Findings[a]	Distinctive Findings[b]	Other Features[c]	Common Findings[d]
Skin	Poikiloderma Lichen planus–like skin changes Skin sclerosis Morphealike features Lichen sclerosis–like skin changes	Depigmentation Papulosquamous lesions	Hypohidrosis Ichthyosis Keratosis pilaris Hypopigmentation Hyperpigmentation	Erythema Maculopapular rash Pruritus
Nails	—	Dystrophy Longitudinal ridging, splitting, or brittle nails Onycholysis Pterygium unguis Nail loss	—	—
Scalp and body hair	—	New-onset scarring or nonscarring alopecia Loss of body hair Scaling	Hair texture changes Patchy thinning of scalp hair Premature graying	—
Mouth	Lichen planus–like changes	Xerostomia Mucoceles Mucosal atrophy Ulcers Pseudomembranes	—	Gingivitis Mucositis Erythema Pain
Genitalia	Lichen planus–like features Lichen sclerosis–like features	Erosions Fissures Ulcers	—	—
Women	Vaginal scarring or clitoral/labial agglutination	—	—	—
Men	Phimosis or urethral/meatus scarring or stenosis	—	—	—

[a] Sufficient to make diagnosis.
[b] Seen in cGVHD, but not diagnostic.
[c] May be part of cGVHD presentation if diagnosis confirmed by other findings.
[d] Seen in both aGVHD and cGVHD.

Adapted from Jagasia, M.H., H.T. Greinix, M. Arora, et al. National Institutes of Health Consensus Development Project on Criteria for Clinical Trials in Chronic Graft-versus-Host Disease: I. The 2014 Diagnosis and Staging Working Group report. Biology of Blood and Marrow Transplantation: journal of the American Society for Blood and Marrow Transplantation 2015;21(3):p. 389–401.e1l; with permission.

Mycophenolate mofetil and calcineurin inhibitor

Mycophenolate mofetil (MMF) may be an effective alternative to MTX for minimizing toxicity associated with MTX use. In a phase II trial, 43 patients received MMF with tacrolimus and 47 patients received MTX plus tacrolimus.[33] MMF plus calcineurin inhibitor (CNI) was similar to the MTX and tacrolimus regimen in incidence of aGVHD II to IV($P = .8$), whereas grade III to IV aGVHD incidence was higher with MMF (19%) than with MTX (4%, $P = .03$).[33] MMF was associated with less early toxicity than MTX. Patients receiving MMF had less severe mucositis than those receiving MTX (21% vs 65%, $P = .008$) and faster engraftment (11 vs 18 days; $P<.001$).[34]

T-cell depletion

aGVHD is in large part caused by immunocompetent T cells in the donor stem cell graft that are

Table 3
Grading of acute graft-versus-host disease

Grade I (A)	Maculopapular rash <25% of body with no liver or GI involvement
Grade 2 (B)	Maculopapular rash 25%–50% of body, diarrhea 500–1500 mL/d, and bilirubin 2–6 mg/dL
Grade 3 (C)	Generalized erythroderma, diarrhea 1500–2000 mL/d, and bilirubin 6.1–15.0 mg/dL
Grade 4 (D)	Generalized erythroderma with bullous formation, diarrhea >2000 mL/d or pain or ileus, bilirubin>15 mg/dL

Data from Glucksberg, H., R. Storb, A. Fefer, et al. Clinical manifestations of graft-versus-host disease in human recipients of marrow from HL-A-matched sibling donors. Transplantation 1974;18(4):p. 295–304; and Rowlings, P.A., D. Przepiorka, J.P. Klein, et al. IBMTR Severity Index for grading acute graft-versus-host disease: retrospective comparison with Glucksberg grade. Br J Haematol 1997;97(4):p. 855–64.

reactive against host tissues. Therefore, depleting these immunocompetent cells may be an effective way to prevent GVHD.[35] In adult leukemic marrow recipients of HLA-identical sibling marrow, 23 patients were randomized to T-cell depletion and 25 received MTX plus CSA. T-cell depletion was associated with a slightly higher incidence of grade II to IV GVHD (23%) compared with the MTX plus CSA regimen (12%) but an overall low incidence of GVHD.[36] There was no significant difference in incidence of cGVHD between the T-cell depletion (51%) and MTX plus CSA groups (23%; $P = .06$).[36]

Prevention of Chronic Graft-Versus-Host Disease

Although extensively studied, most preventive options for cGVHD lack efficacy.[37] However, 2

Table 4
Grading of chronic graft-versus-host disease

Mild	2 or fewer organs/sites with no functional impairment
Moderate	3 or more organs/sites with no clinically significant functional impairment or at least 1 organ/site with clinically functional impairment with no major disability
Severe	Major disability

Data from Filipovich, A.H., D. Weisdorf, S. Pavletic, et al. National Institutes of Health consensus development project on criteria for clinical trials in chronic graft-versus-host disease: I. Diagnosis and staging working group report. Biol Blood Marrow Transplant 2005;11(12):p. 945–56.

options with some efficacy are antithymocyte globulin (ATG) and rituximab.

Antithymocyte globulin

ATG is made of polyclonal antibodies serving an immunomodulatory role through T-cell and B-cell pathways.[38] In a trial of 202 patients receiving HSCT, 202 patients were randomized to receive combination CSA and MTX with or without ATG. ATG use resulted in decreased incidence and severity of aGVHD and cGVHD without a change in relapse frequency or mortality.[39,40] A phase III trial of 161 patients with acute leukemia undergoing HSCT and taking CSA and MTX showed that addition of ATG after 24 months resulted in more than 50% decrease in incidence of cGVHD and more than 50% of patients weaning off CSA. Rates of relapse and mortality were similar between treatment groups.[41]

Rituximab

Rituximab is an anti-CD20 monoclonal antibody that functions via an array of mechanisms to target B cells, which may have a role in the pathophysiology of GVHD.[42] Two phase II trials show the efficacy of rituximab. In the first phase II trial of peripheral blood stream stem cell transplant (8 out of 8 HLA-matched donor or single antigen/allele-mismatch donor) patients receiving rituximab, the 2-year rate of cGVHD and systemic corticosteroid-requiring cGVHD was 48% and 31%, compared with control groups rates of 60% and 49%, respectively.[43] In the other phase II trial of patients receiving transplants (10 of 10 HLA-matched or single antigen/allele-mismatched donor) and treatment with rituximab, the incidence of cGVHD was 20% with non-relapse mortality of 3%.[44]

Treatments for Acute and Chronic Graft-Versus-Host Disease

Treatment of aGVHD and cGVHD can be challenging because it relies on preventive measures and adjusting treatment regimens based on response. Recommendations from the joint working group established by the American Society of Blood and Marrow Transplant (ASBMT), the hemato-oncology subgroup of the British Committee for Standards in Haematology and the British Society for Bone Marrow Transplantation (BSBMT), the EBMT, and the ELN working group, and the German-Austrian-Swiss Consensus Conference are highlighted here.[16,30,45–48] The NIH Ancillary Therapy and Supportive Care Working Group Report is also included.[49] Because the number of available guidelines are limited, additional treatment options not in these guidelines are included to provide a comprehensive overview of therapeutic options.

General treatment principles include topical treatments for mild disease and systemic treatments for severe disease. Large body surface area involvement in mild disease may also benefit from systemic therapy.[16] Emollients, antipruritic agents, antiinfective measures, and avoidance of ultraviolet light exposure should be recommended regardless of severity.[49]

Topical Therapies for Localized Graft-Versus-Host Disease

Localized aGVHD and cGVHD are typically confined to epidermis and can respond well to topical therapies, including corticosteroids and CNIs. BSBMT recommends topical therapies for grade I aGVHD and the German-Austrian-Swiss guidelines recommend them for mild cGVHD.[47,48]

Topical corticosteroids
For mild to moderate skin involvement in aGVHD and cGVHD, topical corticosteroids are recommended.[16,47,48] From the neck down, the German-Austrian-Swiss guidelines recommend high-potency topical steroids.[47] Treatment of the face, axilla, and groin pose challenges given that the thin skin at these locations may be more susceptible to atrophy. German-Austrian-Swiss guidelines recommend a 3-day course of a class II or III topical corticosteroid for patients with lesions in these areas, followed by tapering.[47]

In a double-blind trial, 32 patients were randomized to clobetasol propionate 0.05% solution with nystatin or dexamethasone solution with nystatin. Patients treated with clobetasol had significantly greater improvement than those given dexamethasone ($P = .02$), with 85% of patients experiencing partial response.[50] In an open, multicenter, phase II trial evaluating topical budesonide, patients had a 61% improvement in oral GVHD.[51] In a prospective cohort study, 29.1% of patients using 0.01% dexamethasone solution for 28 days reported symptomatic improvement.[52] Long-term use of topical corticosteroids is not recommended because of adverse effects so alternative agents are recommended, including other topical agents or systemic treatments.

Topical calcineurin inhibitors
CNIs form complexes with cyclophilin to block the action of calcineurin, which decreases production of inflammatory cytokines released by T cells.[53] The most commonly discussed topical CNI in guidelines is tacrolimus.[16,46,47] German-Austrian-Swiss guidelines recommend topical CNIs as first-line therapy for cutaneous cGVHD. However,

they document that evidence for this recommendation is not as strong as that for topical corticosteroids.[45] BSMBT recommends topical CNIs in steroid-resistant cases for aGVHD.[48] In surveying the literature, the evidence for CNI use is mostly derived from case reports and case series. Topical CNIs are useful for sites of skin atrophy but are not ideal for skin involvement with active lesions and erosions. In case series of 18 patients, tacrolimus 0.1% ointment was used in patients with cGVHD with symptoms refractory to systemic corticosteroid therapy,[54] and 72% of patients reported improvement in pruritus and/or erythema. However, all patients required additional treatment to control skin disease. Another case report documented resolution of extensive cutaneous cGVHD in an infant treated with topical pimecrolimus as monotherapy.[55] A particular benefit of topical CNIs is its use in areas of thin skin and long-term use in steroid-dependent individuals.[47]

First-line Systemic Therapies for Graft-Versus-Host Disease

Oral corticosteroids
Corticosteroids are first-line therapy in ASBMT, British Committee for Standards in Haematology and the British Society for Bone Marrow Transplantation (BCSH-BSBMT), EBMT-ELN, and German-Austrian-Swiss guidelines.[16,30,45–48] For grades II to IV aGVHD and moderate to severe cGVHD, systemic corticosteroids are the initial treatment. Their therapeutic effect is a result of lympholytic and antiinflammatory properties. Two studies assessed response to corticosteroids in patients with grades II to IV aGVHD resulting in complete or partial response in 44% of patients.[56] A resolution of aGVHD occurred in 41% of patients after a median time of 21 days on corticosteroids.[8] A retrospective study of 443 patients receiving prednisolone 60 mg/m^2 for 14 days followed by 8-week taper resulted in a complete response (CR) in 35% of patients and partial response in 20% of patients.[57]

There is little consensus on the optimal dose of the corticosteroid. A multicenter trial randomly assigned 95 patients to either low-dose intravenous (IV) 6-methylprednisone (2 mg/kg/d) or high-dose 6-methylprednisone (10 mg/kg/d) for 5 days. Improvement of aGVHD was similar between low-dose and high-dose groups (68% vs 71%, respectively; $P = .9$) and relapse rates were also comparable (17% vs 7%; $P = .1$).[58] Treating with high-dose corticosteroids does not seem to improve response rate compared with low-dose corticosteroids.[58] For less severe forms of aGVHD, treating with a lower dose (1 mg/kg) compared with higher dose (2 mg/kg) resulted in little difference between nonrelapse mortality (15% vs 15%), recurrent malignancy (15% vs 17%), and overall survival (77% vs 76%).[59]

Second-line Therapies for Graft-Versus-Host Disease

BSBMT recommends adding a second-line agent when patients fail to respond to oral corticosteroids by day 5 or have progressive symptoms after 3 days.[48] There are a variety of agents but the data are limited on the efficacy of these agents. Often, the use of second-line therapies varies by institution and there is no consensus on which agent to initiate first among the various guidelines. Second-line therapies include extracorporeal photopheresis (ECP), MMF, mammalian target of rapamycin (mTOR) inhibitors, and Janus kinase (JAK) inhibitors.

Extracorporeal photopheresis
ECP uses ultraviolet A (UVA) to radiate autologous peripheral blood mononuclear cells after their exposure to 8-methoxypsoralen. It is thought to cause apoptosis of white blood cells, release antiinflammatory cytokines by APCs, and produce antigen-specific immunosuppressive Tregs.[60] BSCH-BSBMT guidelines recommend ECP as a second-line treatment in cutaneous, oral, or liver GVHD. In cutaneous cGVHD, ECP provides up to 80% resolution[16] and is advised for use in steroid-refractory cases. In contrast, EBMT-ELN guidelines claim there is no standard second-line treatment of GVHD and that ECP is one of 5 treatment options most commonly used in both aGVHD and cGVHD after first-line measures have been exhausted.[30] ECP is discussed in German-Austrian-Swiss guidelines without formal recommendation for when it should be administered.[47] Numerous clinical trials have been performed to identify when ECP should be administered for GVHD.[60] A multicenter, retrospective analysis of 98 patients with steroid-refractory aGVHD treated with ECP or anticytokine therapy supported the superiority of ECP for CR rates (54% vs 20%).[61] Another study of 21 patient treated with ECP had CRs in 100% and 67% of patients with grade II and III aGVHD, respectively.[62]

Mycophenolate mofetil
MMF is a prodrug of mycophenolic acid, an inhibitor of inosine-5′-monophosphate dehydrogenase, which depletes guanosine nucleotides. It preferentially limits proliferation of T and B lymphocytes, suppressing the immune system.[63] Efficacy of MMF is limited in aGVHD. In a retrospective study of patients with aGVHD treated with MMF, 48% of patients had a response and survival was more

than 50% at 6 and 12 months.[64] A phase III trial comparing corticosteroids with corticosteroids plus MMF did not significantly improve survival (60% vs 50%) or incidence of cGVHD (42% vs 43%).[65] This drug has not been shown to be effective in cGVHD despite its use. In a double-blind, randomized, multicenter trial, combination of MMF or placebo with a regimen already consisting of systemic corticosteroids and CNI showed no difference.[66] Lack of efficacy in the treatment group and higher risk of mortality in the MMF group (presumed to be caused by additional immunosuppression leading to infection), led to early closure of the study.[66] In an open, single-center trial, moderate improvement was seen in 3 out of 6 patients with limited-stage cGVHD. Overall, efficacy of MMF for treatment of GVHD is limited.[67]

Sirolimus and everolimus
mTOR inhibitors sirolimus and everolimus inhibit T cells. mTOR inhibitors may decrease collagen production and inhibit platelet-derived and fibroblast growth factors. Sirolimus (rapamycin) has been used to treat refractory GVHD.[68] A phase II trial of sirolimus plus tacrolimus and methylprednisolone in steroid-refractory cGVHD cases showed a 63% response rate and 17% showed CR.[69] In a phase I/II study of 21 patients with severe aGVHD, 12 patients responded, including 5 with CR and 7 with partial response.[70] Adverse effects included myelosuppression and hemolytic uremic syndrome. A retrospective study in patients with sclerotic cGVHD treated with either sirolimus or everolimus showed a 76% response rate when given with corticosteroids.[71] Two other retrospective studies of combinational systemic treatments with sirolimus showed response rates up to 81%.[72,73]

Ruxolitinib
JAK inhibitors function by blocking the signal transduction and activation of transcription (STAT) pathway, which produces growth factors and inflammatory cytokines.[18] Ruxolitinib is a JAK 1 and 2 inhibitor, whereas tofacitinib is a JAK 3 inhibitor.[74,75] Few studies have shown this class's efficacy.[74,76] The largest study, which was a retrospective analysis of 95 patients with steroid-refractory GVHD receiving ruxolitinib as salvage therapy, showed an overall response rate of 85.4%.[77] A multicenter, retrospective study including 54 adult patients with steroid-refractory grade III/IV aGVHD treated with ruxolitinib resulted in 82% of patients experiencing a response, a low relapse rate (7%), and high survival rate at 6 months (79%).[77] Adverse events include cytopenias and reactivation of cytomegalovirus. Even in

children, the response rate is 45%, and more than 50% were alive at median follow-up of more than 400 days when treated with ruxolitinib.[78]

Phototherapy

Phototherapy exerts antiproliferative effects and decreases cytokine production, cell activation, and antigen presentation.[79] In patients with extensive cutaneous disease, phototherapy may serve as monotherapy or adjunctive therapy.[80] Both BSCH-BSBMT and German-Austrian-Swiss guidelines state that ultraviolet B (UVB; 290–320 nm) is useful in lichenoid or late aGVHD skin disease and is usually administered as narrow-band therapy (311 nm).[16,47] UVA (320–400 nm), a longer wavelength, penetrates deeper than UVB and may be used with oral psoralen, which is effective in treating sclerodermatous lesions of cGVHD.[16,47] A newer modality, UVA-1 (340–400 nm), which is used in an array of sclerotic-type skin disorders, is also effective in sclerodermoid cGVHD.[16,47] Treatment may take weeks to months to produce a response. The number of treatment sessions per week is poorly studied, with recommendations ranging from 2 to 5 sessions per week.[45]

Methotrexate

MTX is a folate analogue that exerts immunosuppressant effects through the action of adenosine.[81] MTX is only discussed in BSCH-BSBMT guidelines as a possible third-line systemic treatment of refractory cGVHD. However, there is some clinical evidence that supports its use, albeit limited. Low-dose MTX has a 90% response rate in cutaneous cGVHD when used as a first-line therapy in conjunction with other immunosuppressants.[82]

Imatinib mesylate

Imatinib mesylate is an inhibitor of several kinases, such as bcr-abl, c-kit, platelet-derived growth factor receptor (PDGFR), and other kinases.[83] Although used in treatment of Philadelphia chromosome–positive chronic myelogenous leukemia and acute lymphoblastic leukemia, its use in sclerotic cGVHD stems from is inhibition of PDGFR.[83] However, PDGFR antibodies in systemic sclerosis and sclerotic cGVHD have not been found. A randomized phase II trial of patients with sclerotic cGVHD showed improvement in skin symptoms and joint motion in 36% of patients randomized to imatinib.[84] Three prospective studies of patients with steroid-refractory cGVHD showed response in 7 out of 14 (50%), 15 out of 19 (79%), and 20 out of 39 (51%) patients treated with imatinib.[85–87] Prophylactic use of imatinib does not prevent sclerotic cGVHD skin changes.[88] Second-generation tyrosine kinase inhibitors, such as nilotinib and dasatinib, have started to be investigated but are lacking sufficient evidence to make recommendations at this time.[89,90]

Rituximab

Rituximab is an anti-CD20 monoclonal antibody that functions via an array of mechanisms to target B cells, which may contribute to GVHD.[91] In a phase II trial of rituximab in steroid-refractory cGVHD, 32 out of 37 (86%) patients responded to treatment with skin and oral mucosal improvement.[92] Similarly, a phase I/II study of 21 patients with steroid-refractory cGVHD undergoing treatment with rituximab showed 70% response rate (only in cutaneous and musculoskeletal sites).[93] Another phase II randomized study of patients with sclerotic cGVHD showed skin or joint motion improvement in 27% of patients treated with rituximab.[84] A large meta-analysis of 111 patients pooled from 3 prospective and 4 retrospective studies showed cutaneous response to rituximab ranging from 0% to 83% for oral disease and 13% to 100% for cutaneous disease. Patients treated with rituximab were able to reduce systemic corticosteroid use.[94]

Emerging Treatments

Acute graft-versus-host disease

Bortezomib is a proteasome inhibitor and potent inhibitor of nuclear factor kappa B, important for T-cell proliferation, activation, and survival.[42] Early-phase studies show that bortezomib is effective in preventing aGVHD.[95] Brentuximab vedotin (BV) is an anti-30 monoclonal antibody potentially useful in treating aGVHD, for patients with a higher percentage of CD30-expressing CD8+ T cells.[42] In a phase I trial, 14.7% and 23.5% of patients using BV achieved complete and partial response, respectively.[96] Tofacitinib is a JAK inhibitor currently being investigated.[42] One animal model GVHD study showed reduced expansion and activation of CD8 T cells along with reduced expression of interferon-gamma by keratinocytes. Mesenchymal stromal cells (MSCs) are pluripotent stem cells that can inhibit B-cell and T-cell activation.[42] Thus far, phase I and II trials evaluating MSC treatment in patients with steroid-resistant aGVHD report response rates of 60% to 75%.[97–100] Further trials assessing these therapies individually and in comparison with other therapies are needed to evaluate their efficacies for GVHD.

Chronic graft-versus-host disease

Treatments currently being studied for cGVHD include spleen tyrosine kinase (Syk) inhibitors, Rho kinase inhibitors, abatacept, ibrutinib, IL-2, and Tregs. Syk inhibitors are necessary for T-cell receptor signaling pathways and are also responsible for activation of proinflammatory cytokines.[42] Syk inhibitors showed promise in animal studies, with decreased incidence of aGVHD and reduced numbers of cytokines.[101] There is currently a phase II trial of Syk inhibitors in combination with systemic corticosteroids for first-line treatment of cGVHD.[42]

Rho-associated protein kinase (ROCK) plays a role in promoting cytokine production of IL-17 and IL-21 and may be useful in GVHD.[42] In 2 murine models, a ROCK inhibitor led to a reversal of cGVHD manifestations.[102] There is currently a phase II trial evaluating its safety and tolerability in treatment of steroid-resistant cGVHD.

Abatacept is composed of cytotoxic T lymphocyte–associated protein-4 (CTLA-4), which inhibits T-cell activation via blockade of costimulatory molecules.[42] In a phase I trial, 44% of patients with steroid-resistant cGVHD had a partial response to abatacept.[103] A phase II trial is currently being planned.

Ibrutinib is an irreversible inhibitor of Bruton tyrosine kinase and IL-2–inducible kinase, which activate B-cell and T-cell receptor signaling pathways, respectively.[104] It was approved in 2017 for use in cGVHD after a multicenter, open-label, phase II clinical trial showed that ibrutinib was effective in steroid-dependent or steroid-resistant cGVHD.[42,105] Multiple organs, including the skin, showed improvement in the study.[105]

IL-2 is a cytokine that is an integral part of immune system signaling. It is essential in the development and function of Tregs, which may control GVHD. Thus far, a phase I study has shown doses higher than 1×106 IU/m^2 produce constitutional symptoms. Eleven of 23 patients had partial improvement in skin, subcutaneous tissue, or both.[106] A phase II study showed clinical response in 20 out of 33 patients (61%) with steroid-refractory cGVHD by week 12.[107] Tregs were increased in patients undergoing treatment with low-dose IL-2.[107]

Tregs are reduced in cGVHD and there are potential therapeutic benefits of an adoptive cell transfer of Tregs. In the first-in-human use of adoptive transfer of ex vivo–expanded Tregs in 1 patient with aGVHD and another patient with cGVHD, there was significant improvement in the patient with cGVHD.[108] Larger, randomized trials are still necessary to determine long-term benefits and outcomes.

Miscellaneous Treatments

Case reports and case series of other treatments provide limited evidence for use and include systemic retinoids, hydroxychloroquine, thalidomide, clofazimine, alefacept, alemtuzumab, and tocilizumab.[109–113]

Skin Transplant

Skin transplant has been used in some cases of skin ulceration in patients with cGVHD after HSCT.[114–116] The transplants are performed with split-thickness transplant from HLA-identical donors. This modality is pursued when conservative wound care management has failed. Ruling out infection and malignancy is important in chronic ulcers/wounds.[83]

Adjunctive Treatment

The NIH Consensus Development Project on Criteria for Clinical Trials in Chronic Graft-versus-Host Disease released 2014 recommendations for the prevention and management of infections, complications of cGVHD, and information for patient education and follow-up. Review of this impressive document is outside the scope of this article but it provides an excellent resource for patients and caregivers, including adjunctive conservative management strategies for cutaneous and mucosal sites.[49]

Treatment Response Assessment

Cutaneous cGVHD lesions can be clinically assessed at follow-up visits. cGVHD is a multisystemic disorder that involves interdisciplinary care in many cases and therefore the NIH Chronic Graft-versus-Host Disease Consensus Response Criteria Working Group developed a classification system to assess clinical response in 2015. Although this guideline is more applicable to clinical trials, it provides insight into how systemic treatments, many of which address internal organ complications as well as skin manifestations, may be affecting patients' overall disease states.

Recommended Follow-up

Depending on clinical manifestation, coordination of care with several specialties (eg, hematology-oncology, gastroenterology, and allergy and immunology) may be considered. Long-term follow-up is more commonly recommended for cGVHD and typically involves laboratory testing and organ function testing (eg, pulmonary function tests) to assess internal organ sequelae.[117] Patients on immunosuppressants should receive annual screening by a dermatologist given their increased risk of skin cancer.[22] Some dermatologists recommend screening annually even after immunosuppressants are stopped.[118] Six-month screening may be advisable in patients with pre-transplant history of cutaneous malignancy.[22,118]

Limitations

Until the last decade, clinical trial data have been limited in evaluating and comparing treatments for aGVHD and cGVHD. Long-term sequelae (eg, organ failure) and high mortality associated with aGVHD and chronic GVHD make conducting prospective trials more difficult. Guidelines often quickly become outdated and lack recommendations based on most recent studies. The committees that develop the guidelines often take years to develop consensus guidelines, which may be outdated when they are published. There are minimal recommendations for combination therapies in GVHD.

SUMMARY

GVHD is a complex and potentially life-threatening disease commonly encountered in HSCT patients. Dermatologists are often involved in the diagnosis and management of these patients. Clinical presentation and skin biopsy are helpful in making the diagnosis. A plethora of treatments are available for aGVHD and cGVHD. For limited GVHD, topical corticosteroids or CNIs can be effective. For moderate to severe GVHD, first-line therapies include oral corticosteroids, which seem to be superior to many other treatments. If patients fail to improve on corticosteroids, there are numerous second-line therapies, including phototherapy, ECP, MTX, monoclonal antibodies, as well as many emerging treatments currently being investigated. Overall, interdisciplinary care coordination plays an important role in cases of GVHD. Future research, including clinical trials, promises additional therapeutic options for this disorder.

REFERENCES

1. Kernan NA, Collins NH, Juliano L, et al. Clonable T lymphocytes in T cell-depleted bone marrow transplants correlate with development of graft-v-host disease. Blood 1986;68(3):770–3.
2. Molaro GL, De Angelis V. [Graft versus host disease after transfusion of blood and its products]. Riv Emoter Immunoematol 1984;31(2):107–23.
3. Fidler C, Klumpp T, Mangan K, et al. Spontaneous graft versus host disease occurring in a patient with multiple myeloma after autologous stem cell transplant. Am J Hematol 2012;87(2):219–21.
4. Murali AR, Chandra S, Stewart Z, et al. Graft versus host disease after liver transplantation in adults: a case series, review of literature, and an approach to management. Transplantation 2016;100(12):2661–70.
5. Ferrara JL, Reddy P. Pathophysiology of graft-versus-host disease. Semin Hematol 2006;43(1):3–10.
6. Jagasia M, Arora M, Flowers ME, et al. Risk factors for acute GVHD and survival after hematopoietic cell transplantation. Blood 2012;119(1):296–307.
7. Atkinson K, Horowitz MM, Gale RP, et al. Risk factors for chronic graft-versus-host disease after HLA-identical sibling bone marrow transplantation. Blood 1990;75(12):2459–64.
8. Weisdorf D, Haake R, Blazar B, et al. Treatment of moderate/severe acute graft-versus-host disease after allogeneic bone marrow transplantation: an analysis of clinical risk features and outcome. Blood 1990;75(4):1024–30.
9. Paralkar VR, Nasta SD, Morrissey K, et al. Allogeneic hematopoietic SCT for primary cutaneous T cell lymphomas. Bone Marrow Transplant 2012;47(7):940–5.
10. Zeiser R, Penack O, Holler E, et al. Danger signals activating innate immunity in graft-versus-host disease. J Mol Med (Berl) 2011;89(9):833–45.
11. Reddy P. Pathophysiology of acute graft-versus-host disease. Hematol Oncol 2003;21(4):149–61.
12. Yu Y, Wang D, Liu C, et al. Prevention of GVHD while sparing GVL effect by targeting Th1 and Th17 transcription factor T-bet and RORgammat in mice. Blood 2011;118(18):5011–20.
13. MacDonald KP, Shlomchik WD, Reddy P. Biology of graft-versus-host responses: recent insights. Biol Blood Marrow Transpl 2013;19(1 Suppl):S10–4.
14. Sung AD, Chao NJ. Acute graft-versus-host disease: are we close to bringing the bench to the bedside? Best practice & research. Clin Haematol 2013;26(3):285–92.
15. Zeiser R, Blazar BR. Pathophysiology of chronic graft-versus-host disease and therapeutic targets. N Engl J Med 2017;377(26):2565–79.
16. Dignan FL, Scarisbrick JJ, Cornish J, et al. Organ-specific management and supportive care in chronic graft-versus-host disease. Br J Haematol 2012;158(1):62–78.
17. Jagasia MH, Greinix HT, Arora M, et al. National Institutes of Health Consensus Development Project on criteria for clinical trials in chronic graft-versus-host disease: I. The 2014 Diagnosis and Staging Working Group report. Biol Blood Marrow Transplant 2015;21(3):389–401.e1.
18. Strong Rodrigues K, Oliveira-Ribeiro C, de Abreu Fiuza Gomes S, et al. Cutaneous graft-versus-host disease: diagnosis and treatment. Am J Clin Dermatol 2018;19(1):33–50.
19. Imanguli MM, Alevizos I, Brown R, et al. Oral graft-versus-host disease. Oral Dis 2008;14(5):396–412.

20. Byun HJ, Yang JI, Kim BK, et al. Clinical differentiation of acute cutaneous graft-versus-host disease from drug hypersensitivity reactions. J Am Acad Dermatol 2011;65(4):726–32.

21. Lerner KG, Kao GF, Storb R, et al. Histopathology of graft-vs.-host reaction (GvHR) in human recipients of marrow from HL-A-matched sibling donors. Transplant Proc 1974;6(4):367–71.

22. Villarreal CD, Alanis JC, Perez JC, et al. Cutaneous graft-versus-host disease after hematopoietic stem cell transplant - a review. An Bras Dermatol 2016; 91(3):336–43.

23. Shulman HM, Cardona DM, Greenson JK, et al. NIH consensus development project on criteria for clinical trials in chronic graft-versus-host disease: II. The 2014 Pathology Working Group Report. Biol Blood Marrow Transpl 2015;21(4): 589–603.

24. Glucksberg H, Storb R, Fefer A, et al. Clinical manifestations of graft-versus-host disease in human recipients of marrow from HL-A-matched sibling donors. Transplantation 1974;18(4):295–304.

25. Rowlings PA, Przepiorka D, Klein JP, et al. IBMTR severity index for grading acute graft-versus-host disease: retrospective comparison with Glucksberg grade. Br J Haematol 1997;97(4):855–64.

26. Filipovich AH, Weisdorf D, Pavletic S, et al. National Institutes of Health consensus development project on criteria for clinical trials in chronic graft-versus-host disease: I. Diagnosis and staging working group report. Biol Blood Marrow Transpl 2005; 11(12):945–56.

27. Paczesny S, Braun TM, Levine JE, et al. Elafin is a biomarker of graft-versus-host disease of the skin. Sci Transl Med 2010;2(13):13ra2.

28. McDonald GB, Tabellini L, Storer BE, et al. Plasma biomarkers of acute GVHD and nonrelapse mortality: predictive value of measurements before GVHD onset and treatment. Blood 2015;126(1):113–20.

29. Ahmed SS, Wang XN, Norden J, et al. Identification and validation of biomarkers associated with acute and chronic graft versus host disease. Bone Marrow Transplant 2015;50(12):1563–71.

30. Ruutu T, Gratwohl A, de Witte T, et al. Prophylaxis and treatment of GVHD: EBMT-ELN working group recommendations for a standardized practice. Bone Marrow Transplant 2014;49(2):168–73.

31. Ringden O, Klaesson S, Sundberg B, et al. Decreased incidence of graft-versus-host disease and improved survival with methotrexate combined with cyclosporin compared with monotherapy in recipients of bone marrow from donors other than HLA identical siblings. Bone Marrow Transplant 1992;9(1):19–25.

32. Ratanatharathorn V, Nash RA, Przepiorka D, et al. Phase III study comparing methotrexate and tacrolimus (prograf, FK506) with methotrexate and cyclosporine for graft-versus-host disease prophylaxis after HLA-identical sibling bone marrow transplantation. Blood 1998;92(7):2303–14.

33. Perkins J, Field T, Kim J, et al. A randomized phase II trial comparing tacrolimus and mycophenolate mofetil to tacrolimus and methotrexate for acute graft-versus-host disease prophylaxis. Biol Blood Marrow Transplant 2010;16(7): 937–47.

34. Bolwell B, Sobecks R, Pohlman B, et al. A prospective randomized trial comparing cyclosporine and short course methotrexate with cyclosporine and mycophenolate mofetil for GVHD prophylaxis in myeloablative allogeneic bone marrow transplantation. Bone Marrow Transplant 2004;34(7):621–5.

35. Hertenstein B, Arseniev L, Novotny J, et al. A comparative review of methods for T cell depletion in the prophylaxis of graft-versus-host disease. BioDrugs 1998;9(2):105–23.

36. Ringden O, Pihlstedt P, Markling L, et al. Prevention of graft-versus-host disease with T cell depletion or cyclosporin and methotrexate. A randomized trial in adult leukemic marrow recipients. Bone Marrow Transplant 1991;7(3):221–6.

37. Lee SJ. New approaches for preventing and treating chronic graft-versus-host disease. Blood 2005; 105(11):4200–6.

38. Mohty M. Mechanisms of action of antithymocyte globulin: T-cell depletion and beyond. Leukemia 2007;21(7):1387–94.

39. Finke J, Bethge WA, Schmoor C, et al. Standard graft-versus-host disease prophylaxis with or without anti-T-cell globulin in haematopoietic cell transplantation from matched unrelated donors: a randomised, open-label, multicentre phase 3 trial. Lancet Oncol 2009;10(9):855–64.

40. Socie G, Schmoor C, Bethge WA, et al. Chronic graft-versus-host disease: long-term results from a randomized trial on graft-versus-host disease prophylaxis with or without anti-T-cell globulin ATG-Fresenius. Blood 2011; 117(23):6375–82.

41. Kröger N, Solano C, Wolschke C, et al. Antilymphocyte globulin for prevention of chronic graft-versus-host disease. N Engl J Med 2016;374(1): 43–53.

42. Hill L, Alousi A, Kebriaei P, et al. New and emerging therapies for acute and chronic graft versus host disease. Ther Adv Hematol 2018;9(1):21–46.

43. Cutler C, Kim HT, Bindra B, et al. Rituximab prophylaxis prevents corticosteroid-requiring chronic GVHD after allogeneic peripheral blood stem cell transplantation: results of a phase 2 trial. Blood 2013;122(8):1510–7.

44. Arai S, Sahaf B, Narasimhan B, et al. Prophylactic rituximab after allogeneic transplantation decreases

B-cell alloimmunity with low chronic GVHD incidence. Blood 2012;119(25):6145–54.

45. Martin PJ, Rizzo JD, Wingard JR, et al. First- and second-line systemic treatment of acute graft-versus-host disease: recommendations of the American Society of Blood and Marrow Transplantation. Biol Blood Marrow Transplant 2012;18(8): 1150–63.

46. Dignan FL, Amrolia P, Clark A, et al. Diagnosis and management of chronic graft-versus-host disease. Br J Haematol 2012;158(1):46–61.

47. Marks C, Stadler M, Hausermann P, et al. German-Austrian-Swiss Consensus Conference on clinical practice in chronic graft-versus-host disease (GVHD): guidance for supportive therapy of chronic cutaneous and musculoskeletal GVHD. Br J Dermatol 2011;165(1):18–29.

48. Dignan FL, Clark A, Amrolia P, et al. Diagnosis and management of acute graft-versus-host disease. Br J Haematol 2012;158(1):30–45.

49. Carpenter PA, Kitko CL, Elad S, et al. National Institutes of Health Consensus Development Project on Criteria for Clinical Trials in Chronic Graft-versus-Host Disease: V. The 2014 Ancillary Therapy and Supportive Care Working Group Report. Biol Blood Marrow Transpl 2015;21(7):1167–87.

50. Noce CW, Gomes A, Shcaira V, et al. Randomized double-blind clinical trial comparing clobetasol and dexamethasone for the topical treatment of symptomatic oral chronic graft-versus-host disease. Biol Blood Marrow Transpl 2014;20(8): 1163–8.

51. Elad S, Zeevi I, Finke J, et al. Improvement in oral chronic graft-versus-host disease with the administration of effervescent tablets of topical budesonide—an open, randomized, multicenter study. Biol Blood Marrow Transplant 2012;18(1):134–40.

52. Park AR, La HO, Cho BS, et al. Comparison of budesonide and dexamethasone for local treatment of oral chronic graft-versus-host disease. Am J Health Syst Pharm 2013;70(16):1383–91.

53. Matsuda S, Koyasu S. Mechanisms of action of cyclosporine. Immunopharmacology 2000;47(2–3):119–25.

54. Choi CJ, Nghiem P. Tacrolimus ointment in the treatment of chronic cutaneous graft-vs-host disease: a case series of 18 patients. Arch Dermatol 2001;137(9):1202–6.

55. Ziemer M, Gruhn B, Thiele JJ, et al. Treatment of extensive chronic cutaneous graft-versus-host disease in an infant with topical pimecrolimus. J Am Acad Dermatol 2004;50(6):946–8.

56. Martin PJ, Schoch G, Fisher L, et al. A retrospective analysis of therapy for acute graft-versus-host disease: initial treatment. Blood 1990;76(8):1464–72.

57. MacMillan ML, Weisdorf DJ, Wagner JE, et al. Response of 443 patients to steroids as primary therapy for acute graft-versus-host disease: comparison of grading systems. Biol Blood Marrow Transpl 2002;8(7):387–94.

58. Van Lint MT, Uderzo C, Locasciulli A, et al. Early treatment of acute graft-versus-host disease with high- or low-dose 6-methylprednisolone: a multicenter randomized trial from the Italian Group for Bone Marrow Transplantation. Blood 1998;92(7): 2288–93.

59. Mielcarek M, Furlong T, Storer BE, et al. Effectiveness and safety of lower dose prednisone for initial treatment of acute graft-versus-host disease: a randomized controlled trial. Haematologica 2015; 100(6):842–8.

60. Hart JW, Shiue LH, Shpall EJ, et al. Extracorporeal photopheresis in the treatment of graft-versus-host disease: evidence and opinion. Ther Adv Hematol 2013;4(5):320–34.

61. Jagasia M, Greinix H, Robin M, et al. Extracorporeal photopheresis versus anticytokine therapy as a second-line treatment for steroid-refractory acute GVHD: a multicenter comparative analysis. Biol Blood Marrow Transpl 2013;19(7):1129–33.

62. Greinix HT, Volc-Platzer B, Kalhs P, et al. Extracorporeal photochemotherapy in the treatment of severe steroid-refractory acute graft-versus-host disease: a pilot study. Blood 2000;96(7): 2426–31.

63. Allison AC. Mechanisms of action of mycophenolate mofetil. Lupus 2005;14(Suppl 1):s2–8.

64. Furlong T, Martin P, Flowers MED, et al. Therapy with mycophenolate mofetil for refractory acute and chronic GVHD. Bone Marrow Transplant 2009;44(11):739–48.

65. Bolanos-Meade J, Logan BR, Alousi AM, et al. Phase 3 clinical trial of steroids/mycophenolate mofetil vs steroids/placebo as therapy for acute GVHD: BMT CTN 0802. Blood 2014;124(22): 3221–7 [quiz 3335].

66. Martin PJ, Storer BE, Rowley SD, et al. Evaluation of mycophenolate mofetil for initial treatment of chronic graft-versus-host disease. Blood 2009; 113(21):5074–82.

67. Basara N, Blau WI, Romer E, et al. Mycophenolate mofetil for the treatment of acute and chronic GVHD in bone marrow transplant patients. Bone Marrow Transplant 1998;22(1):61–5.

68. Park J, Ha H, Ahn HJ, et al. Sirolimus inhibits platelet-derived growth factor-induced collagen synthesis in rat vascular smooth muscle cells. Transpl Proc 2005;37(8):3459–62.

69. Couriel DR, Saliba R, Escalon MP, et al. Sirolimus in combination with tacrolimus and corticosteroids for the treatment of resistant chronic graft-versus-host disease. Br J Haematol 2005;130(3):409–17.

70. Benito AI, Furlong T, Martin PJ, et al. Sirolimus (rapamycin) for the treatment of steroid-refractory

acute graft-versus-host disease. Transplantation 2001;72(12):1924–9.

71. Jedlickova Z, Burlakova I, Bug G, et al. Therapy of sclerodermatous chronic graft-versus-host disease with mammalian target of rapamycin inhibitors. Biol Blood Marrow Transpl 2011;17(5):657–63.

72. Furlong T, Kiem HP, Appelbaum FR, et al. Sirolimus in combination with cyclosporine or tacrolimus plus methotrexate for prevention of graft-versus-host disease following hematopoietic cell transplantation from unrelated donors. Biol Blood Marrow Transpl 2008;14(5):531–7.

73. Jurado M, Vallejo C, Perez-Simon JA, et al. Sirolimus as part of immunosuppressive therapy for refractory chronic graft-versus-host disease. Biol Blood Marrow Transpl 2007;13(6):701–6.

74. Spoerl S, Mathew NR, Bscheider M, et al. Activity of therapeutic JAK 1/2 blockade in graft-versus-host disease. Blood 2014;123(24):3832–42.

75. Okiyama N, Furumoto Y, Villarroel VA, et al. Reversal of CD8 T-cell-mediated mucocutaneous graft-versus-host-like disease by the JAK inhibitor tofacitinib. J Invest Dermatol 2014;134(4): 992–1000.

76. Maffini E, Giaccone L, Festuccia M, et al. Ruxolitinib in steroid refractory graft-vs.-host disease: a case report. J Hematol Oncol 2016;9(1):67.

77. Zeiser R, Burchert A, Lengerke C, et al. Ruxolitinib in corticosteroid-refractory graft-versus-host disease after allogeneic stem cell transplantation: a multicenter survey. Leukemia 2015;29(10):2062–8.

78. Khandelwal P, Teusink-Cross A, Davies SM, et al. Ruxolitinib as salvage therapy in steroid-refractory acute graft-versus-host disease in pediatric hematopoietic stem cell transplant patients. Biol Blood Marrow Transpl 2017;23(7):1122–7.

79. Greinix HT, Socie G, Bacigalupo A, et al. Assessing the potential role of photopheresis in hematopoietic stem cell transplant. Bone Marrow Transplant 2006; 38(4):265–73.

80. Ballester-Sánchez R, Navarro-Mira MÁ, de Unamuno-Bustos B, et al. Análisis retrospectivo del papel de la fototerapia en la enfermedad injerto contra huésped crónica cutánea. Revisión de la literatura. Actas Dermosifiliogr 2015;106(8):651–7.

81. Cutolo M, Sulli A, Pizzorni C, et al. Anti-inflammatory mechanisms of methotrexate in rheumatoid arthritis. Ann Rheum Dis 2001;60(8):729–35.

82. Wang Y, Xu LP, Liu DH, et al. First-line therapy for chronic graft-versus-host disease that includes low-dose methotrexate is associated with a high response rate. Biol Blood Marrow Transpl 2009; 15(4):505–11.

83. Hymes SR, Alousi AM, Cowen EW. Graft-versus-host disease: part I. Pathogenesis and clinical manifestations of graft-versus-host disease. J Am Acad Dermatol 2012;66(4):515.e1-18 [quiz 533–4].

84. Arai S, Pidala J, Pusic I, et al. A randomized phase II crossover study of imatinib or rituximab for cutaneous sclerosis after hematopoietic cell transplantation. Clin Cancer Res 2016;22(2):319–27.

85. Magro L, Mohty M, Catteau B, et al. Imatinib mesylate as salvage therapy for refractory sclerotic chronic graft-versus-host disease. Blood 2009; 114(3):719–22.

86. Olivieri A, Locatelli F, Zecca M, et al. Imatinib for refractory chronic graft-versus-host disease with fibrotic features. Blood 2009;114(3):709–18.

87. Olivieri A, Cimminiello M, Corradini P, et al. Long-term outcome and prospective validation of NIH response criteria in 39 patients receiving imatinib for steroid-refractory chronic GVHD. Blood 2013; 122(25):4111–8.

88. Nakasone H, Kanda Y, Takasaki H, et al. Prophylactic impact of imatinib administration after allogeneic stem cell transplantation on the incidence and severity of chronic graft versus host disease in patients with Philadelphia chromosome-positive leukemia. Leukemia 2010;24(6):1236–9.

89. Breccia M, Cannella L, Stefanizzi C, et al. Efficacy of dasatinib in a chronic myeloid leukemia patient with disease molecular relapse and chronic GVHD after haploidentical BMT: an immunomodulatory effect? Bone Marrow Transplant 2009;44(5): 331–2.

90. Pulanic D, Cowen EW, Baird K, et al. Development of severe sclerotic chronic GVHD during treatment with dasatinib. Bone Marrow Transplant 2010; 45(9):1469–70.

91. Weiner GJ. Rituximab: mechanism of action. Semin Hematol 2010;47(2):115–23.

92. Kim SJ, Lee JW, Jung CW, et al. Weekly rituximab followed by monthly rituximab treatment for steroid-refractory chronic graft-versus-host disease: results from a prospective, multicenter, phase II study. Haematologica 2010;95(11): 1935–42.

93. Cutler C, Miklos D, Kim HT, et al. Rituximab for steroid-refractory chronic graft-versus-host disease. Blood 2006;108(2):756–62.

94. Kharfan-Dabaja MA, Mhaskar AR, Djulbegovic B, et al. Efficacy of rituximab in the setting of steroid-refractory chronic graft-versus-host disease: a systematic review and meta-analysis. Biol Blood Marrow Transpl 2009;15(9):1005–13.

95. Sun K, Welniak LA, Panoskaltsis-Mortari A, et al. Inhibition of acute graft-versus-host disease with retention of graft-versus-tumor effects by the proteasome inhibitor bortezomib. Proc Natl Acad Sci U S A 2004;101(21):8120–5.

96. Chen YB, Perales MA, Li S, et al. Phase 1 multicenter trial of brentuximab vedotin for steroid-refractory acute graft-versus-host disease. Blood 2017;129(24):3256–61.

97. Le Blanc K, Rasmusson I, Sundberg B, et al. Treatment of severe acute graft-versus-host disease with third party haploidentical mesenchymal stem cells. Lancet 2004;363(9419):1439–41.

98. Le Blanc K, Frassoni F, Ball L, et al. Mesenchymal stem cells for treatment of steroid-resistant, severe, acute graft-versus-host disease: a phase II study. Lancet 2008;371(9624):1579–86.

99. von Bonin M, Stolzel F, Goedecke A, et al. Treatment of refractory acute GVHD with third-party MSC expanded in platelet lysate-containing medium. Bone Marrow Transplant 2009;43(3):245–51.

100. Ringden O, Uzunel M, Rasmusson I, et al. Mesenchymal stem cells for treatment of therapy-resistant graft-versus-host disease. Transplantation 2006; 81(10):1390–7.

101. Leonhardt F, Zirlik K, Buchner M, et al. Spleen tyrosine kinase (Syk) is a potent target for GvHD prevention at different cellular levels. Leukemia 2012; 26(7):1617–29.

102. Flynn R, Paz K, Du J, et al. Targeted Rho-associated kinase 2 inhibition suppresses murine and human chronic GVHD through a Stat3-dependent mechanism. Blood 2016;127(17): 2144–54.

103. Nahas MR, Soiffer RJ, Kim HT, et al. Phase 1 clinical trial evaluating abatacept in patients with steroid-refractory chronic graft-versus-host disease. Blood 2018;131(25):2836–45.

104. Ryan CE, Sahaf B, Logan AC, et al. Ibrutinib efficacy and tolerability in patients with relapsed chronic lymphocytic leukemia following allogeneic HCT. Blood 2016;128(25):2899–908.

105. Miklos D, Cutler CS, Arora M, et al. Multicenter open-label phase 2 study of ibrutinib in Chronic Graft Versus Host Disease (cGVHD) after failure of corticosteroids. Blood 2016;128(22). LBA-3-LBA-3.

106. Koreth J, Matsuoka K-i, Kim HT, et al. Interleukin-2 and regulatory T cells in graft-versus-host disease. N Engl J Med 2011;365(22):2055–66.

107. Koreth J, Kim HT, Jones KT, et al. Efficacy, durability, and response predictors of low-dose interleukin-2 therapy for chronic graft-versus-host disease. Blood 2016;128(1):130–7.

108. Trzonkowski P, Bieniaszewska M, Juscinska J, et al. First-in-man clinical results of the treatment of patients with graft versus host disease with human ex vivo expanded CD4+CD25+CD127- T regulatory cells. Clin Immunol 2009;133(1):22–6.

109. Zhou H, Guo M, Bian C, et al. Efficacy of bone marrow-derived mesenchymal stem cells in the treatment of sclerodermatous chronic graft-versus-host disease: clinical report. Biol Blood Marrow Transpl 2010;16(3):403–12.

110. Inamoto Y, Flowers ME. Treatment of chronic graft-versus-host disease in 2011. Curr Opin Hematol 2011;18(6):414–20.

111. Flowers ME, Martin PJ. How we treat chronic graft-versus-host disease. Blood 2015;125(4):606–15.

112. Marcellus DC, Altomonte VL, Farmer ER, et al. Etretinate therapy for refractory sclerodermatous chronic graft-versus-host disease. Blood 1999; 93(1):66–70.

113. de Lavallade H, Mohty M, Faucher C, et al. Low-dose methotrexate as salvage therapy for refractory graft-versus-host disease after reduced-intensity conditioning allogeneic stem cell transplantation. Haematologica 2006; 91(10):1438–40.

114. Ammer J, Prantl L, Holler B, et al. Successful treatment of a refractory skin ulcer in chronic cutaneous GvHD after allogeneic HSCT with split-thickness skin allografting from the stem cell donor. Bone Marrow Transplant 2012;47(10):1368–9.

115. Knobler HY, Sagher U, Peled IJ, et al. Tolerance to donor-type skin in the recipient of a bone marrow allograft. Treatment of skin ulcers in chronic graft-versus-host disease with skin grafts from the bone marrow donor. Transplantation 1985;40(2): 223–5.

116. Crocchiolo R, Dubois V, Nicolini FE, et al. Skin allograft for severe chronic GvHD. Bone Marrow Transplant 2017;52:1060.

117. Palmer J, Williams K, Inamoto Y, et al. Pulmonary symptoms measured by the national institutes of health lung score predict overall survival, nonrelapse mortality, and patient-reported outcomes in chronic graft-versus-host disease. Biol Blood Marrow Transplant 2014;20(3):337–44.

118. Penas PF, Zaman S. Many faces of graft-versus-host disease. Australas J Dermatol 2010;51(1): 1–10 [quiz 11].

Phakomatoses

Benjamin Becker, MD[a],*, Roy E. Strowd III, MD, MEd[a,b,c]

KEYWORDS

- Phakomatoses • Genodermatoses • Neurocutaneous syndromes • Neurofibromatosis
- Tuberous sclerosis

KEY POINTS

- Neurocutaneous syndromes arise from germline mutation in a tumor suppressor gene that predisposes individuals to the development of tumors, with a predilection for neuroectodermally derived tissues.
- Syndromes include neurofibromatosis type 1, neurofibromatosis type 2, schwannomatosis, tuberous sclerosis complex, von Hippel Lindau syndrome, ataxia telangiectasia, and Sturge Weber syndrome.
- Neurofibromatosis type 1, the most common phakomatosis, is an autosomal dominant genetic disease that presents with cutaneous, peripheral and/or central nervous system tumors, and other findings.
- Tuberous sclerosis complex is an autosomal-dominant neurocutaneous syndrome characterized by hypomelanotic macules, shagreen patches, angiofibroma, fibrous cephalic plaques, confetti lesions, and a predisposition to lesions of the brain, kidneys, lung, and heart.

INTRODUCTION

The phakomatoses are a heterogenous group of clinical syndromes characterized by cutaneous, neurologic, and oncologic manifestations. These neurocutaneous syndromes are often first recognized early in childhood, but can be encountered by both pediatric and adult clinicians as manifestations occur throughout an individual's life and often vary by age. Each disorder has a genetic basis often with an autosomal-dominant inheritance pattern. Tumors are a unifying feature of these diseases, which represent prototypical tumor suppressor syndromes. Tumor suppressors are the cellular proteins that function as key negative regulators to inhibit cell growth. Tumors develop as a result of biallelic loss of a tumor suppressor protein, a process that occurs according to Knudson's 2-hit hypothesis.[1] Dermatologists and other clinicians who encounter these individuals

must be aware of the myriad manifestations, common tumor syndromes, variability in presentation by age, surveillance recommendations, and treatment options.

In this article, we review 2 of these syndromes: neurofibromatosis type 1 (NF1) and tuberous sclerosis complex (TSC). These diseases represent 2 of the most commonly encountered of the neurocutaneous syndromes and both have important tumor manifestations and treatments. Other clinically relevant conditions that are not discussed in this article include neurofibromatosis type 2, schwannomatosis, von Hippel Lindau syndrome, ataxia-telangiectasia, and Sturge Weber syndrome; they are reviewed elsewhere.[2] In general, this article is organized by disease type, focusing on NF1 and then TSC. Each section reviews the diagnostic criteria, which are both necessary and sufficient for the diagnosis. The relevant

Disclosure Statement: No actual or potential conflicts of interest.
[a] Department of Neurology, Wake Forest Baptist Health, 1 Medical Center Boulevard, Winston Salem, NC 27157, USA; [b] Department of Internal Medicine, Section on Hematology and Oncology, Wake Forest Baptist Health, Winston Salem, NC 27157, USA; [c] Translational Science Institute, Wake Forest Baptist Health, Winston Salem, NC 27157, USA
* Corresponding author.
E-mail address: BeckerBe@med.umich.edu

Dermatol Clin 37 (2019) 583–606
https://doi.org/10.1016/j.det.2019.05.015

epidemiology, genetics, common cutaneous manifestations, oncologic manifestations, current treatment options, and emerging therapies are also reviewed.

NEUROFIBROMATOSIS TYPE 1
Introduction and Epidemiology

NF1 is the most common neurocutaneous syndrome with estimated annual incidence of 1 in 2700 to 3300 live births,[3–5] and a frequency similar to cystic fibrosis.[6] Estimates of the mutation rate for the *NF1* gene are upwards of 1:10,000, which place it among the highest mutation rates for any known human gene.[7] Although the condition was not formally classified as a syndrome until 1882 by Dr Friedrich Daniel von Recklinghausen,[8] written descriptions of NF1 date back as far as 1000 AD.[9] Men and women are equally affected and there is no reported racial or ethnic predilection.

Pathophysiology and Genetics

NF1 results from mutations within the *NF1* gene on chromosome 17q11.2. The *NF1* gene encodes the tumor suppressor protein neurofibromin, which is a critical negative regulator of the RAS protein within the mitogen-activated protein kinase pathway.[10] NF1 follows an autosomal-dominant inheritance pattern with complete penetrance (ie, all person carrying the germline mutation are affected) but variable expressivity (ie, manifestations differ from individual to individual and even within families). Up to 30% to 50% of individuals with NF1 have no affected relatives and acquire the germline *NF1* gene mutation de novo during embryogenesis.[11–14]

NF1 is an extremely large gene (350 kb).[15] More than 100 different causative mutations have been described,[16] including nonsense (37%), splice site (28%), or frameshift mutations (18%). Approximately 80% of these result in a truncated protein, although a minority of mutations encompass a large portion of the gene (termed microdeletion, about 1.4 mBP) or the whole gene,[17] which corresponds with a more severe phenotype with early cutaneous neurofibromas, more frequent and severe cognitive disability, somatic overgrowth, and dysmorphic facial features.[18–20]

Clinical manifestations in NF1 can arise both from single and biallelic loss of the *NF1* alleles. Germline mutation of 1 *NF1* allele (the first hit) is sufficient to result in minor clinical symptoms (eg, scoliosis, learning disability, etc) owing to a phenomenon termed haploinsufficiency, where 1 functioning *NF1* gene is insufficient to maintain normal cellular function. Over time, cells may acquire the mutation in the single remaining normal *NF1* allele (the second hit). This is termed loss of heterozygosity and leads to the major manifestations of the disease, including dermal and plexiform neurofibromas, malignant peripheral nerve sheath tumors (MPNSTs), astrocytomas, café-au-lait macules (CALMs), glomus tumors, and bony dysplasia with or without pseudoarthrosis.[1,21–25] In NF1 mouse models, loss of heterozygosity is necessary but not sufficient for tumorigenesis, underscoring the role of other microenvironmental factors, including in mast cells, fibroblasts, endothelial cells, and other cells present within these tumors.[26]

Germline mutations in the *NF1* gene result in a whole body predisposition to the disease. Somatic mutations that occur after fertilization result in genetic mosaicism or segmental NF1 where only a portion of the body is affected.[22] Mosaic NF1 is typically milder with clinical manifestations limited to 1 or more regions of the body.[7,22]

Diagnostic Criteria

In 1987, the National Institutes of Health released a consensus statement defining the clinical diagnostic criteria for NF1 (**Table 1**). Studies show that these criteria continue to be highly sensitive and specific.[27,28] Clinical manifestations vary by age. CALMs are the most common first finding and are present in most individuals with NF1 before 2 to 3 years of age.[29] Although 1 or a few CALMs are not uncommon in the normal population, more than 6 CALMs of greater than 5 mm in size (prepubertal) or greater than 15 mm (postpubertal) fulfill the first clinically apparent criterion in most individuals with NF1. The most common second manifestation is intertriginous freckling followed by Lisch nodules.[29] These Lisch nodules, or iris hamartomas, often occur later in life with more than 95% of adult individuals with NF1 harboring a Lisch nodule by age 21. Because symptoms develop over time during childhood, caution must be taken to exclude other diagnoses when evaluating a young child with multiple CALMs (**Table 2**).[7,30–35]

Genetic testing is not required for the diagnosis of NF1, but is often considered in adult individuals for family planning, in young children with affected parents to establish risk, or other instances.[7] Single gene testing identifies 95% of those who meet the National Institutes of Health criteria, as long as gene DNA, compliment DNA, and whole gene or exon copy changes are tested.[31,36–39] Accuracy is lower in individuals who do not fulfill the clinical criteria for NF1.[40]

Table 1
National Institutes of Health 1987 consensus conference neurofibromatosis diagnostic criterion

	Diagnostic Criterion	Details
Must of 2 or more criterion to fulfill diagnostic criteria	Café-au-Lait Macules	• Six or more • Prepubertal: >5 mm in greatest diameter • Postpubertal: >15 mm in greatest diameter
	Neurofibromas	• Two or more dermal neurofibromas OR • One plexiform neurofibroma
	Skin fold freckling	• Located in the axillary or inguinal area
	Optic pathway glioma	
	Two or more Lisch nodules	• Two or more • Consider slit lamp exam
	Osseous lesions	• Sphenoid wing dysplasia or Pseudoarthrosis (thinning of long bone cortex with fracture contributing to "false joint"
	Family History	• First degree relative (Parents, sibling, or offspring) • Diagnosed by other 6 criteria

Data from The Office Medical Applications of Research, National Institutes of Health. Neurofibromatosis. Conference Statement. National Institutes of Health Consensus Development Conference. JAMA Neurology. 1988;45(5):575–578.

Clinical Manifestations

The various manifestations of NF1 can be divided into the following groups: cutaneous manifestations, oncologic manifestations, non-oncologic extracutaneous manifestations, and other findings.

Cutaneous manifestations

Café-au-lait macules CALMs are uniformly pigmented macules that can occur anywhere on the body, although they rarely develop on the scalp, palms, or soles. Typical CALMs are sharply demarcated and ovoid with uniform pigmentation and should be differentiated from atypical CALMs, which have a less distinct and irregular border, inhomogeneous pigmentation, and are uncommon in NF1.[41,42] The number of CALMs is important; 10% to 26% of the general population are found to have between 1 and 5 CALMs[11,43,44]; however, children with 6 or more CALMs have a 75% to 95% chance of a subsequent NF1 diagnosis,[45] often occurring by age 8.[29] CALMs increase in size proportionally with growth, usually do not continue to expand after puberty, and can fade in late adulthood.[46] Larger CALMs with hypertrichosis should be palpated because this may indicate an underlying plexiform neurofibroma.[41,42]

Intertriginous freckling Axillary freckling, also known as Crowe sign, was first described by Dr. Frank Crowe in 1956.[11] Since then freckling has also been noted in the inguinal area and is termed skin-fold freckling, which occurs in about 80% of individuals with NF1.[47,48] Skin-fold freckling is often first noted around 4 to 6 years of age and remains apparent in adolescents and adults.[41,42] Freckling is the second diagnostic criterion used to establish an NF1 diagnosis in 77% of individuals and is particularly useful in the evaluation of young children with multiple CALMs.[49]

Dermal neurofibromas Neurofibromas are the hallmark of NF1 and represent benign tumors of the peripheral nerves. These tumors are thought to arise from proliferation of nonmyelinating Schwann cells in the peripheral nerve but also consist of numerous other cell types including mast cells, fibroblasts, endothelial cells, perineural cells, hair follicles, sweat glands, and others.[50,51] Dermal neurofibromas, unlike plexiform neurofibromas, are restricted to the skin and do not pose a risk of malignant transformation, but can be painful and/or cosmetically disfiguring. Dermal neurofibromas are broadly categorized as cutaneous neurofibromas, which manifest as well-defined pink, tan, or brown papulonodules that have a soft rubbery texture[51] or subcutaneous neurofibromas, which occur deeper in the dermis and tend to be firmer, well circumscribed lesions.[41,42] Cutaneous neurofibromas have been described by their clinical appearance as nascent, flat, sessile, globular, and pedunculated, although these categories do not seem to have prognostic implications.[52] Cutaneous neurofibroma are typically asymptomatic, but can at times become pruritic or cosmetically disfiguring.[53] Subcutaneous neurofibromas are evident

Table 2
Syndromes that present with multiple CALMs

Strong association	NF1
	Multiple familial CALMs
	Legius (NF1-like) syndrome
	McCune-Albright syndrome
	Constitutional mismatch repair deficiency syndrome
	Ring chromosome syndromes
	LEOPARD/multiple lentigines syndrome
	Cowden syndromes (multiple hamartoma syndrome)
	Banayan-Riley-Ruvalcaba syndrome
Weaker association	Ataxia-telangiectasia
	Bloom syndrome
	Fanconi anemia
	Russell-Silver syndrome
	TSC
	Turner syndrome
	Noonan syndrome
	Multiple endocrine neoplasia type 1 syndrome
	Multiple endocrine neoplasia type 2B syndrome
	Johanson-Blizzard syndrome
	Microcephalic osteodysplastic primordial dwarfism, type II
	Nijmegen breakage syndrome
	Rubinstein-Taybi syndrome
	Kabuki syndrome

Syndromes associated with multiple CALMs. The strength of association is determined by how common CALMs are in each disorder; disorders with significantly greater prevalence of CALMs and higher prevalence of greater numbers of CALM compared to the normal population have a strong association and those with lower prevalence and tend to have fewer calm have a weaker association.

Adapted from Shah KN. The diagnostic and clinical significance of cafe-au-lait macules. Pediatric clinics of North America 2010;57(5):1131–1153; with permission.

on palpation and occasionally are more tender or painful when compressed.[54] Males tend to have a greater number of subcutaneous neurofibromas than females.[55] Although dermal neurofibromas have been observed as early as 4 to 5 years of age, particularly in individuals with microdeletions, they typically begin to develop around puberty and can increase in number and size throughout life, and more so during pregnancy.[41,42,46,55–58] Even when cellular atypia is present histopathologically, these tumors are benign and have no malignant potential.[51,59]

Less common cutaneous findings Individuals with NF1 have a slightly greater incidence of juvenile xanthogranulomas, nevus anemicus, and glomus tumors. Juvenile xanthogranulomas are orange papules that occur transiently in children around ages 2 to 3.[60–62] Nevus anemicus is an irregularly shaped macule that is paler than the surrounding skin and becomes red after rubbing.[63,64] Glomus tumors occur on the fingers more often than toes and present with paroxysmal pain, sensitivity to cold, reddish discoloration, and nail dystrophy.[65]

Oncologic manifestations
Cancer is the second most common cause of death in the NF1 population[66] owing to the increased overall risk of cancer,[67] despite the prognosis from individual cancers being slightly better in individuals with NF1.[68] Tumors seen in NF1 include those of the peripheral nervous system, such as benign and MPNST; central nervous system, such as the optic pathway and non-optic pathway gliomas; and tumors outside of the nervous system, such as leukemia, myelodysplastic syndrome,[7] rhabdomyosarcoma,[69] pheochromocytoma,[70] retinal vasoproliferative tumors,[71] gastrointestinal stromal tumors,[72] and early-onset breast cancer.[73–75]

Benign peripheral nerve sheath tumors Peripheral nerve sheath tumors are the prototypical tumor in NF1 and are termed plexiform neurofibromas. Plexiform neurofibromas involve the deep peripheral nerves, plexi, and surrounding tissue. They may be localized to a specific region or diffuse covering a larger region (**Fig. 2A–C, F, G**).[54] Current evidence suggests that these neoplasms are likely congenital in origin, but usually not detected until early adolescence or adulthood.[76] They tend to be tender, firm, and commonly described as a "bag of worms" texture on palpation (**Fig. 1**).[41] Presenting symptoms include pain out of proportion to examination, disfigurement, and neurologic dysfunction owing to nerve compression, as well as incidental findings on imaging. In some cases, deep plexiform neurofibromas extend to the surface causing an overlying area of pigmentation, hypertrichosis, and can resemble a congenital melanocytic nevus.[77] MRI is the method of choice for imaging plexiform neurofibromas[7] and can be used to follow the size and extent of the lesion over time,[78–83] but may not be necessary in the absence of rapid growth, new unexplained neuropathic pain, or new neurologic deficits. Although plexiform neurofibromas may grow steadily throughout life, these signs may herald malignant transformation.[84–86]

Malignant peripheral nerve sheath tumor Malignant transformation of a plexiform neurofibroma is an uncommon but devastating oncologic complication in NF1. MPNSTs are aggressive and often fatal cancers.[87] MPNST is a sarcoma of the nerve sheath cells typically developing

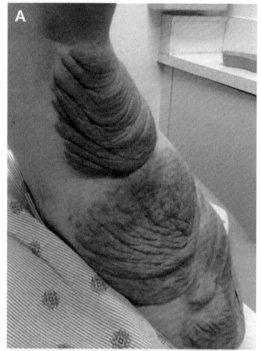

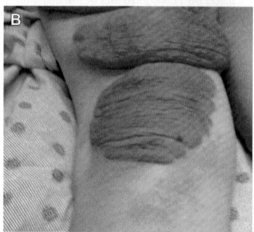

Fig. 1. Cutaneous manifestations of NF1. (*A*) Plexiform neurofibroma. (*B*) Plexiform neurofibroma from a second angle.

within an existing plexiform neurofibroma.[50] It is estimated that between 3% and 15% of individuals with NF1 will develop MPNST[13,47,67,88–91] with the peak incidence occurring between 20 and 35 years of age.[66,89] Risks of developing MPNST include previous radiotherapy, personal or family history of cancer, whole gene or microdeletion of *NF1*, and a high burden of internal plexiform neurofibromas.[20,78,82,92–100] Individuals who report rapid growth of a known plexiform neurofibroma, unexplained persistent pain, or a new neurologic deficit should be evaluated.[41] Differentiating between benign peripheral nerve sheath

tumors and MPNST on imaging has proven challenging.[101–103] Imaging features that suggest a benign biology include a size of less than 5 cm, well-defined margins, homogenous signal density, and an absence of necrosis.[104–106] Emerging studies suggest that the use of diffusion imaging may aid in noninvasively evaluating these individuals with low apparent diffusion coefficient values suggesting the risk for malignancy. In a prior study, tumors less than 4.2 cm in size with an apparent diffusion coefficient value of greater than 1.0×10^3 showed good specificity and sensitivity for BPNST.[106] PET with [18]flurodeoxyglucose has also been explored. Studies support the use of both a standard and delayed 4-hour PET to assess for prolonged tissue clearance of [18]flurodeoxyglucose, which seems to suggest a higher risk of malignancy.[56,83,107–112] Ultimately, prompt evaluation at a large-volume center and use of image-guided percutaneous tissue biopsy may be needed.[113]

Optic pathway glioma Optic pathway gliomas and non-optic gliomas are the second most common neoplasms in NF1.[114–119] Optic pathway gliomas occur in 15% to 20% of children with NF1,[119,120] with a median age at diagnosis of 4.5 years.[114,121,122] It is rare for optic pathway gliomas to develop after the age of 7 and those that do rarely require intervention.[116,123–125] Optic pathway gliomas are slow-growing, benign, pilocytic astrocytomas[119,125–128] that may occur anywhere in the optic pathway, including the optic nerve, chiasm, tract, optic radiations, and adjacent hypothalamus (**Fig. 2**D, E).[125,129,130] Even when present, individuals may never develop symptoms or require treatment and should be followed at least annually with ophthalmologic examinations to evaluate for proptosis, progressive visual compromise, and precocious puberty.[131] Optic pathway gliomas have been shown to spontaneously regress over time after puberty.[119,125,127,128] When symptomatic or progressive, response to treatment is good and outcomes tend to be more favorable than for sporadic optic pathway gliomas.[118,132,133] Extraoptic gliomas are less common and occur in only 5% of individuals with NF1,[48] frequently occurring in the brainstem (49%), cerebral hemisphere (21%), or basal ganglia (14%).[129] These lesions should not be confused with NF1 focal areas of signal intensity, which are benign and often resolve spontaneously.[134–137]

Non-oncologic extracutaneous manifestations or other clinical manifestations

All organ systems can be affected in NF1 with ophthalmologic manifestations, musculoskeletal

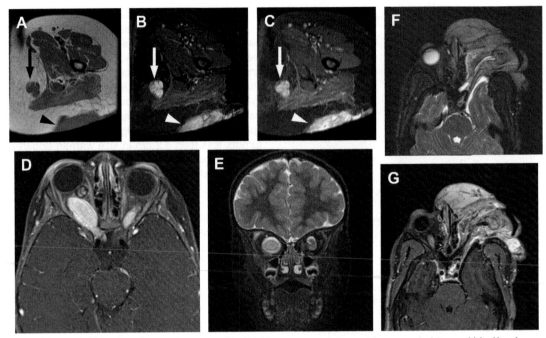

Fig. 2. Radiographic findings in NF1. Localized neurofibromas are shown with arrows (*white and black*), whereas diffuse dermal fibromas shown with arrow heads (*white and black*) (*A*) T1-weighted MRI of the thigh, (*B*) T2-weighted MRI of the thigh, (*C*) T1 contrast-enhanced MRI of the thigh, (*D*) right optic pathway glioma on contrast-enhancing MRI sagittal view, (*E*) right optic pathway glioma on T2-weighted MRI coronal view, (*F*) T2-weighted MRI of a left-sided plexiform dermal fibroma of the face, and (*G*) T1-weighted MRI of a left-sided plexiform dermal fibroma of the face.

abnormalities, cardiovascular affects, neuropsychiatric symptoms, and incidental findings on imaging being common.

Ophthalmologic manifestations Lisch nodules are pigmented hamartomas of the iris. They are usually well-defined, 1- to 2-mm dome-shaped elevations from the iris and are commonly melanotic but can vary from clear, to yellow, to brown in appearance.[41,138] Lisch nodules are best examined via slit lamp examination because this modality helps to distinguish these nodules from nevi of the iris.[138] Lisch nodules are usually not symptomatic and have no known long-term complications.[41,138] Choroidal nodules are a separate finding consisting of ovoidal deposits on the choroidal layer of the eye.[139] These nodules are not apparent on clinical examination,[140] but can be detected by near infrared reflectance imaging.[141,142]

Musculoskeletal abnormalities Two major musculoskeletal findings included in the NF1 diagnostic criteria are pseudoarthrosis and sphenoid wing dysplasia. The term pseudoarthrosis results from long bone dysplasia in which cortical bone thinning and eventual fracture leads to false joint formation, commonly in the tibia or fibula of the lower extremities.[47,76] This finding is thought to be congenital and presents with bowing of the lower leg.[7,143] Early recognition, bracing, and surgical referral is imperative.[7] Sphenoid wing dysplasia is a bony defect in the posterior wall of the orbit[7,47] that may either be incidental or present with strabismus, asymmetry of the orbits, or pulsating exophthalmos in the most advanced cases.[7,47,144] Other musculoskeletal manifestations include osteopenia, scoliosis, dural ectasia with vertebral scalloping, macrocephaly, and others.[41,143,145–148]

Cardiovascular manifestations Cardiac and vascular anomalies are more common in NF1 than the general population. Cardiovascular findings include pulmonic stenosis,[149] congenital heart defects particularly in those with whole gene or microdeletions,[150] pulmonary hypertension, or coarctation of the aorta.[151–154] Cerebral vascular manifestations include moyamoya syndrome and intracranial aneurysms, as well as a slightly higher incidence of stroke. Although individuals with NF1 may develop benign essential hypertension, new or refractory hypertension should prompt an evaluation for secondary causes, including pheochromocytoma or renal artery stenosis.[155,156]

Neurologic and neuropsychiatric manifestations

Severe intellectual disability is uncommon in NF1, although mild intellectual disability or behavioral disorders are extremely common and have been reported in up to 80% of individuals with NF1.[47,148,157–161] Autism, attention deficit hyperactivity disorder, headache disorders, and sleep disturbances are also seen.[47,148,162–166] Seizures are seen in 5% of individuals and can require management with more than 1 antiepileptic drug.[167,168]

The average lifespan in individuals with NF1 has been reported to be 8 years shorter than healthy controls,[14,66] which is mostly attributed to malignancy and vasculopathy.[66,88,169,170] These numbers are improved from previous estimates of a decreased life expectancy by up to 15 years.[169] Irrespective of life expectancy, children and adults report lower quality of life,[171–173] most likely stemming from the cosmetic, medical, social, and behavioral manifestations of NF1.[174]

Surveillance and Treatment

The diverse manifestations associated with NF1 do not lend themselves to a single algorithm for diagnostic assessment and treatment. Guidelines for surveillance and management have been reviewed elsewhere.[7,28,45,175–178] In general, multidisciplinary approaches to evaluation, surveillance, and management are optimal.[179,180] Referral to specialists with experience in NF1 is always preferred, but at the minimum the following specialties should be considered: geneticist, pediatrician, neurologist, and dermatologist.[45,181]

Surveillance

Before diagnosis, surveillance of children presenting with 3 or more CALMs is recommended to screen for other manifestations of NF1 because 1 in 3 of these children will go on to meet the diagnostic criteria.[182,183] At the time of diagnosis, a thorough evaluation should be performed to screen for dermatologic, musculoskeletal, cardiovascular, ophthalmologic (using slit lamp examination), and neurologic manifestations.[7] A thorough family history should not be overlooked. For children who meet the diagnostic criteria, developmental assessment, consultation with clinical geneticist or genetic counselor, and system-specific surveillance should be initiated (**Table 3**).

Treatment

In general, the treatment of NF1 is primarily supportive; however, emerging studies are evaluating symptom-specific disease-modifying treatments.

For CALMs, observation and surgical treatment have been the mainstay of management.

Table 3	
Recommended surveillance for pediatric and adult patients with NF1, organized by clinical examination	
Examination	**Description**
Pediatric	
Dermatologic examination	Complete evaluation annually; disfiguring or painful lesions should be referred to surgery; rapidly growing lesions should be evaluated by PET/CT.
Ophthalmologic examination	Examination and visual assessment annually; visual acuity testing and fundoscopic examination annually from 2 to 7 y of age; MRI orbits as indicated by clinical examination.
Musculoskeletal examination	Evaluation for scoliosis, tibial bowing, and macrocephaly annually; abnormalities referred orthopedic and evaluated by radiography or CT scan.
Developmental survey	Before beginning school and as needed; this may involve formal neurocognitive assessment and/or accommodation with schoolwork (eg, individualized education program).
Endocrine screening	Evaluate if precocious puberty occurs; orbital/brain MRI and endocrine referral.
Blood pressure monitoring	Annually; if hypertensive undergo renal arteriography and 24-h urine catecholamine and metanephrine testing.
Neurologic examination	Complete examination annually; MRI as needed; no evidence for evaluation of asymptomatic lesions.

(continued on next page)

Table 3 (continued)	
Examination	Description
Adult	
Blood pressure monitoring	Annually; if hypertensive repeat in triplicate over 1 mo, if persistent undergo renal arteriography and 24-h urine catecholamine and metanephrine testing.
Breast cancer monitoring	Clinical examination and mammography annually beginning at age 30; Contrast-enhanced breast MRI can be considered between ages 30–50
Neurologic examination	Complete examination annually; MRI as needed; no evidence for evaluation for asymptomatic lesions
Ophthalmologic examination	Screen every 2 y for early onset glaucoma, cataracts,
Neurocognitive examination	Select adult patients may benefit from neurocognitive assessment and/or vocational rehab for developmentally delayed

Data from Refs.[7,28,45,175–178]

The benefits of surgical removal should be balanced against the risk of the procedure, recurrence, and scarring. Typical indications for surgical removal include pain, disfigurement, or symptomatic location (eg, belt or brassiere line). Pruritus can be particularly problematic and responds poorly to antihistamines. Excision and laser treatments are all available, with no clear efficacy advantage of one over the other.[45] Laser treatment has been cited as less laborious when lesions are numerous.[184] Referral to a plastic surgeon may be needed for lesions on the face.[45,185,186] Radiation therapy is avoided owing to the risk of malignant transformation.[7,187]

For progressive plexiform neurofibromas, the landscape for managing these tumors is rapidly changing. Historically, no systemic agents were available for treating these lesions and management was primarily surgical. Surgical removal is most beneficial with superficial plexiform neurofibromas that are small and localized[188] to avoid postoperative neurologic deficits. Complication rates can be high and referral to high-volume centers should be considered.[45] Emerging data support the consideration of targeted therapies for selected progressive and/or symptomatic plexiform neurofibromas. Imatinib, a tyrosine kinase inhibitor, was shown to have modest activity in children with progressive plexiform neurofibromas, particularly in those of the head, neck, and upper airway.[189,190] Selumetinib, a MEK inhibitor, is perhaps one of the most promising emerging therapies. Results of a phase I study of selumetinib for progressive plexiform neurofibroma in children with NF1 showed a remarkable 71% objective response rate and subsequent studies could establish a definitive role in MEK pathway modulation for the treatment of progressive plexiform neurofibromas.[191] As of the writing of this article, several clinical trials are ongoing to further evaluate plexiform neurofibroma treatment with selumetinib (NCT03259633, NCT02407405, NCT03326388), imatinib (NCT02177825), PLX3397 (NCT02390752), binimetinib (NCT03231306), trametinib (NCT03741101, NCT03363217), and cabozantinib (NCT02101736).

The management of MPNSTs is extremely challenging owing to the aggressive nature of these cancers. Currently the best treatment for possible cure includes complete surgical excision with tumor free margins,[93,192,193] which may not be possible in many cases. Radiotherapy and chemotherapy have been used occasionally and have shown mixed results.[193–195] Radiotherapy is commonly used as adjuvant therapy under the following circumstances: MPNST greater than 5 cm, high-grade MPNST, or incompletely excised MPNST.[93] Chemotherapy is commonly used on a palliative treatment basis with the most common regimens including ifosfamide and doxorubicin.[93]

The treatment of optic pathway gliomas is recommended when symptoms become progressive or vision loss occurs.[56] Chemotherapy has been the historical treatment of choice with regimens including carboplatin/vincristine, vinblastine, or carboplatin.[56,131,196–198] Response rates for tumor growth are as high as 60% to 70%.[125,199–203] Radiation therapy is only used if the optic pathway glioma has failed to respond to chemotherapy. Increasingly, targeted agents are being explored and early results have shown promise. Current clinical trials at the time of this writing include selumetinib (NCT03326388, NCT01089101), trametinib (NCT03363217), lenalidomide (NCT01553149), and pomalidomide (NCT02415153).

TUBEROUS SCLEROSIS COMPLEX
Introduction and Epidemiology

TSC is a neurocutaneous condition resulting from hamartomatous growth in major organs including the brain, kidney, lungs, cardiac, and other tissues.[204] The first observations of TSC date back to the mid 1800s when Virchow first described scleromas of the brain and von Recklinghausen reported an individual with scleromas and myomata of the heart.[47] The link between these cutaneous and the neurologic findings were not discovered until Bourneville in the late 1800s.[41] In the early 20th century a triad was described by Campbell and then Vogt, initially termed the Vogt triad, which consisted of intellectual disability, epilepsy, and angiofibromas.[205,206] Ultimately, its genetic link was determined in the mid 1900s. Compared with NF1, TSC is rare with an annual incidence of 1 in 5800 to 10,000 live births.[207-213] There is no ethnic or sex predilection.[212,213]

Pathophysiology and Genetics

Like NF1, TSC follows an autosomal-dominant inheritance pattern. De novo mutations are common with 70% of individuals harboring new germline mutations and lacking a family history.[41,205] Two genes have been identified as causing TSC including TSC1 and TSC2. TSC1 was discovered in the 1980s on chromosome 9q34[41,214] and produces a protein called hamartin. TSC2 was isolated later in 1992 on chromosome 16p13[212,215] and produces a protein called tuberin. Originally, estimates showed an equal prevalence of TSC1 and TSC2[216]; however, recent reports show this is likely only true in familial inherited cases. Like NF1, there is complete penetrance but variable expressivity.[214]

Hamartin and tuberin form a complex[217] that acts as a tumor suppressor GTPase for Rheb.[218-224] By dephosphorylating Rheb-GTP to Rheb-GDP, the TSC1–TSC2 complex inhibits the activation of mTORC1, a driver of cellular growth, and possibly independently inactivates mTORC2.[225] Figures and explanation of this mechanism are shown elsewhere.[225]

Diagnostic Criteria

Diagnostic guidelines were published in 1998 and revised to include genetic testing in 2012 by the International Tuberous Sclerosis Complex Consensus.[204] Identification of a pathogenic mutation for TSC1 or TSC2 from biopsy of normal tissue provides a definitive diagnosis for TSC. However, up to 10% to 25% of individuals with clinical TSC have no identified mutation and the lack of genetic findings should not exclude a diagnosis of TSC.

Clinical diagnostic criteria are divided into major criteria and minor criteria (Table 4). A definitive diagnosis requires fulfilling (1) 2 major criteria, or (2) 1 major criterion and 2 or more minor criteria. A possible diagnosis of TSC can be fulfilled by (1) 1 major criterion, or (2) 2 or more minor criteria. Common first features include cardiac rhabdomyoma (often via antenatal identification), hypopigmented macules, seizures, or infantile spasms

Table 4
Clinical diagnostic criteria for TSC

Features	
Major	
Hypomelanotic macules (Ash leaf spots)	Three or more Five millimeters or more in diameter
Angiofibromas or fibrous cephalic plaque	Three or more angiofibromas One or more fibrous cephalic plaque
Ungal fibromas	Two or more
Shagreen patch	
Retinal hamartomas	Two or more
Cortical tubers (or other cortical dysplasias, ie, whiter matter radial migration lines)	
Subependymal nodules	
Cardiac rhabdomyoma	
Pulmonary lymphangioleiomyoma[a]	
Angiomyolipomas[a]	Two or more
Minor	
Confetti lesions	
Dental enamel pits	Three or more
Intraoral fibromas	Two or more
Retinal achromatic patch	
Multiple renal cysts	
Nonretinal hamartoma	

[a] If lymphangioleiomyoma and angiomyolipomas co-occur, combined they count as 1 major feature, not 2.

Adapted from Northrup H, Krueger DA, International Tuberous Sclerosis Complex Consensus G. Tuberous sclerosis complex diagnostic criteria update: recommendations of the 2012 International Tuberous Sclerosis Complex Consensus Conference. Pediatr Neurol 2013;49(4):243–254; with permission.

in childhood.[214] Other conditions that can mimic TSC include multiple endocrine neoplasia type 1, Birt-Hogg Dube syndrome, acne vulgaris, trichoepitheliomas, idiopathy guttate hypomelanosis, and congenital hypopigmented macules.[41,226]

Clinical manifestations

Similar to NF1, manifestations of TSC vary widely between individuals (ie, variable expressivity) and relate to the presence and location of hamartomas. Hamartomas are benign overgrowths of normal tissue. They can be found in almost any organ system, but most prominently occur in the skin, brain, kidneys, lungs, and heart of individuals with TSC.

Cutaneous manifestations

Cutaneous manifestations are seen in approximately 90% of individuals with TSC and are a common reason to seek medical attention.[227]

Hypomelanotic macules Originally termed Ash leaf spots owing to the common appearance of a round side with contralateral tapering to a sharp edge shape, these characteristics findings are present in 90% of those with skin lesions.[41,42,214] Three or more hypopigmented lesions greater than 5 mm in diameter is one of the most specific diagnostic findings.[204,228] Hypomelanotic macules are seen in only 1% to 4% of healthy infants, and more than 3 lesions have not been reported in a healthy child.[229–231] These lesions are typically present at birth or in early infancy[41,232,233] and are a valuable early diagnostic marker. A woods lamp examination may be useful in evaluating individuals with light-colored skin.

Shagreen patch Shagreen patches are collagenoma-like lesions found on the lumbosacral area with an orange peel appearance.[41,42,214] The prevalence is estimated to be as high as 50% in those with TSC and often occur in the first decade of life.[204,228] The patches may be hypopigmented, hyperpigmented, or skin colored. Similar collagenomas are seen in other TSC mimickers: multiple endocrine neoplasia type 1, Birt-Hugg Dube syndrome, and Cowden syndrome.[204]

Angiofibromas Angiofibromas are cutaneous lesions occurring on the face (facial angiofibromas) and hands (ungal fibromas). Although 1 or 2 fibromas are common in the general healthy population, 3 or more is rare and fulfills a major diagnostic criterion.[204] Ungal fibromas may be periungual and subungual, appearing as fleshy fibromatous lesions in the proximal and lateral nailfolds (**Fig. 3**), where they manifest as red streaks

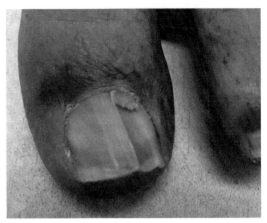

Fig. 3. Cutaneous manifestations of TSC. Ungal angiofibroma.

with proximal narrowing or red comets.[41] If seen close to the matrix of the nail, longitudinal ridging is commonly seen.[205] These lesions commonly occur in the second decade and are more common in females.[233–235] Facial angiofibromas are similar in appearance to ungal fibromas but are located in the centrofacial area and occur earlier in life. They often begin as an erythematous macule and progress to red/red-brown smooth shiny papules on the bilateral malar area, nasal dorsum, nasolabial folds, forehead, and chin.[41,212,236] Facial fibromas are not usually present at birth, but begin to manifest in the first decade and increase in number with adolescence.[214,237]

Fibrous cephalic plaque Fibrous cephalic plaques are large variants of angiofibromas located on the forehead, scalp, and face in almost equal frequencies.[238] They are found in 20% to 36% of individuals[204,228,238] appearing as firm, yellow or brown, and are slow growing (eg, commonly <5 cm).[41,238]

Confetti lesions These hypomelanotic lesions are smaller in size (<5 cm) than Ash leaf spots. Often appearing in groups or clusters, these hypomelanotic lesions often develop in the first decade of life.[204] Later onset in adulthood has been described in 58% of adults.[233,237] Commonly confused with guttate leukoderma, it is essential to remember than confetti lesions are asymmetric and appear in childhood.[205]

Oral lesions Oral lesions seen in TSC include intraoral fibromas and dental enamel pits. Intraoral fibromas are normal or violaceous in color and located in the gingiva, buccal mucosa, labial mucosa, or tongue.[204,229,239,240] The prevalence of these intraoral fibromas have been reported to be between 20% and 70% of people with TSC.[229,232,233,239–241] Dental enamel pitting is seen in virtually all people with diagnosed TSC.[242] Of note, the clinical usefulness of this finding is in question, because it has been found in the healthy population between 7% and 70% of the time.[242]

Oncologic manifestations
Tumorous growths in TSC most frequently occur in the nervous system, cardiovascular system, renal system, pulmonary system, and others.

Nervous system oncologic manifestations Nervous system lesions include subependymal nodules subependymal giant cell astrocytoma (SEGA), cortical tubers, and retinal hamartomas. Subependymal nodules are benign overgrowths of the ependymal tissue lining the ventricles in the brain (**Fig. 4**A).[131,204] These tumors are often present at birth (80% of 2-year-olds) with an increased prevalence with advancing age.[214,237,243] There is a tendency for these nodules to calcify over time leading to visible findings on imaging.[41,131] Subependymal nodules rarely enlarge, do not enhance with gadolinium contrast (**Fig. 4**C), and are typically not symptomatic. SEGAs also arise along the ependymal surface of the ventricles and are considered a benign tumor that can grow, enhance with gadolinium contrast on MRI (**Fig. 4**A, B) and can contribute to morbidity and rarely mortality. SEGAs are present in 5% to 15% of individuals with TSC, are more common during childhood, and rarely seen after 20 years of age.[243,244] Findings that herald SEGA growth include ventriculomegaly and obstructive hydrocephalus.[204,205,245] Cortical tubers are the neuropathologic hallmark of the disease. These glioneuronal hamartomas are regions of dysplastic neural proliferation, form during fetal development, and are seen in the cortex (cortical nodule or tuber)

(see **Fig. 4**A) and subcortex (subcortical nodule or tuber). They have no malignant potential.[204,237] Multiple cortical tubers are seen in up to 90% of individuals with TSC and are rare in the general population.[204] Retinal hamartomas are flat translucent or mulberry-like lesions seen in 30% to 50% of individuals with TSC[41,214] and are rarely symptomatic.[214] Epilepsy occurs in 70% to 90% of those with TSC.[41,211,214] Seizures are thought to arise in the vicinity of cortical tubers and can be reduced with surgical resection of an offending tuber, but multiple mechanisms may be involved in TSC-associated epilepsy.

Cardiovascular system oncologic manifestations Rhabdomyoma, or benign tumors of the cardiac muscle, can be an early sign of TSC and are often discovered within the cardiac ventricle[204,246] on prenatal echocardiogram after the 20th week of gestation.[246] The presence of multiple cardiac rhabdomyomas at birth confers a 75% to 80% chance of a subsequent TSC diagnosis.[214,247–249] Although usually asymptomatic, manifestations may range from ventricular dysfunction, valvular dysfunction, cardiomegaly, arrhythmia, nonimmune hydrops fetalis, and death.[204,214] Cardiac rhabdomyomas can resolve spontaneously with age.[250]

Renal system oncologic manifestations Angiomyolipomas are benign tumors composed of vascular cells, immature smooth muscle cells, and adipose tissue. The presence of 2 angiomyolipomas fulfills a major diagnostic criterion and is present in up to 80% of the individuals with TSC.[214] Angiomyolipomas commonly present as asymptomatic kidney lesions,[251] but can result in hematuria, loss of kidney function, and in rare cases hemorrhage, dialysis, or need for transplantation, particularly with larger lesions.[204,214] Angiomyolipomas tend to develop in childhood and slowly enlarge until early adulthood. Growth ceases in

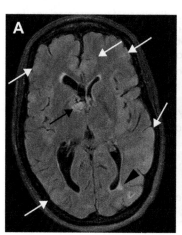
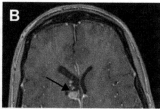
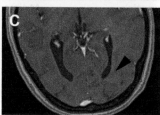

Fig. 4. Radiographic findings in TSC, including (A) fluid-attenuated inversion recovery MRI showing SEGA (*black arrow*), subependymal nodules (*black arrowhead*), and multiple cortical tubers (*white arrows*), (B) contrasted MRI study showing enhancing SEGA (*black arrow*), and (C) contrasted MRI showing nonenhancing subependymal nodule (*black arrowhead*).

up to 30% of adults.[252,253] Angiomyolipomas in the liver are rarer, reported in 10% to 25% of individuals,[254–256] and do contribute to the major diagnostic criteria.[204] Renal cell carcinoma can occur and is more common in TSC than the general population. Few studies have determined the prognostic and therapeutic implications of renal cell carcinoma in this population.[257,258]

Pulmonary system oncologic manifestations
Lymphangioleiomyomatosis (LAM) of the lung arises from benign interstitial expansion of the smooth muscle cells of the lung.[259,260] Unlike other findings, there is a female predominance affecting 30% to 80% of females and 10% to 12% of males[41,252,261–264] with TSC. LAM typically presents in the third to fourth decade[204] with symptoms of worsening dyspnea and recurrent pneumothoraces. High-resolution CT shows cystic pulmonary lesions.[41] Confirmation by pathologic examination can be necessary when other clinical diagnostic features are not present. To facilitate noninvasive diagnosis, the European Respiratory Society established diagnostic criteria by high resolution CT scan[259] that include (1) profusion of more than 4 cysts, no confounding comorbidities/exposures and at least 1 other major or 2 minor criteria for TSC (outside of angiomyolipoma), or (2) one of the following: abdominal or thoracic LAM, chylous pleural effusion, or chylous ascites.[204]

Table 5
Surveillance recommendations for TSC

System	Description	Frequency
Dental	Dental examination – Oral fibroma and dental enamel pits	Every 6 mo (as general population).
Neuropsychiatric	Screen for behavior problems and intellectual disability – TS-associated neuropsychiatric disorder	Annually.
	Comprehensive neuropsychiatric screening – TS-associated neuropsychiatric disorder	Once during the following age ranges: 0–3, 3–6, 6–9, 12–16, 18–25.
Neurologic	EEG – Epileptiform activity	At time of diagnosis; 24-h monitoring as needed after suspected seizure activity, behavioral change, or positive comprehensive neuropsychiatric screening.
	Brain MRI with and without contrast – Cortical tubers and SEGA	At time of diagnosis; repeat every 1–3 y or more often is suspected/known SEGA.
Cardiovascular	Echocardiogram – Rhabdomyoma	At time of diagnosis if <3 old; repeat for asymptomatic lesions every 1–3 y until regression; referral to cardiology if symptomatic.
	ECG – Arrhythmias	At time of diagnosis.
	Blood pressure monitoring	Annually.
Pulmonary	High resolution CT scan, 6-min walk test, pulmonary function testing – LAM	At time of diagnosis if symptomatic or if a woman ≥18 y old; repeat every 5–10 y if asymptomatic; repeat every 2–3 y if symptomatic.
Renal	Abdominal MRI (ultrasound or CT can be done but less sensitive) – Angiomyolipoma and renal cysts	At time of diagnosis; repeat every 1–3 y.
	Glomerular filtration rate	Annually.
Dermatologic	Complete skin examination – Hypomelanotic macules, shagreen patches, angiofibromas, fibrous cephalic plaques, confetti lesions, oral lesions	At time of diagnosis and annually.
Ophthalmologic	Dilated fundoscopic examination – Retinal hamartomas or eye lesion	At time of diagnosis; annually if known lesion.

Data from Refs.[214,251,269]

Extracutaneous non-oncologic or other manifestations

Epilepsy is common and occurs in 70% to 90% of individuals with TSC.[214] Infantile spasms are the most common type of seizure to develop in individuals with TSC less than 1 year old; other seizure types occur in older individuals.[265] Other disorders termed TS-associated neuropsychiatric disorders are seen in 30% to 50% of the TSC population[245,252] and include intellectual disability, autism, attention deficit hyperactivity disorder, aggressive behaviors, anxiety, depression, sleep disorders, learning difficulties, and other biopsychosocial difficulties.[245,266,267]

Surveillance and Treatment

Surveillance

Recommendations for diagnosis and surveillance have been extensively reviewed[214,251,268,269] (Table 5). At the time of diagnosis, a full history of dermatologic symptoms, seizures, intellectual disability, behavior abnormalities, pulmonary symptoms, cardiac symptoms, and renal or genitourinary symptoms should be conducted; first-degree relatives should be offered a clinical assessment for a possible TSC diagnosis. A 3-generation family history is imperative. Genetic testing and genetic counseling should be offered.

Treatment

The cutaneous manifestations of TSC usually do not need to be actively managed unless they are disfiguring or have a high bleeding risk.[269] The current therapies include surgery, laser therapy, and topical mammalian target of rapamycin (mTOR) inhibitors. Procedural interventions such as electrosurgery, dermabrasion, and ablative fraction pulsed dye laser lead to variable results; however, they tend to be painful and have high recurrence rates with possible hypertrophic scarring.[205,270,271] Ungal fibromas are especially known to recur.[205] Topical mTOR inhibitors have shown benefit for angiofibroma, fibrous plaques, and hypomelanotic macules.[213,236,272–274] A twin study even showed a possible prophylactic benefit to mTOR inhibitors in preventing angiofibroma formation,[275] which may counter the current guidance to only treat fibromas after adolescence.[214] Intraoral fibromas may be excised if symptomatic or interfere with oral hygiene. Those with a high cavity risk and dental pits may undergo restorative treatment.

Historically, surgery has been the mainstay treatment of symptomatic SEGA with indications including acute hydrocephalus, increased seizure burden, or a rapid increase in the tumor growth rate[276–280]; however, prophylactic intervention is currently being investigated.[281,282] The International TSC Consensus Conference suggested good surgical candidates with unilateral singular SEGA undergo surgery and all other candidates should consider medical therapy[269,283] owing to adverse effects of surgical intervention.[131,277,278] Gamma knife surgery, reserved only for recurrent SEGA,[284] has shown benefit.[276,285] The mTOR inhibitors are considered first line for medical therapy, particularly everolimus[283,286–289], however, there is concern of SEGA recurrence with discontinuation. The mTOR inhibitors have also shown benefit with seizures[290–292] and possibly for TS-associated neuropsychiatric disorder.[269] Treatment for symptomatic and asymptomatic epileptic activity is suggested[293–295] with no medical therapy showing specific advantage except vigabatrin for infantile spasm[296,297] and vagal nerve stimulator for children at risk of regression.[269] Cannabidiol is currently being investigated for seizure control[298] (NCT02544763). Acute neurologic symptom onset should prompt emergent imaging for possible surgical resection or cerebrospinal fluid diversion should be undergone.

Treatment of angiomyolipomas is reserved for tumors more than 3 cm in diameter[269] owing to the risk of hemorrhage.[299] The first-line therapy is an mTOR inhibitor,[300,301] with either embolization followed by steroids, kidney-sparing resection, or ablation (considered second line).[269] If hemorrhage does occur, embolization followed by corticosteroid therapy is preferred.[269] Should screening reveal growth of 0.5 cm or more per year, then a biopsy should be obtained to rule out renal cell carcinoma.[269] Like many other manifestations, LAM has shown good benefit from mTOR inhibitors,[300,302,303] with lung transplant reserved for treatment-resistant cases.[269]

SUMMARY

The neurocutaneous syndromes are a heterogeneous group of conditions that have cutaneous, oncologic, neurologic, and other manifestations which dermatologists should be aware. NF1 should be suspected in children presenting with 6 or more CALMs and intertriginous freckling or Lisch nodules; monitoring is required for dermatologic or neurologic changes that may herald underlying oncologic disease. TSC has diverse manifestations resulting from hamartoma formation in various systems including the brain, kidney, lung, heart, and skin; surveillance includes screening for complications of these hamartomas as well as TS-associated neuropsychiatric disorder. Novel therapies, especially MEK inhibitors for selected NF1 tumors and mTOR inhibitors for

TSC, are showing promise in controlling the dermatologic, oncologic, and other organ manifestations of these tumor suppressor neurocutaneous syndromes.

REFERENCES

1. Emmerich D, Zemojtel T, Hecht J, et al. Somatic neurofibromatosis type 1 (NF1) inactivation events in cutaneous neurofibromas of a single NF1 patient. Eur J Hum Genet 2015;23(6):870–3.

2. Islam MP, Roach ES. Neurocutaneous syndromes. Handb Clin Neurol 2016;135:565–89.

3. Friedman JM. Epidemiology of neurofibromatosis type 1. Am J Med Genet 1999;89(1):1–6.

4. Lammert M, Friedman JM, Kluwe L, et al. Prevalence of neurofibromatosis 1 in German children at elementary school enrollment. Arch Dermatol 2005;141(1):71–4.

5. Evans DG, Howard E, Giblin C, et al. Birth incidence and prevalence of tumor-prone syndromes: estimates from a UK family genetic register service. Am J Med Genet A 2010;152A(2):327–32.

6. O'Sullivan BP, Freedman SD. Cystic fibrosis. Lancet 2009;373(9678):1891–904.

7. Friedman JM. Neurofibromatosis 1. 1998 Oct 2. In: Adam MP, Ardinger HH, Pagon RA, et al, editors. GeneReviews® [Internet]. Seattle (WA): University of Washington, Seattle; 1993-2019. Available at: https://www.ncbi.nlm.nih.gov/books/NBK1109/.

8. Antonio JR, Goloni-Bertollo EM, Tridico LA. Neurofibromatosis: chronological history and current issues. An Bras Dermatol 2013;88(3):329–43.

9. Zanca A, Zanca A. Antique illustrations of neurofibromatosis. Int J Dermatol 1980;19(1):55–8.

10. Wigler MH. Oncoproteins. GAPs in understanding ras. Nature 1990;346(6286):696–7.

11. Crowe FW. A clinical, pathological, and genetic study of multiple neurofibromatosis. Springfield (IL): Charles C Thomas Publishers; 1956.

12. Samuelsson B, Axelsson R. Neurofibromatosis. A clinical and genetic study of 96 cases in Gothenburg, Sweden. Acta Derm Venereol Suppl (Stockh) 1981;95:67–71.

13. Huson SM, Compston DA, Clark P, et al. A genetic study of von Recklinghausen neurofibromatosis in south east Wales. I. Prevalence, fitness, mutation rate, and effect of parental transmission on severity. J Med Genet 1989;26(11):704–11.

14. Wilding A, Ingham SL, Lalloo F, et al. Life expectancy in hereditary cancer predisposing diseases: an observational study. J Med Genet 2012;49(4):264–9.

15. Heim RA, Silverman LM, Farber RA, et al. Screening for truncated NF1 proteins. Nat Genet 1994;8(3):218–9.

16. Abernathy CR, Rasmussen SA, Stalker HJ, et al. NF1 mutation analysis using a combined heteroduplex/SSCP approach. Hum Mutat 1997;9(6):548–54.

17. Kluwe L, Siebert R, Gesk S, et al. Screening 500 unselected neurofibromatosis 1 patients for deletions of the NF1 gene. Hum Mutat 2004;23(2):111–6.

18. Mautner VF, Kluwe L, Friedrich RE, et al. Clinical characterisation of 29 neurofibromatosis type-1 patients with molecularly ascertained 1.4 Mb type-1 NF1 deletions. J Med Genet 2010;47(9):623–30.

19. Pasmant E, Sabbagh A, Spurlock G, et al. NF1 microdeletions in neurofibromatosis type 1: from genotype to phenotype. Hum Mutat 2010;31(6):E1506–18.

20. Kehrer-Sawatzki H, Cooper DN. NF1 microdeletions and their underlying mutational mechanisms. In: Upadhyaya M, Cooper DN, editors. Neurofibromatosis type 1. Berlin: Springer-Verlag; 2012. p. 187–209.

21. Colman SD, Williams CA, Wallace MR. Benign neurofibromas in type 1 neurofibromatosis (NF1) show somatic deletions of the NF1 gene. Nat Genet 1995;11(1):90–2.

22. Maertens O, De Schepper S, Vandesompele J, et al. Molecular dissection of isolated disease features in mosaic neurofibromatosis type 1. Am J Hum Genet 2007;81(2):243–51.

23. De Schepper S, Maertens O, Callens T, et al. Somatic mutation analysis in NF1 cafe au lait spots reveals two NF1 hits in the melanocytes. J Invest Dermatol 2008;128(4):1050–3.

24. Upadhyaya M, Chuzhanova N, Cooper DN. The somatic mutational spectrum of the NF1 gene. In: Upadhyaya M, Cooper DN, editors. Neurofibromatosis type 1. Berlin: Springer-Verlag; 2012. p. 211–33.

25. Kobus K, Hartl D, Ott CE, et al. Double NF1 inactivation affects adrenocortical function in NF1Prx1 mice and a human patient. PLoS One 2015;10(3):e0119030.

26. Yang FC, Ingram DA, Chen S, et al. Nf1-dependent tumors require a microenvironment containing Nf1+/– and c-kit-dependent bone marrow. Cell 2008;135(3):437–48.

27. Ferner R, Huson S, Evans DG. Neurofibromatoses in clinical practice. London: Springer; 2011.

28. Ferner RE, Gutmann DH. Neurofibromatosis type 1 (NF1): diagnosis and management. Handb Clin Neurol 2013;115:939–55.

29. Nunley KS, Gao F, Albers AC, et al. Predictive value of cafe au lait macules at initial consultation in the diagnosis of neurofibromatosis type 1. Arch Dermatol 2009;145(8):883–7.

30. Brems H, Pasmant E, Van Minkelen R, et al. Review and update of SPRED1 mutations causing Legius syndrome. Hum Mutat 2012;33(11):1538–46.

31. Evans DG, Bowers N, Burkitt-Wright E, et al. Comprehensive RNA analysis of the NF1 gene in classically affected NF1 affected individuals meeting NIH criteria has high sensitivity and mutation negative testing is reassuring in isolated cases with pigmentary features only. EBioMedicine 2016; 7:212–20.

32. Wimmer K, Rosenbaum T, Messiaen L. Connections between constitutional mismatch repair deficiency syndrome and neurofibromatosis type 1. Clin Genet 2017;91(4):507–19.

33. Stevens CA, Chiang PW, Messiaen LM. Cafe-au-lait macules and intertriginous freckling in piebaldism: clinical overlap with neurofibromatosis type 1 and Legius syndrome. Am J Med Genet A 2012; 158a(5):1195–9.

34. Merker VL, Esparza S, Smith MJ, et al. Clinical features of schwannomatosis: a retrospective analysis of 87 patients. Oncologist 2012;17(10): 1317–22.

35. Colley A, Donnai D, Evans DG. Neurofibromatosis/ Noonan phenotype: a variable feature of type 1 neurofibromatosis. Clin Genet 1996;49(2):59–64.

36. Wimmer K, Yao S, Claes K, et al. Spectrum of single- and multiexon NF1 copy number changes in a cohort of 1,100 unselected NF1 patients. Genes Chromosomes Cancer 2006;45(3):265–76.

37. Messiaen L, Wimmer K. NF1 mutational spectrum. In: Kaufmann D, editor. Neurofibromatoses monographs in human genetics, vol. 16. Basel (Switzerland): Karger; 2008. p. 63–77.

38. Valero MC, Martin Y, Hernandez-Imaz E, et al. A highly sensitive genetic protocol to detect NF1 mutations. J Mol Diagn 2011;13(2):113–22.

39. Sabbagh A, Pasmant E, Imbard A, et al. NF1 molecular characterization and neurofibromatosis type I genotype-phenotype correlation: the French experience. Hum Mutat 2013;34(11):1510–8.

40. Stella A, Lastella P, Loconte DC, et al. Accurate classification of NF1 gene variants in 84 Italian patients with neurofibromatosis type 1. Genes (Basel) 2018;9(4) [pii:E216].

41. Tsao H, Luo S. Neurofibromatosis and tuberous sclerosis complex. In: Bolognia J, Schaffer J, Cerroni L, editors. Dermatology. 4th edition; 2018. p. 985–1003.

42. Strowd RE, Strowd LC, Blakeley JO. Cutaneous manifestations in neuro-oncology: clinically relevant tumor and treatment associated dermatologic findings. Semin Oncol 2016;43(3):401–7.

43. Whitehouse D. Diagnostic value of the cafe-au-lait spot in children. Arch Dis Child 1966;41(217): 316–9.

44. Burwell RG, James NJ, Johnston DI. Cafe-au-lait spots in schoolchildren. Arch Dis Child 1982; 57(8):631–2.

45. Ferner RE, Huson SM, Thomas N, et al. Guidelines for the diagnosis and management of individuals with neurofibromatosis 1. J Med Genet 2007; 44(2):81–8.

46. Duong TA, Bastuji-Garin S, Valeyrie-Allanore L, et al. Evolving pattern with age of cutaneous signs in neurofibromatosis type 1: a cross-sectional study of 728 patients. Dermatology 2011;222(3): 269–73.

47. Pivnick EK, Riccardi V. The neurofibromatoses. In: Freedberg IM, Eisen AZ, Wolff K, et al, editors. Fitzpatrick's dermatology in general medicine. 6th edition. New York: McGraw-Hill; 2003. p. 1825–33.

48. McGaughran JM, Harris DI, Donnai D, et al. A clinical study of type 1 neurofibromatosis in north west England. J Med Genet 1999;36(3):197–203.

49. Korf BR. Diagnostic outcome in children with multiple cafe au lait spots. Pediatrics 1992;90(6):924–7.

50. Woodruff JM. Pathology of tumors of the peripheral nerve sheath in type 1 neurofibromatosis. Am J Med Genet 1999;89(1):23–30.

51. Jouhilahti EM, Peltonen S, Callens T, et al. The development of cutaneous neurofibromas. Am J Pathol 2011;178(2):500–5.

52. Riccardi V. An overview of NF-1: dysplasia and neoplasia. In: Riccardi VM, editor. Neurofibromatosis: phenotype, natural history, and pathogenesis. Baltimore (MD): The Johns Hopkins University Press; 1992. p. 28–33.

53. Brenaut E, Nizery-Guermeur C, Audebert-Bellanger S, et al. Clinical characteristics of pruritus in neurofibromatosis 1. Acta Derm Venereol 2016;96(3):398–9.

54. Korf BR. Plexiform neurofibromas. Am J Med Genet 1999;89(1):31–7.

55. Sbidian E, Duong TA, Valeyrie-Allanore L, et al. Neurofibromatosis type 1: neurofibromas and sex. Br J Dermatol 2016;174(2):402–4.

56. Plotkin SR, Wick A. Neurofibromatosis and schwannomatosis. Semin Neurol 2018;38(1):73–85.

57. Dugoff L, Sujansky E. Neurofibromatosis type 1 and pregnancy. Am J Med Genet 1996;66(1):7–10.

58. Roth TM, Petty EM, Barald KF. The role of steroid hormones in the NF1 phenotype: focus on pregnancy. Am J Med Genet A 2008;146A(12):1624–33.

59. Beert E, Brems H, Daniels B, et al. Atypical neurofibromas in neurofibromatosis type 1 are premalignant tumors. Genes Chromosomes Cancer 2011; 50(12):1021–32.

60. Cambiaghi S, Restano L, Caputo R. Juvenile xanthogranuloma associated with neurofibromatosis 1: 14 patients without evidence of hematologic malignancies. Pediatr Dermatol 2004;21(2):97–101.

61. Ferrari F, Masurel A, Olivier-Faivre L, et al. Juvenile xanthogranuloma and nevus anemicus in the diagnosis of neurofibromatosis type 1. JAMA Dermatol 2014;150(1):42–6.

62. Fenot M, Stalder JF, Barbarot S. Juvenile xanthogranulomas are highly prevalent but transient in

young children with neurofibromatosis type 1. J Am Acad Dermatol 2014;71(2):389–90.

63. Marque M, Roubertie A, Jaussent A, et al. Nevus anemicus in neurofibromatosis type 1: a potential new diagnostic criterion. J Am Acad Dermatol 2013;69(5):768–75.

64. Hernandez-Martin A, Garcia-Martinez FJ, Duat A, et al. Nevus anemicus: a distinctive cutaneous finding in neurofibromatosis type 1. Pediatr Dermatol 2015;32(3):342–7.

65. Brems H, Park C, Maertens O, et al. Glomus tumors in neurofibromatosis type 1: genetic, functional, and clinical evidence of a novel association. Cancer Res 2009;69(18):7393–401.

66. Evans DG, O'Hara C, Wilding A, et al. Mortality in neurofibromatosis 1: in North West England: an assessment of actuarial survival in a region of the UK since 1989. Eur J Hum Genet 2011;19(11):1187–91.

67. Walker L, Thompson D, Easton D, et al. A prospective study of neurofibromatosis type 1 cancer incidence in the UK. Br J Cancer 2006;95(2):233–8.

68. Huttner AJ, Kieran MW, Yao X, et al. Clinicopathologic study of glioblastoma in children with neurofibromatosis type 1. Pediatr Blood Cancer 2010;54(7):890–6.

69. Crucis A, Richer W, Brugieres L, et al. Rhabdomyosarcomas in children with neurofibromatosis type I: a national historical cohort. Pediatr Blood Cancer 2015;62(10):1733–8.

70. Gorgel A, Cetinkaya DD, Salgur F, et al. Coexistence of gastrointestinal stromal tumors (GISTs) and pheochromocytoma in three cases of neurofibromatosis type 1 (NF1) with a review of the literature. Intern Med 2014;53(16):1783–9.

71. Shields JA, Pellegrini M, Kaliki S, et al. Retinal vasoproliferative tumors in 6 patients with neurofibromatosis type 1. JAMA Ophthalmol 2014;132(2):190–6.

72. Valencia E, Saif MW. Neurofibromatosis type 1 and GIST: is there a correlation? Anticancer Res 2014;34(10):5609–12.

73. Madanikia SA, Bergner A, Ye X, et al. Increased risk of breast cancer in women with NF1. Am J Med Genet A 2012;158A(12):3056–60.

74. Wang X, Levin AM, Smolinski SE, et al. Breast cancer and other neoplasms in women with neurofibromatosis type 1: a retrospective review of cases in the Detroit metropolitan area. Am J Med Genet A 2012;158A(12):3061–4.

75. Seminog OO, Goldacre MJ. Age-specific risk of breast cancer in women with neurofibromatosis type 1. Br J Cancer 2015;112(9):1546–8.

76. Gutmann DH, Collins F. Neurofibromatosis type 1. In: Vogelstein B, Kinzler KW, editors. The genetic basis of human cancer. New York: McGraw-Hill; 1998. p. 423–42.

77. Riccardi VM. Pathophysiology of neurofibromatosis. IV. Dermatologic insights into heterogeneity and pathogenesis. J Am Acad Dermatol 1980;3(2):157–66.

78. Mautner VF, Asuagbor FA, Dombi E, et al. Assessment of benign tumor burden by whole-body MRI in patients with neurofibromatosis 1. Neuro Oncol 2008;10(4):593–8.

79. Cai W, Kassarjian A, Bredella MA, et al. Tumor burden in patients with neurofibromatosis types 1 and 2 and schwannomatosis: determination on whole-body MR images. Radiology 2009;250(3):665–73.

80. Matsumine A, Kusuzaki K, Nakamura T, et al. Differentiation between neurofibromas and malignant peripheral nerve sheath tumors in neurofibromatosis 1 evaluated by MRI. J Cancer Res Clin Oncol 2009;135(7):891–900.

81. Van Meerbeeck SF, Verstraete KL, Janssens S, et al. Whole body MR imaging in neurofibromatosis type 1. Eur J Radiol 2009;69(2):236–42.

82. Plotkin SR, Bredella MA, Cai W, et al. Quantitative assessment of whole-body tumor burden in adult patients with neurofibromatosis. PLoS One 2012;7(4):e35711.

83. Hirbe AC, Gutmann DH. Neurofibromatosis type 1: a multidisciplinary approach to care. Lancet Neurol 2014;13(8):834–43.

84. Dombi E, Solomon J, Gillespie AJ, et al. NF1 plexiform neurofibroma growth rate by volumetric MRI: relationship to age and body weight. Neurology 2007;68(9):643–7.

85. Tucker T, Friedman JM, Friedrich RE, et al. Longitudinal study of neurofibromatosis 1 associated plexiform neurofibromas. J Med Genet 2009;46(2):81–5.

86. Nguyen R, Dombi E, Widemann BC, et al. Growth dynamics of plexiform neurofibromas: a retrospective cohort study of 201 patients with neurofibromatosis 1. Orphanet J Rare Dis 2012;7:75.

87. Storm FK, Eilber FR, Mirra J, et al. Neurofibrosarcoma. Cancer 1980;45(1):126–9.

88. Rasmussen SA, Yang Q, Friedman JM. Mortality in neurofibromatosis 1: an analysis using U.S. death certificates. Am J Hum Genet 2001;68(5):1110–8.

89. Evans DG, Baser ME, McGaughran J, et al. Malignant peripheral nerve sheath tumours in neurofibromatosis 1. J Med Genet 2002;39(5):311–4.

90. Friedrich RE, Hartmann M, Mautner VF. Malignant peripheral nerve sheath tumors (MPNST) in NF1-affected children. Anticancer Res 2007;27(4A):1957–60.

91. McCaughan JA, Holloway SM, Davidson R, et al. Further evidence of the increased risk for malignant peripheral nerve sheath tumour from a Scottish

cohort of patients with neurofibromatosis type 1. J Med Genet 2007;44(7):463–6.

92. Khosrotehrani K, Bastuji-Garin S, Zeller J, et al. Clinical risk factors for mortality in patients with neurofibromatosis 1: a cohort study of 378 patients. Arch Dermatol 2003;139(2):187–91.

93. Ferner RE, Gutmann DH. International consensus statement on malignant peripheral nerve sheath tumors in neurofibromatosis. Cancer Res 2002;62(5): 1573–7.

94. Sharif S, Ferner R, Birch JM, et al. Second primary tumors in neurofibromatosis 1 patients treated for optic glioma: substantial risks after radiotherapy. J Clin Oncol 2006;24(16):2570–5.

95. De Raedt T, Brems H, Wolkenstein P, et al. Elevated risk for MPNST in NF1 microdeletion patients. Am J Hum Genet 2003;72(5):1288–92.

96. Khosrotehrani K, Bastuji-Garin S, Riccardi VM, et al. Subcutaneous neurofibromas are associated with mortality in neurofibromatosis 1: a cohort study of 703 patients. Am J Med Genet A 2005;132A(1): 49–53.

97. Ferner RE, Hughes RA, Hall SM, et al. Neurofibromatous neuropathy in neurofibromatosis 1 (NF1). J Med Genet 2004;41(11):837–41.

98. Kluwe L, Friedrich RE, Peiper M, et al. Constitutional NF1 mutations in neurofibromatosis 1 patients with malignant peripheral nerve sheath tumors. Hum Mutat 2003;22(5):420.

99. Tucker T, Wolkenstein P, Revuz J, et al. Association between benign and malignant peripheral nerve sheath tumors in NF1. Neurology 2005;65(2): 205–11.

100. Nguyen R, Jett K, Harris GJ, et al. Benign whole body tumor volume is a risk factor for malignant peripheral nerve sheath tumors in neurofibromatosis type 1. J Neurooncol 2014;116(2):307–13.

101. Bhargava R, Parham DM, Lasater OE, et al. MR imaging differentiation of benign and malignant peripheral nerve sheath tumors: use of the target sign. Pediatr Radiol 1997;27(2):124–9.

102. Kehrer-Sawatzki H, Kluwe L, Funsterer C, et al. Extensively high load of internal tumors determined by whole body MRI scanning in a patient with neurofibromatosis type 1 and a non-LCR-mediated 2-Mb deletion in 17q11.2. Hum Genet 2005;116(6):466–75.

103. Kosucu P, Ahmetoglu A, Cobanoglu U, et al. Mesenteric involvement in neurofibromatosis type 1: CT and MRI findings in two cases. Abdom Imaging 2003;28(6):822–6.

104. Wasa J, Nishida Y, Tsukushi S, et al. MRI features in the differentiation of malignant peripheral nerve sheath tumors and neurofibromas. AJR Am J Roentgenol 2010;194(6):1568–74.

105. Frassica FJ, Khanna JA, McCarthy EF. The role of MR imaging in soft tissue tumor evaluation: perspective of the orthopedic oncologist and musculoskeletal pathologist. Magn Reson Imaging Clin N Am 2000;8(4):915–27.

106. Demehri S, Belzberg A, Blakeley J, et al. Conventional and functional MR imaging of peripheral nerve sheath tumors: initial experience. AJNR Am J Neuroradiol 2014;35(8):1615–20.

107. Ferner RE, Lucas JD, O'Doherty MJ, et al. Evaluation of (18)fluorodeoxyglucose positron emission tomography ((18)FDG PET) in the detection of malignant peripheral nerve sheath tumours arising from within plexiform neurofibromas in neurofibromatosis 1. J Neurol Neurosurg Psychiatr 2000; 68(3):353–7.

108. Combemale P, Valeyrie-Allanore L, Giammarile F, et al. Utility of 18F-FDG PET with a semi-quantitative index in the detection of sarcomatous transformation in patients with neurofibromatosis type 1. PLoS One 2014;9(2):e85954.

109. Salamon J, Veldhoen S, Apostolova I, et al. 18F-FDG PET/CT for detection of malignant peripheral nerve sheath tumours in neurofibromatosis type 1: tumour-to-liver ratio is superior to an SUVmax cut-off. Eur Radiol 2014;24(2):405–12.

110. Chirindel A, Chaudhry M, Blakeley JO, et al. 18F-FDG PET/CT qualitative and quantitative evaluation in neurofibromatosis type 1 patients for detection of malignant transformation: comparison of early to delayed imaging with and without liver activity normalization. J Nucl Med 2015;56(3):379–85.

111. Salamon J, Papp L, Toth Z, et al. Nerve sheath tumors in neurofibromatosis type 1: assessment of whole-body metabolic tumor burden using F-18-FDG PET/CT. PLoS One 2015;10(12):e0143305.

112. Van Der Gucht A, Zehou O, Djelbani-Ahmed S, et al. Metabolic tumour burden measured by 18F-FDG PET/CT predicts malignant transformation in patients with neurofibromatosis type-1. PLoS One 2016;11(3):e0151809.

113. Brahmi M, Thiesse P, Ranchere D, et al. Diagnostic accuracy of PET/CT-guided percutaneous biopsies for malignant peripheral nerve sheath tumors in neurofibromatosis type 1 patients. PLoS One 2015;10(10):e0138386.

114. Prada CE, Hufnagel RB, Hummel TR, et al. The use of magnetic resonance imaging screening for optic pathway gliomas in children with neurofibromatosis type 1. J Pediatr 2015;167(4):851–6.e1.

115. Blanchard G, Lafforgue MP, Lion-Francois L, et al. Systematic MRI in NF1 children under six years of age for the diagnosis of optic pathway gliomas. Study and outcome of a French cohort. Eur J Paediatr Neurol 2016;20(2):275–81.

116. Friedrich RE, Nuding MA. Optic pathway glioma and cerebral focal abnormal signal intensity in patients with neurofibromatosis type 1: characteristics, treatment choices and follow-up in

134 affected individuals and a brief review of the literature. Anticancer Res 2016;36(8):4095–121.

117. Parkhurst E, Abboy S. Optic gliomas in neurofibromatosis type 1. J Pediatr Ophthalmol Strabismus 2016;53(6):334–8.

118. Sellmer L, Farschtschi S, Marangoni M, et al. Non-optic glioma in adults and children with neurofibromatosis 1. Orphanet J Rare Dis 2017; 12(1):34.

119. Sellmer L, Farschtschi S, Marangoni M, et al. Serial MRIs provide novel insight into natural history of optic pathway gliomas in patients with neurofibromatosis 1. Orphanet J Rare Dis 2018;13(1):62.

120. Lewis RA, Gerson LP, Axelson KA, et al. von Recklinghausen neurofibromatosis. II. Incidence of optic gliomata. Ophthalmology 1984;91(8):929–35.

121. Listernick R, Charrow J, Greenwald M, et al. Natural history of optic pathway tumors in children with neurofibromatosis type 1: a longitudinal study. J Pediatr 1994;125(1):63–6.

122. Listernick R, Charrow J, Greenwald MJ, et al. Optic gliomas in children with neurofibromatosis type 1. J Pediatr 1989;114(5):788–92.

123. Listernick R, Louis DN, Packer RJ, et al. Optic pathway gliomas in children with neurofibromatosis 1: consensus statement from the NF1 Optic Pathway Glioma Task Force. Ann Neurol 1997; 41(2):143–9.

124. Listernick R, Ferner RE, Piersall L, et al. Late-onset optic pathway tumors in children with neurofibromatosis 1. Neurology 2004;63(10):1944–6.

125. Listernick R, Ferner RE, Liu GT, et al. Optic pathway gliomas in neurofibromatosis-1: controversies and recommendations. Ann Neurol 2007; 61(3):189–98.

126. Freret M, Gutmann DH. Understanding vision loss from optic pathway glioma in neurofibromatosis type 1. Ann Neurol 2007;61(3):189–98.

127. Shamji MF, Benoit BG. Syndromic and sporadic pediatric optic pathway gliomas: review of clinical and histopathological differences and treatment implications. Neurosurg Focus 2007;23(5):E3.

128. Nicolin G, Parkin P, Mabbott D, et al. Natural history and outcome of optic pathway gliomas in children. Pediatr Blood Cancer 2009;53(7):1231–7.

129. Guillamo JS, Creange A, Kalifa C, et al. Prognostic factors of CNS tumours in Neurofibromatosis 1 (NF1): a retrospective study of 104 patients. Brain 2003;126(Pt 1):152–60.

130. Liu GT, Brodsky MC, Phillips PC, et al. Optic radiation involvement in optic pathway gliomas in neurofibromatosis. Am J Ophthalmol 2004;137(3): 407–14.

131. Strowd RE, Blakeley J. Genetic syndromes associated with brain tumors. In: Richard Winn H, editor. Youmans neurological surgery. 7th edition. New York: Saunders, Elsevier Inc; 2017. p. 916–22.

132. Mandiwanza T, Kaliaperumal C, Khalil A, et al. Suprasellar pilocytic astrocytoma: one national centre's experience. Childs Nerv Syst 2014;30(7): 1243–8.

133. Ullrich NJ, Raja AI, Irons MB, et al. Brainstem lesions in neurofibromatosis type 1. Neurosurgery 2007;61(4):762–6 [discussion: 766–7].

134. Duffner PK, Cohen ME, Seidel FG, et al. The significance of MRI abnormalities in children with neurofibromatosis. Neurology 1989;39(3):373–8.

135. Kraut MA, Gerring JP, Cooper KL, et al. Longitudinal evolution of unidentified bright objects in children with neurofibromatosis-1. Am J Med Genet A 2004;129A(2):113–9.

136. DiPaolo DP, Zimmerman RA, Rorke LB, et al. Neurofibromatosis type 1: pathologic substrate of high-signal-intensity foci in the brain. Radiology 1995;195(3):721–4.

137. Gonen O, Wang ZJ, Viswanathan AK, et al. Three-dimensional multivoxel proton MR spectroscopy of the brain in children with neurofibromatosis type 1. AJNR Am J Neuroradiol 1999;20(7):1333–41.

138. Lubs M-LE, Bauer MS, Formas ME, et al. Lisch nodules in Neurofibromatosis type 1. N Engl J Med 1991;324(18):1264–6.

139. Woog JJ, Albert DM, Craft J, et al. Choroidal ganglioneuroma in neurofibromatosis. Graefes Arch Clin Exp Ophthalmol 1983;220(1):25–31.

140. Kumar V, Singh S. Multimodal imaging of choroidal nodules in neurofibromatosis type-1. Indian J Ophthalmol 2018;66(4):586–8.

141. Tadini G, Milani D, Menni F, et al. Is it time to change the neurofibromatosis 1 diagnostic criteria? Eur J Intern Med 2014;25(6):506–10.

142. Vagge A, Nelson LB, Capris P, et al. Choroidal freckling in pediatric patients affected by neurofibromatosis type 1. J Pediatr Ophthalmol Strabismus 2016;53(5):271–4.

143. Elefteriou F, Kolanczyk M, Schindeler A, et al. Skeletal abnormalities in neurofibromatosis type 1: approaches to therapeutic options. Am J Med Genet A 2009;149a(10):2327–38.

144. Friedrich RE, Stelljes C, Hagel C, et al. Dysplasia of the orbit and adjacent bone associated with plexiform neurofibroma and ocular disease in 42 NF-1 patients. Anticancer Res 2010;30(5): 1751–64.

145. Tucker T, Schnabel C, Hartmann M, et al. Bone health and fracture rate in individuals with neurofibromatosis 1 (NF1). J Med Genet 2009;46(4):259–65.

146. Tsirikos AI, Ramachandran M, Lee J, et al. Assessment of vertebral scalloping in neurofibromatosis type 1 with plain radiography and MRI. Clin Radiol 2004;59(11):1009–17.

147. White AK, Smith RJ, Bigler CR, et al. Head and neck manifestations of neurofibromatosis. Laryngoscope 1986;96(7):732–7.

148. Riccardi V, Eichner J. Neurofibromatosis: phenotype, natural history, and pathogenesis. Baltimore (MD): Johns Hopkins University Press; 1986. p. 29–36.

149. Lin AE, Birch PH, Korf BR, et al. Cardiovascular malformations and other cardiovascular abnormalities in neurofibromatosis 1. Am J Med Genet 2000; 95(2):108–17.

150. Nguyen R, Mir TS, Kluwe L, et al. Cardiac characterization of 16 patients with large NF1 gene deletions. Clin Genet 2013;84(4):344–9.

151. Kimura M, Kakizaki S, Kawano K, et al. Neurofibromatosis type 1 complicated by atypical coarctation of the thoracic aorta. Case Rep Pediatr 2013;2013: 458543.

152. Mavani G, Kesar V, Devita MV, et al. Neurofibromatosis type 1-associated hypertension secondary to coarctation of the thoracic aorta. Clin Kidney J 2014;7(4):394–5.

153. Omeje I, Christov G, Khambadkone S, et al. Cor triatriatum dexter and coarctation of the aorta–a rare association in a 7-year-old child with type 1 neurofibromatosis. Cardiol Young 2015;25(2): 308–11.

154. Veean S, Thakkar N, Gupta S, et al. A case of coarctation of the abdominal aorta and renal artery stenosis due to neurofibromatosis type 1. Postgrad Med J 2017;93(1098):235–6.

155. Walther MM, Herring J, Enquist E, et al. von Recklinghausen's disease and pheochromocytomas. J Urol 1999;162(5):1582–6.

156. Fossali E, Signorini E, Intermite RC, et al. Renovascular disease and hypertension in children with neurofibromatosis. Pediatr Nephrol 2000;14(8–9): 806–10.

157. Pride N, North K. The cognitive profile of NF1 children: therapeutic implications. In: Upadhyaya M, Cooper DN, editors. Neurofibromatosis type 1. Berlin: Springer-Verlag; 2012. p. 55–69.

158. Lehtonen A, Howie E, Trump D, et al. Behaviour in children with neurofibromatosis type 1: cognition, executive function, attention, emotion, and social competence. Dev Med Child Neurol 2013;55(2): 111–25.

159. Ferner RE, Hughes RA, Weinman J. Intellectual impairment in neurofibromatosis 1. J Neurol Sci 1996;138(1–2):125–33.

160. North KN, Riccardi V, Samango-Sprouse C, et al. Cognitive function and academic performance in neurofibromatosis. 1: consensus statement from the NF1 Cognitive Disorders Task Force. Neurology 1997;48(4):1121–7.

161. Ozonoff S. Cognitive impairment in neurofibromatosis type 1. Am J Med Genet 1999;89(1):45–52.

162. Leschziner GD, Golding JF, Ferner RE. Sleep disturbance as part of the neurofibromatosis type 1 phenotype in adults. Am J Med Genet A 2013; 161A(6):1319–22.

163. Licis AK, Vallorani A, Gao F, et al. Prevalence of sleep disturbances in children with neurofibromatosis type 1. J Child Neurol 2013;28(11):1400–5.

164. Marana Perez AI, Duat Rodriguez A, Soto Insuga V, et al. Prevalence of sleep disorders in patients with neurofibromatosis type 1. Neurologia 2015;30(9): 561–5.

165. Pinho RS, Fusao EF, Paschoal J, et al. Migraine is frequent in children and adolescents with neurofibromatosis type 1. Pediatr Int 2014;56(6):865–7.

166. Afridi SK, Leschziner GD, Ferner RE. Prevalence and clinical presentation of headache in a national neurofibromatosis 1 service and impact on quality of life. Am J Med Genet A 2015;167a(10):2282–5.

167. Ostendorf AP, Gutmann DH, Weisenberg JL. Epilepsy in individuals with neurofibromatosis type 1. Epilepsia 2013;54(10):1810–4.

168. Gales J, Prayson RA. Hippocampal sclerosis and associated focal cortical dysplasia-related epilepsy in neurofibromatosis type I. J Clin Neurosci 2017;37:15–9.

169. Zoller M, Rembeck B, Akesson HO, et al. Life expectancy, mortality and prognostic factors in neurofibromatosis type 1. A twelve-year follow-up of an epidemiological study in Goteborg, Sweden. Acta Derm Venereol 1995;75(2):136–40.

170. Masocco M, Kodra Y, Vichi M, et al. Mortality associated with neurofibromatosis type 1: a study based on Italian death certificates (1995-2006). Orphanet J Rare Dis 2011;6:11.

171. Vranceanu AM, Merker VL, Park E, et al. Quality of life among adult patients with neurofibromatosis 1, neurofibromatosis 2 and schwannomatosis: a systematic review of the literature. J Neurooncol 2013;114(3):257–62.

172. Merker VL, Bredella MA, Cai W, et al. Relationship between whole-body tumor burden, clinical phenotype, and quality of life in patients with neurofibromatosis. Am J Med Genet A 2014;164a(6):1431–7.

173. Vranceanu AM, Merker VL, Park ER, et al. Quality of life among children and adolescents with neurofibromatosis 1: a systematic review of the literature. J Neurooncol 2015;122(2):219–28.

174. Cohen JS, Levy HP, Sloan J, et al. Depression among adults with neurofibromatosis type 1: prevalence and impact on quality of life. Clin Genet 2015;88(5):425–30.

175. Hersh JH. Health supervision for children with neurofibromatosis. Pediatrics 2008;121(3):633–42.

176. Dunning-Davies BM, Parker AP. Annual review of children with neurofibromatosis type 1. Arch Dis Child Educ Pract Ed 2016;101(2):102–11.

177. Stewart DR, Korf BR, Nathanson KL, et al. Care of adults with neurofibromatosis type 1: a clinical practice resource of the American College of Medical Genetics and Genomics (ACMG). Genet Med 2018;20(7):671–82.

178. Daly MB, Pilarski R, Berry M, et al. NCCN guidelines insights: genetic/familial high-risk assessment: breast and ovarian, version 2.2017. J Natl Compr Cancer Netw 2017;15(1):9–20.

179. National Institutes of Health Consensus Development Conference Statement: neurofibromatosis. Bethesda, Md., USA, July 13-15, 1987. Neurofibromatosis 1988;1(3):172–8.

180. Gutmann DH, Aylsworth A, Carey JC, et al. The diagnostic evaluation and multidisciplinary management of neurofibromatosis 1 and neurofibromatosis 2. JAMA 1997;278(1):51–7.

181. Williams VC, Lucas J, Babcock MA, et al. Neurofibromatosis type 1 revisited. Pediatrics 2009;123(1):124–33.

182. Landau M, Krafchik BR. The diagnostic value of cafe-au-lait macules. J Am Acad Dermatol 1999;40(6 Pt 1):877–90 [quiz: 891–2].

183. Tekin M, Bodurtha JN, Riccardi VM. Cafe au lait spots: the pediatrician's perspective. Pediatr Rev 2001;22(3):82–90.

184. Meni C, Sbidian E, Moreno JC, et al. Treatment of neurofibromas with a carbon dioxide laser: a retrospective cross-sectional study of 106 patients. Dermatology 2015;230(3):263–8.

185. Becker DW Jr. Use of the carbon dioxide laser in treating multiple cutaneous neurofibromas. Ann Plast Surg 1991;26(6):582–6.

186. Levine SM, Levine E, Taub PJ, et al. Electrosurgical excision technique for the treatment of multiple cutaneous lesions in neurofibromatosis type I. J Plast Reconstr Aesthet Surg 2008;61(8):958–62.

187. Evans DG, Birch JM, Ramsden RT, et al. Malignant transformation and new primary tumours after therapeutic radiation for benign disease: substantial risks in certain tumour prone syndromes. J Med Genet 2006;43(4):289–94.

188. Friedrich RE, Schmelzle R, Hartmann M, et al. Resection of small plexiform neurofibromas in neurofibromatosis type 1 children. World J Surg Oncol 2005;3(1):6.

189. Robertson KA, Nalepa G, Yang F-C, et al. Imatinib mesylate for plexiform neurofibromas in patients with neurofibromatosis type 1: a phase 2 trial. Lancet Oncol 2012;13(12):1218–24.

190. Demestre M, Herzberg J, Holtkamp N, et al. Imatinib mesylate (Glivec) inhibits Schwann cell viability and reduces the size of human plexiform neurofibroma in a xenograft model. J Neurooncol 2010;98(1):11–9.

191. Dombi E, Baldwin A, Marcus LJ, et al. Activity of selumetinib in neurofibromatosis type 1-related plexiform neurofibromas. N Engl J Med 2016;375(26):2550–60.

192. Dunn GP, Spiliopoulos K, Plotkin SR, et al. Role of resection of malignant peripheral nerve sheath tumors in patients with neurofibromatosis type 1. J Neurosurg 2013;118(1):142–8.

193. Valentin T, Le Cesne A, Ray-Coquard I, et al. Management and prognosis of malignant peripheral nerve sheath tumors: the experience of the French Sarcoma Group (GSF-GETO). Eur J Cancer 2016;56:77–84.

194. Chaudhary N, Borker A. Metronomic therapy for malignant peripheral nerve sheath tumor in neurofibromatosis type 1. Pediatr Blood Cancer 2012;59(7):1317–9.

195. Zehou O, Fabre E, Zelek L, et al. Chemotherapy for the treatment of malignant peripheral nerve sheath tumors in neurofibromatosis 1: a 10-year institutional review. Orphanet J Rare Dis 2013;8:127.

196. Mahoney DH Jr, Cohen ME, Friedman HS, et al. Carboplatin is effective therapy for young children with progressive optic pathway tumors: a Pediatric Oncology Group phase II study. Neuro Oncol 2000;2(4):213–20.

197. Packer RJ, Ater J, Allen J, et al. Carboplatin and vincristine chemotherapy for children with newly diagnosed progressive low-grade gliomas. J Neurosurg 1997;86(5):747–54.

198. Packer RJ, Lange B, Ater J, et al. Carboplatin and vincristine for recurrent and newly diagnosed low-grade gliomas of childhood. J Clin Oncol 1993;11(5):850–6.

199. Dalla Via P, Opocher E, Pinello ML, et al. Visual outcome of a cohort of children with neurofibromatosis type 1 and optic pathway glioma followed by a pediatric neuro-oncology program. Neuro Oncol 2007;9(4):430–7.

200. Dodgshun AJ, Elder JE, Hansford JR, et al. Long-term visual outcome after chemotherapy for optic pathway glioma in children: site and age are strongly predictive. Cancer 2015;121(23):4190–6.

201. Fisher MJ, Loguidice M, Gutmann DH, et al. Visual outcomes in children with neurofibromatosis type 1-associated optic pathway glioma following chemotherapy: a multicenter retrospective analysis. Neuro Oncol 2012;14(6):790–7.

202. Shofty B, Ben-Sira L, Freedman S, et al. Visual outcome following chemotherapy for progressive optic pathway gliomas. Pediatr Blood Cancer 2011;57(3):481–5.

203. Moreno L, Bautista F, Ashley S, et al. Does chemotherapy affect the visual outcome in children with optic pathway glioma? A systematic review of the evidence. Eur J Cancer 2010;46(12):2253–9.

204. Northrup H, Krueger DA, International Tuberous Sclerosis Complex Consensus Group. Tuberous sclerosis complex diagnostic criteria update: recommendations of the 2012 International Tuberous Sclerosis Complex Consensus Conference. Pediatr Neurol 2013;49(4):243–54.

205. Rodrigues DA, Gomes CM, Costa IM. Tuberous sclerosis complex. An Bras Dermatol 2012;87(2): 184–96.

206. Hinton RB, Prakash A, Romp RL, et al. Cardiovascular manifestations of tuberous sclerosis complex and summary of the revised diagnostic criteria and surveillance and management recommendations from the International Tuberous Sclerosis Consensus Group. J Am Heart Assoc 2014;3(6): e001493.

207. Osborne JP, Fryer A, Webb D. Epidemiology of tuberous sclerosis. Ann N Y Acad Sci 1991;615: 125–7.

208. Wiederholt WC, Gomez MR, Kurland LT. Incidence and prevalence of tuberous sclerosis in Rochester, Minnesota, 1950 through 1982. Neurology 1985; 35(4):600–3.

209. O'Callaghan FJ, Clarke AC, Joffe H, et al. Tuberous sclerosis complex and Wolff-Parkinson-White syndrome. Arch Dis Child 1998;78(2):159–62.

210. Sampson JR, Scahill SJ, Stephenson JB, et al. Genetic aspects of tuberous sclerosis in the west of Scotland. J Med Genet 1989;26(1):28–31.

211. Curatolo P, Bombardieri R, Jozwiak S. Tuberous sclerosis. Lancet 2008;372(9639):657–68.

212. Sadowski K, Kotulska K, Schwartz RA, et al. Systemic effects of treatment with mTOR inhibitors in tuberous sclerosis complex: a comprehensive review. J Eur Acad Dermatol Venereol 2016;30(4): 586–94.

213. DiMario FJ Jr, Sahin M, Ebrahimi-Fakhari D. Tuberous sclerosis complex. Pediatr Clin North Am 2015; 62(3):633–48.

214. Portocarrero LKL, Quental KN, Samorano LP, et al. Tuberous sclerosis complex: review based on new diagnostic criteria. An Bras Dermatol 2018;93(3): 323–31.

215. Kandt RS, Haines JL, Smith M, et al. Linkage of an important gene locus for tuberous sclerosis to a chromosome 16 marker for polycystic kidney disease. Nat Genet 1992;2(1):37–41.

216. Povey S, Burley MW, Attwood J, et al. Two loci for tuberous sclerosis: one on 9q34 and one on 16p13. Ann Hum Genet 1994;58(2):107–27.

217. van Slegtenhorst M, Nellist M, Nagelkerken B, et al. Interaction between hamartin and tuberin, the TSC1 and TSC2 gene products. Hum Mol Genet 1998;7(6):1053–7.

218. Garami A, Zwartkruis FJ, Nobukuni T, et al. Insulin activation of Rheb, a mediator of mTOR/S6K/4E-BP signaling, is inhibited by TSC1 and 2. Mol Cell 2003;11(6):1457–66.

219. Inoki K, Li Y, Xu T, et al. Rheb GTPase is a direct target of TSC2 GAP activity and regulates mTOR signaling. Genes Dev 2003;17(15):1829–34.

220. Stocker H, Radimerski T, Schindelholz B, et al. Rheb is an essential regulator of S6K in controlling cell growth in Drosophila. Nat Cell Biol 2003;5(6): 559–65.

221. Tee AR, Fingar DC, Manning BD, et al. Tuberous sclerosis complex-1 and -2 gene products function together to inhibit mammalian target of rapamycin (mTOR)-mediated downstream signaling. Proc Natl Acad Sci U S A 2002;99(21):13571–6.

222. Tee AR, Manning BD, Roux PP, et al. Tuberous sclerosis complex gene products, Tuberin and Hamartin, control mTOR signaling by acting as a GTPase-activating protein complex toward Rheb. Curr Biol 2003;13(15):1259–68.

223. Zhang Y, Gao X, Saucedo LJ, et al. Rheb is a direct target of the tuberous sclerosis tumour suppressor proteins. Nat Cell Biol 2003;5(6):578–81.

224. Lamb RF, Roy C, Diefenbach TJ, et al. The TSC1 tumour suppressor hamartin regulates cell adhesion through ERM proteins and the GTPase Rho. Nat Cell Biol 2000;2(5):281–7.

225. Huang J, Dibble CC, Matsuzaki M, et al. The TSC1-TSC2 complex is required for proper activation of mTOR complex 2. Mol Cell Biol 2008;28(12): 4104–15.

226. Toro JR, Wei MH, Glenn GM, et al. BHD mutations, clinical and molecular genetic investigations of Birt-Hogg-Dube syndrome: a new series of 50 families and a review of published reports. J Med Genet 2008;45(6):321–31.

227. Wheless JW, Almoazen H. A novel topical rapamycin cream for the treatment of facial angiofibromas in tuberous sclerosis complex. J Child Neurol 2013; 28(7):933–6.

228. Jozwiak S, Schwartz RA, Janniger CK, et al. Skin lesions in children with tuberous sclerosis complex: their prevalence, natural course, and diagnostic significance. Int J Dermatol 1998;37(12):911–7.

229. Hurwitz S, Braverman IM. White spots in tuberous sclerosis. J Pediatr 1970;77(4):587–94.

230. Debard A, Richardet JM. Letter: significance of achromic spots in the infant. Nouv Presse Med 1975;4(33):2405 [in French].

231. Vanderhooft SL, Francis JS, Pagon RA, et al. Prevalence of hypopigmented macules in a healthy population. J Pediatr 1996;129(3):355–61.

232. Webb DW, Clarke A, Fryer A, et al. The cutaneous features of tuberous sclerosis: a population study. Br J Dermatol 1996;135(1):1–5.

233. Au KS, Williams AT, Roach ES, et al. Genotype/phenotype correlation in 325 individuals referred for a diagnosis of tuberous sclerosis complex in the United States. Genet Med 2007;9(2): 88–100.

234. Dabora SL, Jozwiak S, Franz DN, et al. Mutational analysis in a cohort of 224 tuberous sclerosis patients indicates increased severity of TSC2, compared with TSC1, disease in multiple organs. Am J Hum Genet 2001;68(1):64–80.

235. Aldrich CS, Hong CH, Groves L, et al. Acral lesions in tuberous sclerosis complex: insights into pathogenesis. J Am Acad Dermatol 2010;63(2):244–51.

236. Haemel AK, O'Brian AL, Teng JM. Topical rapamycin: a novel approach to facial angiofibromas in tuberous sclerosis. Arch Dermatol 2010;146(7):715–8.

237. Jozwiak S, Schwartz RA, Janniger CK, et al. Usefulness of diagnostic criteria of tuberous sclerosis complex in pediatric patients. J Child Neurol 2000;15(10):652–9.

238. Oyerinde O, Buccine D, Treichel A, et al. Fibrous cephalic plaques in tuberous sclerosis complex. J Am Acad Dermatol 2018;78(4):717–24.

239. Sparling JD, Hong CH, Brahim JS, et al. Oral findings in 58 adults with tuberous sclerosis complex. J Am Acad Dermatol 2007;56(5):786–90.

240. Flanagan N, O'Connor WJ, McCartan B, et al. Developmental enamel defects in tuberous sclerosis: a clinical genetic marker? J Med Genet 1997;34(8):637–9.

241. Lygidakis NA, Lindenbaum RH. Oral fibromatosis in tuberous sclerosis. Oral Surg Oral Med Oral Pathol 1989;68(6):725–8.

242. Mlynarczyk G. Enamel pitting: a common symptom of tuberous sclerosis. Oral Surg Oral Med Oral Pathol 1991;71(1):63–7.

243. Crino P, Mehta R, Vinters HV. Pathogenesis of TSC in the brain. In: Kwiatkowsi D, Whittemore V, Thiele E, editors. Tuberous sclerosis complex: genes, clinical features, and therapeutics. Weinheim (Germany): Wiley-Blackwell; 2010. p. 285–309.

244. Roth J, Roach ES, Bartels U, et al. Subependymal giant cell astrocytoma: diagnosis, screening, and treatment. Recommendations from the International Tuberous Sclerosis Complex Consensus Conference 2012. Pediatr Neurol 2013;49(6):439–44.

245. Curatolo P, Moavero R, de Vries PJ. Neurological and neuropsychiatric aspects of tuberous sclerosis complex. Lancet Neurol 2015;14(7):733–45.

246. Ng KH, Ng SM, Parker A. Annual review of children with tuberous sclerosis. Arch Dis Child Educ Pract Ed 2015;100(3):114–21.

247. Beghetti M, Gow RM, Haney I, et al. Pediatric primary benign cardiac tumors: a 15-year review. Am Heart J 1997;134(6):1107–14.

248. Harding CO, Pagon RA. Incidence of tuberous sclerosis in patients with cardiac rhabdomyoma. Am J Med Genet 1990;37(4):443–6.

249. Holley DG, Martin GR, Brenner JI, et al. Diagnosis and management of fetal cardiac tumors: a multicenter experience and review of published reports. J Am Coll Cardiol 1995;26(2):516–20.

250. Sciacca P, Giacchi V, Mattia C, et al. Rhabdomyomas and tuberous sclerosis complex: our experience in 33 cases. BMC Cardiovasc Disord 2014;14:66.

251. Roach ES, DiMario FJ, Kandt RS, et al. Tuberous sclerosis consensus conference: recommendations for diagnostic evaluation. National tuberous sclerosis association. J Child Neurol 1999;14(6):401–7.

252. Kingswood JC, Bruzzi P, Curatolo P, et al. TOSCA - first international registry to address knowledge gaps in the natural history and management of tuberous sclerosis complex. Orphanet J Rare Dis 2014;9:182.

253. Bhatt JR, Richard PO, Kim NS, et al. Natural history of renal angiomyolipoma (AML): most patients with large AMLs >4cm can be offered active surveillance as an initial management strategy. Eur Urol 2016;70(1):85–90.

254. Fricke BL, Donnelly LF, Casper KA, et al. Frequency and imaging appearance of hepatic angiomyolipomas in pediatric and adult patients with tuberous sclerosis. AJR Am J Roentgenol 2004;182(4):1027–30.

255. Nakhleh R. Angiomyolipoma of the liver. Pathol Case Rev 2009;14:47–9.

256. Jeong A. Tuberous sclerosis complex: a roadmap for future research. Pediatr Neurol Briefs 2016;30(7):32.

257. Kakkar A, Vallonthaiel AG, Sharma MC, et al. Composite renal cell carcinoma and angiomyolipoma in a patient with Tuberous sclerosis: a diagnostic dilemma. Can Urol Assoc J 2015;9(7–8):E507–10.

258. Lam HC, Nijmeh J, Henske EP. New developments in the genetics and pathogenesis of tumours in tuberous sclerosis complex. J Pathol 2017;241(2):219–25.

259. Johnson SR, Cordier JF, Lazor R, et al. European Respiratory Society guidelines for the diagnosis and management of lymphangioleiomyomatosis. Eur Respir J 2010;35(1):14–26.

260. McCormack FX, Henske EP. Lymphangioleiomyomatosis and pulmonary disease in TSC. In: Kwiatkowsi D, Whittemore V, Thiele E, editors. Tuberous sclerosis complex: genes, clinical features, and therapeutics. Weinheim (Germany): Wiley-Blackwell; 2010. p. 345–8.

261. Moss J, Avila NA, Barnes PM, et al. Prevalence and clinical characteristics of lymphangioleiomyomatosis (LAM) in patients with tuberous sclerosis complex. Am J Respir Crit Care Med 2001;164(4):669–71.

262. Adriaensen ME, Schaefer-Prokop CM, Duyndam DA, et al. Radiological evidence of lymphangioleiomyomatosis in female and male patients with tuberous sclerosis complex. Clin Radiol 2011;66(7):625–8.

263. Muzykewicz DA, Black ME, Muse V, et al. Multifocal micronodular pneumocyte hyperplasia: computed tomographic appearance and follow-up in

tuberous sclerosis complex. J Comput Assist To-mogr 2012;36(5):518–22.

264. Cudzilo CJ, Szczesniak RD, Brody AS, et al. Lym-phangioleiomyomatosis screening in women with tuberous sclerosis. Chest 2013;144(2):578–85.

265. Friedman E, Pampiglione G. Prognostic implica-tions of electroencephalographic findings of hyp-sarrhythmia in first year of life. Br Med J 1971; 4(5783):323–5.

266. Hunt A, Dennis J. Psychiatric disorder among chil-dren with tuberous sclerosis. Dev Med Child Neurol 1987;29(2):190–8.

267. Smalley SL, Tanguay PE, Smith M, et al. Autism and tuberous sclerosis. J Autism Dev Disord 1992; 22(3):339–55.

268. Yates JR, Maclean C, Higgins JN, et al. The Tuber-ous sclerosis 2000 study: presentation, initial as-sessments and implications for diagnosis and management. Arch Dis Child 2011;96(11):1020–5.

269. Krueger DA, Northrup H, International Tuberous Sclerosis Complex Consensus Group. Tuberous sclerosis complex surveillance and management: recommendations of the 2012 International Tuber-ous Sclerosis Complex Consensus Conference. Pediatr Neurol 2013;49(4):255–65.

270. Weiss ET, Geronemus RG. New technique using combined pulsed dye laser and fractional resurfac-ing for treating facial angiofibromas in tuberous sclerosis. Lasers Surg Med 2010;42(5):357–60.

271. Koenig MK, Hebert AA, Roberson J, et al. Topical rapamycin therapy to alleviate the cutaneous man-ifestations of tuberous sclerosis complex: a double-blind, randomized, controlled trial to eval-uate the safety and efficacy of topically applied ra-pamycin. Drugs R D 2012;12(3):121–6.

272. Mutizwa MM, Berk DR, Anadkat MJ. Treatment of facial angiofibromas with topical application of oral rapamycin solution (1mgmL(-1)) in two pa-tients with tuberous sclerosis. Br J Dermatol 2011;165(4):922–3.

273. Malissen N, Vergely L, Simon M, et al. Long-term treatment of cutaneous manifestations of tuberous sclerosis complex with topical 1% sirolimus cream: a prospective study of 25 patients. J Am Acad Der-matol 2017;77(3):464–72.e3.

274. Wataya-Kaneda M, Nakamura A, Tanaka M, et al. Efficacy and safety of topical sirolimus therapy for facial angiofibromas in the tuberous sclerosis com-plex: a randomized clinical trial. JAMA Dermatol 2017;153(1):39–48.

275. Bissler JJ, Kingswood JC. Optimal treatment of tu-berous sclerosis complex associated renal angio-myolipomata: a systematic review. Ther Adv Urol 2016;8(4):279–90.

276. Frerebeau P, Benezech J, Segnarbieux F, et al. Intraventricular tumors in tuberous sclerosis. Childs Nerv Syst 1985;1(1):45–8.

277. Cuccia V, Zuccaro G, Sosa F, et al. Subependymal giant cell astrocytoma in children with tuberous sclerosis. Childs Nerv Syst 2003;19(4):232–43.

278. Jiang T, Jia G, Ma Z, et al. The diagnosis and treat-ment of subependymal giant cell astrocytoma com-bined with tuberous sclerosis. Childs Nerv Syst 2011;27(1):55–62.

279. Berhouma M. Management of subependymal giant cell tumors in tuberous sclerosis complex: the neu-rosurgeon's perspective. World J Pediatr 2010; 6(2):103–10.

280. Moavero R, Pinci M, Bombardieri R, et al. The man-agement of subependymal giant cell tumors in tu-berous sclerosis: a clinician's perspective. Childs Nerv Syst 2011;27(8):1203–10.

281. Goh S, Butler W, Thiele EA. Subependymal giant cell tumors in tuberous sclerosis complex. Neurology 2004;63(8):1457–61.

282. de Ribaupierre S, Dorfmuller G, Bulteau C, et al. Subependymal giant-cell astrocytomas in pediatric tuberous sclerosis disease: when should we oper-ate? Neurosurgery 2007;60(1):83–9 [discussion: 89–90].

283. Kingswood JC, d'Augeres GB, Belousova E, et al. TuberOus SClerosis registry to increase disease awareness (TOSCA) - baseline data on 2093 pa-tients. Orphanet J Rare Dis 2017;12(1):2.

284. Matsumura H, Takimoto H, Shimada N, et al. Glio-blastoma following radiotherapy in a patient with tuberous sclerosis. Neurol Med Chir (Tokyo) 1998; 38(5):287–91.

285. Park KJ, Kano H, Kondziolka D, et al. Gamma Knife surgery for subependymal giant cell astrocytomas. Clinical article. J Neurosurg 2011;114(3):808–13.

286. Franz DN, Leonard J, Tudor C, et al. Rapamycin causes regression of astrocytomas in tuberous sclerosis complex. Ann Neurol 2006;59(3): 490–8.

287. Krueger DA, Care MM, Holland K, et al. Everolimus for subependymal giant-cell astrocytomas in tuber-ous sclerosis. N Engl J Med 2010;363(19): 1801–11.

288. Campen CJ, Porter BE. Subependymal giant cell astrocytoma (SEGA) treatment update. Curr Treat Options Neurol 2011;13(4):380–5.

289. Franz DN, Belousova E, Sparagana S, et al. Effi-cacy and safety of everolimus for subependymal giant cell astrocytomas associated with tuberous sclerosis complex (EXIST-1): a multicentre, rando-mised, placebo-controlled phase 3 trial. Lancet 2013;381(9861):125–32.

290. Kotulska K, Chmielewski D, Borkowska J, et al. Long-term effect of everolimus on epilepsy and growth in children under 3 years of age treated for subependymal giant cell astrocytoma associ-ated with tuberous sclerosis complex. Eur J Pae-diatr Neurol 2013;17(5):479–85.

291. Franz DN, Agricola K, Mays M, et al. Everolimus for subependymal giant cell astrocytoma: 5-year final analysis. Ann Neurol 2015;78(6):929–38.

292. French JA, Lawson JA, Yapici Z, et al. Adjunctive everolimus therapy for treatment-resistant focal-onset seizures associated with tuberous sclerosis (EXIST-3): a phase 3, randomised, double-blind, placebo-controlled study. Lancet 2016; 388(10056):2153–63.

293. Bombardieri R, Pinci M, Moavero R, et al. Early control of seizures improves long-term outcome in children with tuberous sclerosis complex. Eur J Paediatr Neurol 2010;14(2):146–9.

294. Curatolo P, Jozwiak S, Nabbout R. Management of epilepsy associated with tuberous sclerosis complex (TSC): clinical recommendations. Eur J Paediatr Neurol 2012;16(6):582–6.

295. Jozwiak S, Kotulska K, Domanska-Pakiela D, et al. Antiepileptic treatment before the onset of seizures reduces epilepsy severity and risk of mental retardation in infants with tuberous sclerosis complex. Eur J Paediatr Neurol 2011;15(5):424–31.

296. Parisi P, Bombardieri R, Curatolo P. Current role of vigabatrin in infantile spasms. Eur J Paediatr Neurol 2007;11(6):331–6.

297. Camposano SE, Major P, Halpern E, et al. Vigabatrin in the treatment of childhood epilepsy: a retrospective chart review of efficacy and safety profile. Epilepsia 2008;49(7):1186–91.

298. Hess EJ, Moody KA, Geffrey AL, et al. Cannabidiol as a new treatment for drug-resistant epilepsy in tuberous sclerosis complex. Epilepsia 2016;57(10): 1617–24.

299. Dickinson M, Ruckle H, Beaghler M, et al. Renal angiomyolipoma: optimal treatment based on size and symptoms. Clin Nephrol 1998;49(5): 281–6.

300. Bissler JJ, Kingswood JC, Radzikowska E, et al. Everolimus for angiomyolipoma associated with tuberous sclerosis complex or sporadic lymphangioleiomyomatosis (EXIST-2): a multicentre, randomised, double-blind, placebo-controlled trial. Lancet 2013; 381(9869):817–24.

301. Nathan N, Wang JA, Li S, et al. Improvement of tuberous sclerosis complex (TSC) skin tumors during long-term treatment with oral sirolimus. J Am Acad Dermatol 2015;73(5):802–8.

302. Bissler JJ, McCormack FX, Young LR, et al. Sirolimus for angiomyolipoma in tuberous sclerosis complex or lymphangioleiomyomatosis. N Engl J Med 2008;358(2):140–51.

303. McCormack FX, Inoue Y, Moss J, et al. Efficacy and safety of sirolimus in lymphangioleiomyomatosis. N Engl J Med 2011;364(17):1595–606.

Hereditary Tumor Syndromes with Skin Involvement

Ramiz N. Hamid, MD, MPH*, Zeynep M. Akkurt, MD

KEYWORDS

- Genodermatoses • Hereditary tumor syndrome • Gorlin-Goltz syndrome
- Xeroderma pigmentosum

KEY POINTS

- Cutaneous findings in childhood may be the first sign of a hereditary tumor syndrome.
- Early detection of genodermatoses allows the patient and at-risk family members to be screened for associated malignancies.
- Advances in molecular-based therapy have spurred development of novel treatments for xeroderma pigmentosum and Gorlin-Goltz syndrome.

INTRODUCTION

The genodermatoses are a group of hereditary syndromes with skin manifestations. Many of these conditions are associated with increased risk for specific cancers. Cutaneous anomalies in childhood may be the first sign of a disorder. A 2011 review article by Karalis and colleagues[1] offers a classification system for genodermatoses based on the type of genetic defect that results in pathology. The 4 categories are DNA repair defects, signaling pathway defects, primary immunodeficiency syndromes, and other syndromes. The authors use this classification system to organize the disorders covered here, which include hereditary disorders that present with tumor and skin findings. In this article, the authors provide a brief description of the pathogenesis and clinical manifestations of each disorder along with any treatment updates. Accordingly, this article devotes additional attention to novel treatments for these hereditary tumor syndromes.

DNA REPAIR DEFECTS
Lynch Syndrome

Lynch syndrome, also known has hereditary nonpolyposis colorectal cancer (HNPCC), is a common colorectal cancer predisposition that is inherited in an autosomal-dominant manner. Mutations in DNA mismatch repair (MMR) genes including mutL homologue 1 (MLH1), mutS homologue 2 (MSH2), mutS homologue 6 (MSH6), and postmeiotic segregation increased 2 (PMS2) are associated with this disorder. Errors in the genome proofreading and editing system cause accumulation of mutations that manifest as microsatellite instability. Patients with Lynch syndrome are at increased risk for a variety of malignancies, especially colorectal, endometrial, and ovarian cancers. Classic treatment options have included surgical removal of cancers, chemotherapy, and radiation. Commonly used chemotherapeutic agents include 5-fluorouracil and irinotecan. Initial studies suggest that aspirin may have a long-term chemopreventive effect on colorectal cancers.[2]

Disclosure Statement: The authors have nothing to disclose.
Department of Dermatology, Wake Forest School of Medicine, Medical Center Boulevard, Winston-Salem, NC, USA
* Corresponding author.
E-mail address: rhamid@wakehealth.edu

Dermatol Clin 37 (2019) 607–613
https://doi.org/10.1016/j.det.2019.05.016

derm.theclinics.com

Treatment with celecoxib showed resolution of adenomatous polyps but was associated with cardiac adverse effects.[3]

Muir-Torre Syndrome

Muir-Torre syndrome (MTS) is a rare variant of Lynch syndrome with dermatologic features. Although most cases have an autosomal-dominant inheritance pattern, a second subtype of MTS displays microsatellite stability and has autosomal-recessive inheritance. Patients present with the classic visceral malignancies (colorectal, endometrial, and ovarian adenocarcinoma) in conjunction with cutaneous sebaceous neoplasms and other skin tumors. Sebaceous neoplasms seen in MTS patients include adenomas, epitheliomas, carcinomas, and cystic sebaceous tumors. Basal cell carcinomas and keratoacanthomas with sebaceous differentiation are also observed. Additional clinical features include sebaceous hyperplasia and ectopic sebaceous glands (Fordyce spots) on the oral mucosa. Noncutaneous malignancies in MTS patients affect the small bowel, pancreas, hepatobiliary tract, brain, upper uroepithelial tract, breast, lung, cervix, bone marrow, and connective tissues. Most cutaneous cancers are excised, although sebaceous carcinomas require wide local excision with 5 mm margins with adjuvant radiation or Mohs micrographic surgery. Chemotherapy with 5-fluorouracil in conjunction with platinum agents and imiquimod may be another option. Use of aminoglycosides and negamycin to target genetic abnormalities is a potential treatment strategy, but it is limited by the risk of adverse effects. Oral isotretinoin, sometimes in conjunction with interferon-alpha, has shown some success in prevention of skin lesions.[4] MTS patients who are transplant recipients should receive sirolimus for immunosuppression in order to reduce tumor incidence.[5]

Constitutional Mismatch Repair Deficiency Syndrome

Constitutional mismatch repair deficiency syndrome (CMMRD) results from inheritance of biallelic mutations in an MMR gene, as opposed to the single-allele mutation that causes Lynch syndrome. Patients often present with multiple café-au-lait macules with ragged-edge, irregular borders. This syndrome is associated with brain tumors, hematologic malignancy, rhabdomyosarcoma, and early onset gastrointestinal (GI) cancers.[1] Chemotherapy is often unsuccessful in CMMRD patients. Treatment strategies combining immune checkpoint inhibitors and neoantigen-based vaccines are being explored.[6] Long-term daily use of aspirin may reduce cancer risk in children with CMMRD.[7]

Xeroderma Pigmentosum

Xeroderma pigmentosum (XP) is an autosomal-recessive disease that falls into the category of DNA repair defects. Prevalence varies around the world from 1 case per 2 million patients to 1 case per 22,000 patients. XP has higher prevalence in Japan, the Middle East, and North Africa. There is not a single gene defect that causes the disease; instead, different proteins involved in nucleotide excision repair or translesion synthesis may be affected. Patients are classified into complementation groups according to the defect they have (XP-A to G and XP-V). The most common genes that are mutated include DDB2, ERCC1, ERCC2, ERCC3, ERCC4, ERCC5, POLH, XPA, or XPC. Clinical presentation depends on the patient's specific genetic abnormality.[8–10]

Clinical features of XP include accelerated photoaging, which manifests on sun-exposed areas of the body as freckling, lentigines, telangiectasia, and hyper- and hypopigmented macules. The risk of acquiring nonmelanoma skin cancer is over 10,000 times greater, and the risk for melanoma is over 2000 times greater. Freckling may be seen as early as 2 years of age, and many patients develop skin cancer within the first decade of life. Patients may display findings of severe sunburn with blistering or persistent erythema with minimal sun exposure. Over time, the skin becomes dry and parchment-like with increased pigmentation. Ocular involvement caused by sun exposure manifests itself as photophobia, severe keratitis that may lead to corneal opacification, and atrophy of the eyelid skin. The incidence of ocular surface tumors is greatly increased.[8–10]

Neurologic deficits can be seen in about a quarter of patients. Neurologic forms of XP can be classified into 3 relatively distinct groups: XP neurologic disease, XP with trichothiodystrophy, and xeroderma pigmentosum-Cockayne syndrome complex. Common symptoms include ataxia, progressive sensorineural hearing loss, and impaired intelligence. The presence of neurologic symptoms predicts a shorter life expectancy. The median age to death is 37 years in XP without neurodegeneration and about 10 years earlier in patients with neurologic symptoms. Skin cancer is the most common cause of death for XP patients, followed by neurologic degeneration and internal cancers, including hematologic malignancies. Glioma, leukemia, and cancers of the lung, uterus, breast, and GI tract have been reported in patients with XP.[8–11]

General precautions in the management of XP include prevention of skin cancers through use of sunscreen, sun-protective clothing, and UV filters on windows. Follow-up with dermatology and ophthalmology, as well as with neurology and otolaryngology if needed, is recommended every 3 to 6 months. Premalignant lesions are treated with cryotherapy, 5-fluorouracil, or imiquimod. Skin cancers are treated by electrodessication and curettage, surgical excision, or Mohs micrographic surgery. Oral isotretinoin or acitretin may be used to prevent the development of skin cancers. Corneal transplantation may help treat keratitis, and hearing aids can improve hearing loss. More recently, vismodegib and pembrolizumab have been used to treat basal cell carcinomas and melanomas in patients with XP. Experimental work on medications that may increase the resistance of XP cells to UV damage is ongoing, and there have been some promising results with acetohexamide and the bacterial DNA repair enzyme T4 endonuclease V.[8,9,12]

Rothmund-Thomson Syndrome

Rothmund–Thomson syndrome (RTS), also termed congenital poikiloderma, is caused by mutations in RECQL4, the DNA helicase gene. This disorder displays an autosomal recessive inheritance pattern. Between the ages of 3 and 6 months, RTS patients develop an erythematous rash with swelling of the face, buttocks, and extremities. This rash gradually progresses to poikiloderma and one-third of individuals also develop hyperkeratotic lesions. Other clinical features include sparse hair, juvenile cataracts, dental anomalies, premature skin aging, short stature, and skeletal abnormalities. Patients are at increased risk for osteosarcoma. Treatment of manifestations include surgery for cataracts, pulsed dye laser for telangiectasias, and standard cancer therapy.[13]

Bloom Syndrome

Bloom syndrome is an autosomal-recessive chromosomal breakage disorder caused by a mutation in the BLM gene that codes for RECQL3 helicase. It is most common in families of Ashkenazi Jewish descent. Patients are at increased risk for multiple hematologic and solid organ malignancies, especially lymphoma, acute myelogenous leukemia, GI tumors, and skin cancer. Additional findings are narrow facial features, high-pitched voice, short stature, elongated limbs, immunodeficiency, photosensitivity, poikiloderma, pigmentary abnormalities, and telangiectatic erythema. Patients

receive standard cancer treatments and are recommended to avoid sun exposure.[14]

Werner Syndrome

Werner syndrome (progeria) is an autosomal-recessive disorder resulting from a mutation in the WRN gene that codes for a protein in the RECQ DNA helicase family. The disease first presents at puberty with lack of a growth spurt. Patients proceed to develop skin ulcers, hair graying and loss, cataracts, hypogonadism, rapid deterioration of muscle mass, and scleroderma-like appearance of the skin. Skeletal, metabolic, and cardiovascular abnormalities are also common. Individuals affected by Werner syndrome have a 10% lifetime risk of cancer, especially soft tissue sarcomas, meningiomas, thyroid carcinomas, and melanoma. The goal of treatment is symptomatic relief and management of secondary organ dysfunction. The endothelin receptor antagonist bosentan can be used to treat cutaneous ulcers, and sodium etidronate may improve soft tissue calcification.[15]

Fanconi Anemia

Fanconi anemia is a predominately autosomal-recessive disorder with 1 rare X-linked variant. It is the result of mutations in FA complementation group genes that code for proteins involved in the S phase of the growth cycle. The syndrome consists of a triad of physical malformations, hematopoietic abnormalities, and increased risk of solid tumors in adulthood. Pigmentary abnormalities in patients with Fanconi anemia include café-au-lait macules, hyperpigmented mottling, hypopigmented patches, and oral hyperpigmentation. Vitiligo, progeroid appearance, seborrheic dermatitis, eczema, follicular keratosis, xerosis, and hirsutism have been reported. Bone marrow failure, leukemias, and lymphomas are also associated with this disorder.[1] Stem cell transplantation improves life span in patients who develop these hematopoietic abnormalities.[16] A combination of atorvastatin and celecoxib may be a chemoprevention strategy in Fanconi anemia.[17]

Ataxia Telangiectasia

Ataxia telangiectasia is an autosomal-recessive cerebellar ataxia caused by deficiency in the ATM gene involved in DNA repair and cell cycle control. Ataxia appears in the toddler stage and typically stops progressing after the age of 15.[18] Patients may display choreoathetosis, immunodeficiency, premature aging, poor growth and development, and predisposition to cancers, especially lymphoma and leukemia. Cutaneous signs include oculocutaneous telangiectasias, café-au-lait macules, poikiloderma, seborrheic dermatitis, eczema, follicular keratosis, xerosis, vitiligo, and hirsutism. Treatment is typically supportive and based on symptoms.[1]

SIGNALING PATHWAYS DEFECTS
Gorlin-Goltz Syndrome

Gorlin-Goltz syndrome, also termed nevoid basal cell carcinoma syndrome, is a rare autosomal-dominant genetic disorder resulting from a mutation in the PTCH1 tumor suppressor gene. A minority of cases may occur sporadically. Multiple basal cell carcinomas (BCCs) appear at an early age, usually on the face, chest, and back. Risk of medulloblastoma, cardiac fibromas, and ovarian fibromas is increased. Odontogenic keratocysts of the jaw, palmar/plantar pits, calcifications of the falx cerebri, and rib anomalies are common. Other features include macrocephaly, cleft lip or palate, coarse features, hypertelorism, Sprengel deformity, pectus deformity, and syndactyly.[1]

Although there is no gold standard treatment for Gorlin syndrome, the array of therapeutic options has expanded over the last several years. Odontogenic keratocysts may be surgically removed, but the rate of recurrence is unclear. There are few adequately powered studies that investigate topical 5-fluorouracil or modified Carnoy solution as adjuvant treatment options following enucleation and peripheral ostectomy. Basal cell carcinomas can be treated with cryotherapy, surgical excision, Mohs micrographic surgery, photodynamic therapy, laser therapy, or topical imiquimod.[19]

Because PTCH1 is a sonic hedgehog (SHH) antagonist, new molecular-based therapies target this signaling pathway. Vismodegib is the first SHH pathway inhibitor approved by the US Food and Drug Administration (FDA) for treatment of advanced basal cell carcinomas. In a multicenter, randomized, double-blind, placebo-controlled, phase 2 trial, vismodegib at a dose of 150 mg for 3 months reduced tumor burden by over 30 surgically eligible BCCs per patient per year. Vismodegib treatment also reduced the size of odontogenic keratocysts. Adverse effects such as weight loss and muscle cramps caused interruption of treatment in some patients, which resulted in recurrence of BCCs.[20] Sonidegib is another FDA-approved SHH pathway inhibitor for treatment of advanced, recurrent BCCs. Use of this drug is limited by muscle toxicity.[21] Celecoxib may also prevent BCCs in patients with PTCH1 mutation, but the cardiovascular risk limits its usage.[22] Results from a randomized, double-blind, vehicle-controlled trial suggest that topical retinoids like tazarotene do not have a chemopreventive effect.[23] Recent reports suggest that some cases of Gorlin syndrome are associated with mutations in the SUFU (suppressor of fused homolog) gene instead of PTCH1. These patients may respond well to treatment with the antiprogrammed death-1 antibody pembrolizumab.[24]

Costello Syndrome

Costello syndrome is caused by sporadic mutations in HRAS, which is involved in the Ras-mitogen-activated protein kinase (MAPK) pathway. Patients can have skin redundancy, palmoplantar keratoderma, curly and fine hair, acanthosis nigricans, keratosis pilaris, and cutaneous papillomas. They may also exhibit failure to thrive, developmental delay, diffuse hypotonia, coarse facial features, and cardiac abnormalities. Costello syndrome is associated with increased risk for neuroblastoma, rhabdomyosarcoma, and transitional cell carcinoma of the bladder.[1] Oral acitretin may improve severe palmoplantar keratoderma.[25]

Legius Syndrome

Legius syndrome is the result of mutations in SPRED1, a gene involved in the Ras-MAPK pathway, which produce a similar phenotype to neurofibromatosis type 1. Dermatologic findings include café-au-lait macules, axillary and inguinal freckling, neurofibromas, and lipomas. Macrocephaly, attention-deficit/hyperactivity disorder (ADHD), and developmental delays are also features of this disorder. Legius syndrome is linked to increased risk for childhood leukemia. Management consists of screening for developmental delays and treating manifestations.[26]

Li-Fraumeni Syndrome

Li-Fraumeni syndrome is a rare disorder with autosomal-dominant inheritance that is also known as sarcoma, breast, leukemia, and adrenal gland (SBLA) cancer syndrome. Malignancies of the lung, pancreas, and GI tract, as well as lymphoma, germ cell tumors, Wilms tumor, and melanoma have also been reported. The genetic cause for Li-Fraumeni syndrome is mutation in the TP53 tumor suppressor gene, leading to increased cell proliferation and invasion. Malignancies associated with this disorder typically occur earlier in life than expected. Treatment is no different than for any other cancer, with the exception that radiation is avoided because of the high incidence of radiation-associated secondary cancers. There are no specific drugs that target the TP53 mutation.[27]

Multiple Endocrine Neoplasia

Multiple endocrine neoplasia (MEN) is a class of autosomal-dominant syndromes associated with endocrine tumors. MEN type 1 is caused by mutations in the MEN1 tumor suppressor gene. It is characterized by tumors of the parathyroid gland, pancreas, and pituitary gland along with café-au-lait macules, lipomas, collagenomas, and facial angiofibromas. MEN type 2A results from activating mutations of the RET proto-oncogene. Findings include primary hyperparathyroidism. pheochromocytoma, medullary thyroid carcinoma, itchy lesions, cutaneous neuromas, and amyloidosis. MEN type 2B is also caused by RET mutations and is characterized by pheochromocytoma, medullar thyroid carcinoma, marfanoid habitus, café-au-lait macules, and mucosal neuromas.[1] MEN-associated hyperparathyroidism can be treated with parathyroidectomy.

Carney Complex

Carney complex is caused by an inactivating mutation in the protein kinase A (PKA) regulatory subunit-1a gene (PRKAR1A), which is essential in cAMP signaling. It is inherited in an autosomal-dominant manner. Multiple tumors are characteristic of this syndrome including cutaneous and cardiac myxomas, as well as thyroid, pancreatic, ovarian, and colon cancers. Other skin findings include café-au-lait macules, blue nevi, and lentigines.[1] Cardiac myxomas require surgical removal, while treatment of other manifestations may vary.[28]

Beckwith-Wiedemann Syndrome

Beckwith-Wiedemann syndrome (BWS) is an imprinted disorder caused by overexpression of paternal IGF2 growth factor gene or underexpression of maternal CDKN1C growth regulator gene. The characteristic features of this disorder are linear indentation of the ear lobe and posterior helical pits. Macroglossia, hemihypertrophy, zosteriform rash, nevus flammeus, and hemangiomas are also seen. Children with BWS tend to develop the following tumors: hepatoblastoma, Wilms tumor, neuroblastoma, and rhabdomyosarcoma. BWS patients require management of complications and tumor surveillance.[1]

PRIMARY IMMUNODEFICIENCY SYNDROMES
Wiskott-Aldrich Syndrome

Wiskott-Aldrich syndrome is an X-linked recessive immune disorder resulting from mutations in the WASP gene, which codes for proteins that regulate signaling in bone marrow cells. Clinical manifestations include eczema, microthrombocytopenia, immunodeficiency, autoimmunity, and cancer predisposition. Patients must receive a bone marrow transplant for survival past childhood.[1]

Chediak-Higashi Syndrome

Chediak-Higashi syndrome (CHS) is an autosomal-recessive disorder that causes interference in vesicle transport because of a mutation in the CHS1/Lyst gene. Hypopigmentation or partial albinism, immunodeficiency, coagulopathy, and neurologic dysfunction can be seen in CHS. Patients are at increased risk for acute lymphoblastic leukemia and T-cell lymphoma. Hematopoietic cell transplantation can correct hematological and immune dysfunction but does not treat neurologic symptoms.[29]

X-linked Agammaglobulinemia

X-linked agammaglobulinemia is characterized by immune dysfunction caused by a mutation in the BTK gene resulting in failure to produce B lymphocytes. Features of the syndrome include eczema, cellulitis, dermatomyositis-like syndrome, and predisposition for gastric cancer.[1] Intravenous immunoglobulin (IVIG) therapy and hematopoietic stem cell transplantation are potential treatment strategies for this disorder. Patients should also receive antibiotics for active infections.[30]

OTHER SYNDROMES
Neuroblastoma

Neuroblastoma is the most common childhood malignancy, arising from neural crest cells. It is inherited in an autosomal-dominant manner and is associated with café-au-lait macules and cutaneous metastases. Surgery and chemotherapy are the classic treatments for neuroblastoma. Newer therapies include immunotherapy, meta-iodobenzylguanidine (I-MIBG), angiogenesis inhibitors, and epigenetic targeting.[31]

Nail Patella Syndrome

Nail patella syndrome is an autosomal-dominant condition caused by mutations in the gene that encodes transcription factor LMX1B. Patients have dysplastic nails and absent patellae. They may also develop elbow, renal, and ocular abnormalities. Surgery may be required to correct patellar instability.[32]

SUMMARY

The skin manifestations of various syndromes have distinctive qualities despite overlapping features such as café-au-lait macules. Often, the size, shape, and distribution of lesions will provide hints to their etiology. Identifying these subtle differences requires careful examination by discerning eyes. Dermatologists must remain aware of the characteristic cutaneous findings for hereditary tumor syndromes, so patients can receive timely diagnoses and appropriate malignancy work-up. Early identification of at-risk families allows initiation of genetic counseling and screening for family members also.

Genetic screening technology has progressed tremendously in recent years, elucidating the molecular defects in genodermatoses. A growing understanding of the molecular bases of these disorders fosters development of new drugs targeting the specific defects. Management of most hereditary tumor syndromes has remained relatively stable over the last decade. However, novel molecular therapies have revolutionized treatment of XP and Gorlin-Goltz syndrome. Vismodegib is an SHH signaling pathway inhibitor that has shown promise in preventing and treating BCCs, while pembrolizumab may also be an effective option in patients with SUFU-mutated Gorlin syndrome. Further adequately powered studies will provide more definitive evidence of the efficacy of these new therapies for patients with genodermatoses.

REFERENCES

1. Karalis A, Tischkowitz M, Millington GW. Dermatological manifestations of inherited cancer syndromes in children. Br J Dermatol 2011;164(2): 245–56.
2. Lynch HT, Snyder CL, Shaw TG, et al. Milestones of Lynch syndrome: 1895-2015. Nat Rev Cancer 2015; 15(3):181–94.
3. Agarwal R, Liebe S, Turski ML, et al. Targeted therapy for hereditary cancer syndromes: hereditary breast and ovarian cancer syndrome, Lynch syndrome, familial adenomatous polyposis, and Li-Fraumeni syndrome. Discov Med 2014;18(101): 331–9.
4. Graefe T, Wollina U, Schulz H, et al. Muir-Torre syndrome - treatment with isotretinoin and interferon alpha-2a can prevent tumour development. Dermatology 2000;200(4):331–3.
5. John AM, Schwartz RA. Muir-Torre syndrome (MTS): an update and approach to diagnosis and management. J Am Acad Dermatol 2016;74(3):558–66.
6. Westdorp H, Kolders S, Hoogerbrugge N, et al. Immunotherapy holds the key to cancer treatment and prevention in constitutional mismatch repair deficiency (CMMRD) syndrome. Cancer Lett 2017; 403:159–64.
7. Leenders EKSM, Westdorp H, Brüggemann RJ, et al. Cancer prevention by aspirin in children with Constitutional Mismatch Repair Deficiency (CMMRD). Eur J Hum Genet 2018;26(10): 1417–23.
8. Weon JL, Glass DA II. Novel therapeutic approaches to xeroderma pigmentosum. Br J Dermatol 2018. https://doi.org/10.1111/bjd.17253.
9. Kraemer KH, DiGiovanna JJ. Xeroderma pigmentosum. In: Adam MP, Ardinger HH, Pagon RA, et al, editors. GeneReviews. Seattle (WA): University of Washington, Seattle; 2003. p. 1993–2018.
10. Natale V, Raquer H. Xeroderma pigmentosum-Cockayne syndrome complex. Orphanet J Rare Dis 2017;12:65.
11. Kaliki S, Jajapuram SD, Maniar A, et al. Ocular and periocular tumors in xeroderma pigmentosum: a study of 120 Asian Indian patients. Am J Ophthalmol 2018. https://doi.org/10.1016/j.ajo.2018.10.011.
12. Soura E, Plaka M, Dessinioti C, et al. Use of vismodegib for the treatment of multiple basal cell carcinomas in a patient with xeroderma pigmentosum. Pediatr Dermatol 2018;35:e334–6.
13. Wang LL, Plon SE. Rothmund-Thomson Syndrome. In: Adam MP, Ardinger HH, Pagon RA, et al., editors. GeneReviews® [Internet]. Seattle (WA): University of Washington, Seattle; 1993-2019. Available at https://www.ncbi.nlm.nih.gov/books/NBK1237/
14. Arora H, Chacon AH, Choudhary S, et al. Bloom syndrome. Int J Dermatol 2014;53(7):798–802.
15. Sickles CK, Gross GP. Progeria (Werner Syndrome). In: StatPearls [Internet]. Treasure Island (FL): StatPearls Publishing; 2019 Jan. Available from: https://www.ncbi.nlm.nih.gov/books/NBK507797/?report=classic
16. Ebens CL, MacMillan ML, Wagner JE. Hematopoietic cell transplantation in Fanconi anemia: current evidence, challenges and recommendations. Expert Rev Hematol 2017;10(1):81–97.
17. Zhang QS, Deater M, Phan N, et al. Combination therapy with atorvastatin and celecoxib delays tumor formation in a Fanconi anemia mouse model. Pediatr Blood Cancer 2018;66(1):e27460.
18. Rothblum-Oviatt C, Wright J, Lefton-Greif MA, et al. Ataxia telangiectasia: a review. Orphanet J Rare Dis 2016;11(1):159.
19. Akbari M, Chen H, Guo G, et al. Basal cell nevus syndrome (Gorlin syndrome): genetic insights, diagnostic challenges, and unmet milestones. Pathophysiology 2018;25(2):77–82.
20. Tang JY, Ally MS, Chanana AM, et al. Inhibition of the hedgehog pathway in patients with basal-cell nevus syndrome: final results from the multicentre, randomised, double-blind, placebo-controlled, phase 2 trial. Lancet Oncol 2016;17(12):1720–31.
21. Jain S, Song R, Xie J. Sonidegib: mechanism of action, pharmacology, and clinical utility for advanced

basal cell carcinomas. Onco Targets Ther 2017;10: 1645–53.

22. Tang JY, Aszterbaum M, Athar M. Basal cell carcinoma chemoprevention with nonsteroidal anti-inflammatory drugs in genetically predisposed PTCH1+/- humans and mice. Cancer Prev Res (Phila) 2010;3(1):25–34.

23. Tang JY, Chiou AS, Mackay-Wiggan JM. Tazarotene: randomized, double-blind, vehicle-controlled, and open-label concurrent trials for basal cell carcinoma prevention and therapy in patients with basal cell nevus syndrome. Cancer Prev Res (Phila) 2014; 7(3):292–9.

24. Moreira A, Kirchberger MC, Toussaint F. Effective anti-programmed death-1 therapy in a SUFU-mutated patient with Gorlin-Goltz syndrome. Br J Dermatol 2018;179(3):747–9.

25. Marukian NV, Levinsohn JL, Craiglow BG, et al. Palmoplantar keratoderma in costello syndrome responsive to acitretin. Pediatr Dermatol 2017; 34(2):160–2.

26. Stevenson D, Viskochil D, Mao R. Legius Syndrome. In: Adam MP, Ardinger HH, Pagon RA, et al., editors. GeneReviews® [Internet]. Seattle (WA): University of Washington, Seattle; 1993-2019. Available at https://www.ncbi.nlm.nih.gov/books/NBK47312/

27. Vogel WH. Li-Fraumeni syndrome. J Adv Pract Oncol 2017;8(7):742–6.

28. Bertherat J. Carney complex (CNC). Orphanet J Rare Dis 2006;1:21.

29. Ajitkumar A, Ramphul K. Chediak Higashi Syndrome. In: StatPearls [Internet]. Treasure Island (FL): StatPearls Publishing; 2019 Jan-. Available at: https://www.ncbi.nlm.nih.gov/books/NBK507881/

30. Taneja A, Chhabra A. Bruton Agammaglobulinemia. In: StatPearls [Internet]. Treasure Island (FL): StatPearls Publishing. Available at: https://www.ncbi.nlm.nih.gov/books/NBK448170/

31. Davidoff AM. Neuroblastoma. Semin Pediatr Surg 2012;21(1):2–14.

32. Witzgall R. Nail-patella syndrome. Pflugers Arch 2017;469(7–8):927–36.

UNITED STATES POSTAL SERVICE ® Statement of Ownership, Management, and Circulation (All Periodicals Publications Except Requester Publications)

1. Publication Title	2. Publication Number	3. Filing Date
DERMATOLOGIC CLINICS	000 – 705	9/18/2019

4. Issue Frequency	5. Number of Issues Published Annually	6. Annual Subscription Price
JAN, APR, JUL, OCT	4	$404.00

7. Complete Mailing Address of Known Office of Publication (Not printer) (Street, city, county, state, and ZIP+4®)
ELSEVIER INC.
230 Park Avenue, Suite 800
New York, NY 10169

Contact Person
STEPHEN R. BUSHING

Telephone (Include area code)
215-239-3688

8. Complete Mailing Address of Headquarters or General Business Office of Publisher (Not printer)
ELSEVIER INC.
230 Park Avenue, Suite 800
New York, NY 10169

9. Full Names and Complete Mailing Addresses of Publisher, Editor, and Managing Editor (Do not leave blank)
Publisher (Name and complete mailing address)
TAYLOR BALL, ELSEVIER INC.
1600 JOHN F KENNEDY BLVD. SUITE 1800
PHILADELPHIA, PA 19103-2899

Editor (Name and complete mailing address)
JESSICA MCCOOL, ELSEVIER INC.
1600 JOHN F KENNEDY BLVD. SUITE 1800
PHILADELPHIA, PA 19103-2899

Managing Editor (Name and complete mailing address)
PATRICK MANLEY, ELSEVIER INC.
1600 JOHN F KENNEDY BLVD. SUITE 1800
PHILADELPHIA, PA 19103-2899

10. Owner (Do not leave blank. If the publication is owned by a corporation, give the name and address of the corporation immediately followed by the names and addresses of all stockholders owning or holding 1 percent or more of the total amount of stock. If not owned by a corporation, give the names and addresses of the individual owners. If owned by a partnership or other unincorporated firm, give its name and address as well as those of each individual owner. If the publication is published by a nonprofit organization, give its name and address.)

Full Name	Complete Mailing Address
WHOLLY OWNED SUBSIDIARY OF REED/ELSEVIER, US HOLDINGS	1600 JOHN F KENNEDY BLVD. SUITE 1800 PHILADELPHIA, PA 19103-2899

11. Known Bondholders, Mortgagees, and Other Security Holders Owning or Holding 1 Percent or More of Total Amount of Bonds, Mortgages, or Other Securities. If none, check box ► ☐ None

Full Name	Complete Mailing Address
N/A	

12. Tax Status (For completion by nonprofit organizations authorized to mail at nonprofit rates) (Check one)
The purpose, function, and nonprofit status of this organization and the exempt status for federal income tax purposes:
☒ Has Not Changed During Preceding 12 Months
☐ Has Changed During Preceding 12 Months (Publisher must submit explanation of change with this statement)

PS Form 3526, July 2014 [Page 1 of 4 (see instructions page 4)] PSN: 7530-01-000-9931 PRIVACY NOTICE: See our privacy policy on www.usps.com.

13. Publication Title	14. Issue Date for Circulation Data Below
DERMATOLOGIC CLINICS	JULY 2019

15. Extent and Nature of Circulation			Average No. Copies Each Issue During Preceding 12 Months	No. Copies of Single Issue Published Nearest to Filing Date
a. Total Number of Copies (Net press run)			148	159
b. Paid Circulation (By Mail and Outside the Mail)	(1)	Mailed Outside-County Paid Subscriptions Stated on PS Form 3541 (Include paid distribution above nominal rate, advertiser's proof copies, and exchange copies)	55	64
	(2)	Mailed In-County Paid Subscriptions Stated on PS Form 3541 (Include paid distribution above nominal rate, advertiser's proof copies, and exchange copies)	0	0
	(3)	Paid Distribution Outside the Mails Including Sales Through Dealers and Carriers, Street Vendors, Counter Sales, and Other Paid Distribution Outside USPS®	40	56
	(4)	Paid Distribution by Other Classes of Mail Through the USPS (e.g., First-Class Mail®)	0	0
c. Total Paid Distribution (Sum of 15b (1), (2), (3), and (4))		►	95	120
d. Free or Nominal Rate Distribution (By Mail and Outside the Mail)	(1)	Free or Nominal Rate Outside-County Copies included on PS Form 3541	39	21
	(2)	Free or Nominal Rate In-County Copies Included on PS Form 3541	0	0
	(3)	Free or Nominal Rate Copies Mailed at Other Classes Through the USPS (e.g., First-Class Mail)	0	0
	(4)	Free or Nominal Rate Distribution Outside the Mail (Carriers or other means)	0	0
e. Total Free or Nominal Rate Distribution (Sum of 15d (1), (2), (3) and (4))		►	39	21
f. Total Distribution (Sum of 15c and 15e)		►	134	141
g. Copies not Distributed (See Instructions to Publishers #4 (page 83))		►	14	18
h. Total (Sum of 15f and g)		►	148	159
i. Percent Paid (15c divided by 15f times 100)		►	70.9%	85.11%

* If you are claiming electronic copies, go to line 16 on page 3. If you are not claiming electronic copies, skip to line 17 on page 3.

16. Electronic Copy Circulation		Average No. Copies Each Issue During Preceding 12 Months	No. Copies of Single Issue Published Nearest to Filing Date
a. Paid Electronic Copies	►		
b. Total Paid Print Copies (Line 15c) + Paid Electronic Copies (Line 16a)	►		
c. Total Print Distribution (Line 15f) + Paid Electronic Copies (Line 16a)	►		
d. Percent Paid (Both Print & Electronic Copies) (16b divided by 16c × 100)	►		

☒ I certify that 50% of all my distributed copies (electronic and print) are paid above a nominal price.

17. Publication of Statement of Ownership
☒ If the publication is a general publication, publication of this statement is required. Will be printed
in the OCTOBER 2019 issue of this publication. ☐ Publication not required.

18. Signature and Title of Editor, Publisher, Business Manager, or Owner

STEPHEN R. BUSHING – INVENTORY DISTRIBUTION CONTROL MANAGER   Date 9/18/2019

I certify that all information furnished on this form is true and complete. I understand that anyone who furnishes false or misleading information on this form or who omits material or information requested on the form may be subject to criminal sanctions (including fines and imprisonment) and/or civil sanctions (including civil penalties).

PS Form 3526, July 2014 (Page 3 of 4)   PRIVACY NOTICE: See our privacy policy on www.usps.com

Moving?

Make sure your subscription moves with you!

To notify us of your new address, find your **Clinics Account Number** (located on your mailing label above your name), and contact customer service at:

Email: journalscustomerservice-usa@elsevier.com

800-654-2452 (subscribers in the U.S. & Canada)
314-447-8871 (subscribers outside of the U.S. & Canada)

Fax number: 314-447-8029

Elsevier Health Sciences Division
Subscription Customer Service
3251 Riverport Lane
Maryland Heights, MO 63043

*To ensure uninterrupted delivery of your subscription, please notify us at least 4 weeks in advance of move.